TIPS AND TRICKS IN

INFERTILITY AND IVF

A Comprehensive Q&A Guide for Reproductive Medicine

First Edition 2026

Author

DR. AHMED REFAAT ADLY

Consultant in IVF and Infertility

Important Notice:
To access the detailed answers and explanations for this book, a paid subscription to the Arab Association for Education and Training application (ARABAS) is required.
For subscription and app download details, contact us via WhatsApp: +201097982895.

تنويه هام:
للحصول على الإجابات التفصيلية والشرح لأسئلة هذا الكتاب، يُرجى الاشتراك في تطبيق المؤسسة العربية للتعليم والتدريب بعد سداد رسوم الاشتراك للاشتراك وتحميل التطبيق، التواصل عبر واتساب: 201097982895+

For permission, contact:
arabas.org@gmail.com

First Edition, 2026
This book is printed in Egypt

Legal Deposit No.: 2026/2946
ISBN: 978-633-99705-9-7

Medad Al-alaliaa
for Publishing and Printing

Dedication

To my Colleagues around the world,

With deep respect and admiration for your relentless dedication, your pursuit of knowledge, and your tireless efforts to bring hope and healing to patients everywhere.

To my beloved daughter Alice,

for filling my life with joy and inspiration
This book is also dedicated to you, with all my heart.

Ahmed Refaat Adly
2026

About the Author :Dr. Ahmed Refaat Adly

- Consultant in IVF and Infertility
- Diploma in Reproductive Medicine & Surgery, Birmingham Women's Hospital, United Kingdom
- President of the Arab Association for Education and Training (ARABAS), CPD Accredited
- Official Website: www.arabas.org
- Certified International Trainer in Infertility and IVF (TOT)
- International Conferences Speaker
- Owner and Director of Al-Adly Medical Center for Infertility and OB. GYNE, Egypt
- Author of "Tips and Tricks in ICSI & IVF"
- Program Director of the Advanced Professional Diploma in Infertility and IVF (APROF) Training Course, CPD Certified
- Member of the European Society of Human Reproduction and Embryology (ESHRE)
- Dedicated to advancing education, training, and clinical excellence in reproductive medicine worldwide

Preface

This book, Tips and Tricks in Infertility and IVF: A Comprehensive Q&A Guide for Reproductive Medicine, is designed primarily for specialists in Infertility and Assisted Reproductive Technologies (ARTs), while also serving as a valuable resource for obstetricians and gynecologists in general.

It is particularly intended for candidates preparing for examinations in any fellowship or diploma related to reproductive medicine.

The book aims to train candidates to become familiar with exam-style questions and formats, offering an effective tool for self-assessment, focused revision, and building exam confidence.

Beyond exam preparation, the book also provides concise, practical, and evidence-based insights drawn from years of clinical experience, teaching, and collaboration with colleagues worldwide.

Ultimately, this work is intended to serve as both a quick reference and a practical companion for Infertility and IVF/ICSI specialists worldwide, supporting their efforts to advance knowledge, refine practice, and improve patient care in reproductive medicine.

Ahmed Refaat Adly
Sohag, Egypt
January 2026

Table of Contents

Volume 1: INFERTILITY

PART 1: SBA & MCQs

PART 2: TRUE/FALSE QUESTIONS

PART 3: EMQs

PART 4: CASE-BASED & SHORT ESSAY QUESTIONS

Volume 2: IVF/ICSI

PART 1: SBA & MCQs

PART 2: TRUE/FALSE QUESTIONS

PART 3: EMQs

PART 4: CASE-BASED & SHORT ESSAY QUESTIONS

VOLUME 1

INFERTILITY

PART 1

SINGLE BEST ANSWERS (SBAs) & MULTIPLE CHOICE QUESTIONS (MCQs) IN INFERTILITY

1. INFERTILITY WORKUP & OPTIMIZING NATURAL FERTILITY

1. A 25-year-old woman presents to your clinic because she and her husband have been trying to conceive. She reports having regular menstrual cycles every 28–30 days. They have been having unprotected intercourse about twice weekly. They have no significant past medical history. She has no symptoms of pelvic pain, dysmenorrhea, or abnormal vaginal discharge. Her husband is healthy and has no known urological problems. They started trying for a pregnancy 8 months ago.
What is the most appropriate next step?

A. Begin infertility workup now

B. Advise timed intercourse and reassess after 4 months

C. Begin empiric ovulation induction

D. Refer to reproductive endocrinology immediately

E. Order Hysterosalpingography now

2. A 37-year-old woman with regular menses has been trying to conceive for 4 months. Which is the most accurate statement?

A. She meets the definition of infertility

B. She should wait 12 months before any investigation

C. Age has no impact on timing of investigation

D. She should be referred only after 2 years

E. She should be investigated after 6 months of unprotected regular intercourse

3. A 32-year-old woman has been married for 3 months. She has a history of irregular menstrual cycles and facial hair growth.
What is the most appropriate next step in evaluating her infertility?

A. Wait until 12 months of marriage before starting the work-up

B. Proceed directly to hysterosalpingography (HSG)

C. Start ovulation induction without further evaluation

D. Begin infertility evaluation immediately because there is a suspected cause

E. Refer directly for in-vitro fertilization (IVF)

4. A 33-year-old woman with regular cycles asks how to maximize timing of intercourse. What is the most accurate advice about the fertile window?

A. Fertility is highest on the day of ovulation only

B. Fertile window is the 24 hours after ovulation

C. Fertile window is ~5 days before ovulation and day of ovulation

D. Fertile window is in the luteal phase after ovulation

E. Best to time intercourse based on cervical mucus in luteal phase

5. A 28-year-old woman presents after 6 months of trying to conceive. Her cycles are regular every 29 days. Her BMI is 33. Her partner is healthy and does not smoke. What is the single most important lifestyle advice to improve her chances of natural conception?

A. Start low-dose aspirin

B. Reduce BMI to < 30 through diet & exercise

C. Take antioxidant vitamin supplements

D. Increase intercourse frequency to daily

E. Avoid caffeine completely

6. A couple presents to the clinic with 14 months of regular, unprotected intercourse without conception. Both partners have no significant past medical history. What is the most appropriate initial approach to their infertility work-up?

A. Start evaluating the female partner only, since women are more likely to have infertility causes

B. Begin with hysterosalpingography (HSG) in the female

C. Begin evaluation of both partners simultaneously

D. Perform semen analysis only and proceed based on results

E. Refer the couple directly for assisted reproductive techniques

7. Among female factors causing infertility, which is the most common?

A. Uterine anomalies

B. Tubal disease

C. Cervical mucus problems

D. Ovulatory disorders

E. Endometrial polyps

8. Which of the following is part of the basic infertility workup?

A. Ovulation assessment

B. Tubal patency test

C. Semen Analysis

D. All of the above

E. None of the above

9- What is the approximate fecundability in healthy young couples?

A. 5%

B. 10%

C. 20–25%

D. 40–50%

E. > 60%

10- A healthy couple in their 20s has been having regular unprotected intercourse for 1 year. What proportion of couples in this situation would be expected to conceive within the first year?

A. 40–50%

B. 60–70%

C. 80–85%

D. 90–95%

E. > 95%

11- According to the NICE Guidelines (2013), what is the recommended frequency of sexual intercourse for couples trying to conceive naturally?

A. Once a week

B. Only on the predicted day of ovulation

C. Twice daily during the fertile window

D. Every 4–5 days

E. Every 2–3 days

12- What is the approximate global prevalence of infertility among couples of reproductive ages, according to WHO estimates?

A. 2–3%

B. 5–7%

C. 10–15%

D. 20–25%

E. > 30

2. ASSESMENT OF OVUALTION & OVARIAN RESERVE TESTS

13- Which of the following Could be used to confirm ovulation in the current cycle?

A. Day 3 FSH level

B. Serum progesterone on day 21

C. Transvaginal ultrasound on day 3

D. Serum AMH level

E. Antral follicle count (AFC)

14- In a woman with subfertility, when should serum progesterone be measured to assess ovulation?

A. Day 3

B. Day 7

C. Day 14

D. Day 21 (or ~7 days before expected menses)

E. Day 28

15- What mid-luteal serum progesterone suggests ovulation has occurred?

A. ≥ 1 ng/mL

B. ≥ 3 ng/mL

C. ≥ 10 ng/mL

D. ≥ 15 ng/mL

E. ≥ 20 ng/mL

16. Which endometrial feature is most favourable before ovulation?

A. Thin echogenic lining

B. Homogeneous hyperechoic lining

C. Trilaminar pattern $\geq 8 - 14$ mm

D. Hypoechoic lining < 6 mm

E. None of the above

17. All of the following are indications for using urinary LH surge kits EXCEPT:

A. Timing intercourse in natural cycles

B. Predicting ovulation in IUI cycles

C. Guiding hCG trigger timing

D. Diagnosing premature ovarian failure

E. Detecting the LH surge to predict imminent ovulation

18. All of the following are US findings suggestive of ovulation EXCEPT:

A. Collapse of dominant follicle

B. Free fluid in pouch of Douglas

C. Compact secretory endometrium

D. Endometrium thickness less than 6 mm

E. Prescence of C.L

19- What is the expected dominant follicle size just before ovulation in most normal cycles?

A. 12–14 mm

B. 14–16 mm

C. 18–25 mm

D. 28–30 mm

E. > 30 mm

20- In a natural cycle, what is the normal growth rate of the dominant follicle in the late follicular phase?

A. 0.5 mm/day

B. 1–2 mm/day

C. 3–4 mm/day

D. >5 mm/day

E. No consistent rate

21- In a 28-day cycle, the optimal day to begin folliculometry to predict ovulation with minimal scans is:

A. Day 5

B. Day 7

C. Day 9–10

D. Day 14

E. Day 21

22. Which of the following is the initial test for assessing tubal patency in most women with no high risk for pelvic disease?

A. Hysterosalpingography

B. Diagnostic laparoscopy

C. Saline infusion sonography

D. MRI pelvis

E. Abdominal US

23- A 27-year-old woman presents with 1 year of infertility. She has regular 28-day menstrual cycles, no significant medical history, and a normal physical examination. As part of her evaluation, the junior doctor orders a full baseline hormonal profile (FSH, LH, estradiol, prolactin, TSH, and androgens). What is the most appropriate comment regarding this request?

A. Appropriate - all women with infertility should have basal hormonal testing

B. Appropriate - confirms ovulation in women with regular cycles

C. Not routinely indicated - only needed if cycles are irregular or suggest ovulatory dysfunction

D. Not indicated - should never be ordered in infertility workup

E. Should only be done after hysterosalpingography

24- A 38-year-old woman has been trying to conceive for 6 months. Cycles are regular. Which is the most appropriate reason to order ovarian reserve testing now?

A. Age over 35 years with > 6 months infertility

B. Regular cycles regardless of age

C. Only if irregular cycles present

D. Only after failed IVF

E. Never in women with regular cycles

25- Which test is considered the best for assessing ovarian reserve?

A. LH/FSH ratio

B. Day 21 progesterone level

C. AMH (Anti-Müllerian Hormone) or Antral follicle Count (AFC)

D. Clomiphene challenge test

E. Day 3 estradiol level

26- A 42-year-old woman has difficulty conceiving for 1 year. She has regular 28-day cycles. Her investigations show: Day 3 FSH: 8 IU/L AMH: 0.5 ng/mL, AFC: 3. What is the most appropriate interpretation?

A. Normal ovarian reserve for age

B. Suggests hypothalamic anovulation

C. Likely premature ovarian insufficiency

D. Suggests PCOS

E. Indicates diminished ovarian reserve despite regular cycles

3. ANOVULATION

27. A 28-year-old woman presents to your fertility clinic with 2 years of primary infertility. She reports irregular, infrequent menstrual cycles occurring every 3–6 months since menarche. She has a BMI of 19 kg/m², no hirsutism or acne. She reports long distance running and heavy exercise 5 days a week, along with recent weight loss due to strict dieting. Hormonal workup shows: FSH: 2 IU/L, LH: 1 IU/L, Estradiol: 15 pg/mL Prolactin: normal, TSH: normal AMH: 3 ng/mL, Transvaginal ultrasound shows small uterus and thin endometrial lining, with normal antral follicle count. What is the most likely diagnosis?

A. Turner's Syndrome

B. POI

C. PCOS

D. Hypogonadotropic Hypoestrogenic Anovulation

E. Hyperprolactinemia

28. A 33-year-old woman, married for 7 years, presents to your fertility clinic complaining of secondary infertility and inability to breastfeed after her last delivery 4 years ago. She reports that after the delivery - which was complicated by severe postpartum hemorrhage requiring transfusion she never produced adequate breast milk and noticed her periods did not return for 6 months. Since then, she has only occasional light spotting every few months. Laboratory results show: FSH: 2 IU/L, LH: 1.5 IU/L Estradiol: 18 pg/mL, Prolactin: 3.5, TSH: 0.5. What is the most likely diagnosis:

A. Hypergonadotropic Hypoestrogenic Anovulation

B. Hyperprolactinemia

C. Pituitary Tumours

D. Normogonadotropic Normoestrogenic Anovulation

E. Hypogonadotropic Hypoestrogenic Anovulation

29- Induction of ovulation for a case of Hypogonadotropic Hypoestrogenic Anovulation by:

A. FSH only

B. LH

C. Letrozole

D. FSH + LH or Pulsatile GnRH Pump

E. Recombinant FSH

30- What is the type of trigger in cases of Hypogonadotropic Hypoestrogenic Anovulation:

A. hCG trigger

B. GnRH agonist

C. Dual trigger

D. Double trigger

E. No trigger

31. What is the recommended IVF protocol for a patient with Hypogonadotropic Hypogonadism Anovulation?

A. Antagonist Protocol

B. Long Protocol

C. Gonadotropins only protocol

D. PPOS Protocol

E. Double Stimulation Protocol

32. Premature ovarian insufficiency is defined as loss of ovarian function before which age?

A. 35 years

B. 40 years

C. 45 years

D. 50 years

E. 55 years

33. A 32-year-old woman presents with amenorrhea for 6 months and hot flashes. Which lab result is most consistent with premature ovarian insufficiency?

A. Low FSH, low estrogen

B. High FSH, low estrogen

C. High LH, high estrogen

D. Normal FSH, high prolactin

E. High FSH only

34. Which karyotype is commonly associated with Turner's Syndrome?

A. 46, XX

B. 47, XXX

C. 45, X

D. 46, XY

E. 45 XXX

35. The first-line investigation in a young woman with amenorrhea suspected to have POI is:

A. Prolactin level

B. Serum estrogen

C. Serum FSH

D. DEXA scan

E. TSH level

36. Hormone Replacement Therapy (HRT) in women with POI is indicated to:

A. Induce ovulation

B. Prevent multiple pregnancy

C. Lower blood pressure

D. Prevent osteoporosis and relieve vasomotor symptoms

E. Postpone menopause

37. Which of the following is TRUE about fertility in POI patients?

A. They can never conceive spontaneously

B. Assisted reproductive techniques & ovulation induction are effective

C. Oocyte donation is an option but Prohibited in many Countries.

D. Menstrual cycles are always absent

E. PRP is effective treatment

38. Which of the following is the most common cause of chronic anovulation?

A. Hyperprolactinemia

B. Polycystic Ovary Syndrome (PCOS)

C. Thyroid dysfunction

D. Premature ovarian insufficiency

E. Anorexia nervosa

39. A 28-year-old woman presents with secondary amenorrhea and infertility. Her FSH and LH levels are elevated, estradiol is low, and her karyotype is normal (46, XX). Ultrasound shows normal ovaries with multiple small follicles. Which of the following is the most likely diagnosis?

A. Premature ovarian insufficiency

B. Hypothalamic amenorrhea

C. Polycystic ovary syndrome

D. Resistant ovary syndrome

E. Sheehan's syndrome

40. In resistant ovary syndrome, the primary defect lies in:

A. Ovarian follicle responsiveness to gonadotropins

B. Pituitary secretion of FSH and LH

C. Hypothalamic GnRH release

D. Autoimmune damage to the ovary

E. Structural abnormalities in the uterus

41. Which of the following hormone profiles is most consistent with resistant ovary syndrome?

A. High FSH, High LH, Low estradiol

B. Low FSH, Low LH, Low estradiol

C. Normal FSH, Normal LH, High estradiol

D. High FSH, High LH, High estradiol

E. Low FSH, High LH, Normal estradiol

42. What is the typical finding on ovarian ultrasound in a patient with resistant ovary syndrome?

A. Ovarian atrophy

B. Polycystic-appearing ovaries

C. Normal-sized ovaries with multiple small follicles

D. Hemorrhagic cyst

E. Absent ovaries

43. Which of the following is the most effective fertility treatment for a woman diagnosed with resistant ovary syndrome who wishes to conceive?

A. Clomiphene citrate

B. Gonadotropin injections

C. Pulsatile GnRH therapy

D. Oocyte donation

E. Metformin therapy

44. What distinguishes resistant ovary syndrome from premature ovarian insufficiency?

A. Presence of high estradiol levels

B. Irreversibility of the ovarian failure

C. Normal ovarian reserve on ultrasound

D. High gonadotropins with absent follicles

E. Normal karyotype

45. A 28-year-old woman presents with amenorrhea for 8 months and galactorrhea. A pregnancy test is negative. Serum prolactin level is

significantly elevated (180 ng/ml). Which of the following is the most appropriate initial investigation?

A. Liver function tests

B. MRI of the brain

C. CT scan of the abdomen

D. Pelvic ultrasound

E. Endometrial biopsy

46. A 35-year-old woman is found to have elevated serum prolactin on routine blood tests. She denies visual symptoms. Which of the following drugs is most likely to cause this condition?

A. Amlodipine

B. Omeprazole

C. Risperidone

D. Aspirin

E. Metformin

47- A 25-year-old female with confirmed hyperprolactinemia due to a 4 mm pituitary microadenoma is planning to get pregnant. What is the first-line treatment?

A. Transsphenoidal surgery

B. Chemotherapy

C. Radiotherapy

D. Cabergoline

E. Observation only

48- 33-year-old woman presents with bitemporal hemianopia and high serum prolactin. MRI reveals a 2.5 cm pituitary mass. What is the most likely diagnosis?

A. Pituitary apoplexy

B. Craniopharyngioma

C. Macroprolactinoma

D. Meningioma

E. Rathke's cleft cyst

49- A 32-year-old woman presents with secondary amenorrhea and milky nipple discharge. Her prolactin level is mildly elevated. Which of the following should be ruled out before making a diagnosis of prolactinoma?

A. Pregnancy

B. Diabetes insipidus

C. Hyperaldosteronism

D. Adrenal insufficiency

E. Pheochromocytoma

50- A 29-year-old woman has a serum prolactin level of 320 ng/mL (normal < 20 ng/mL). What is the most likely cause?

A. Stress

B. Macroprolactinoma

C. Severe Diet

D. PCOS

E. Chest wall trauma

51- Which of the following is a common side effect of dopamine agonist therapy used in hyperprolactinemia?

A. Hypoglycemia

B. Pulmonary fibrosis

C. Hyperkalemia

D. Orthostatic hypotension

E. Bradycardia

52. A 38-year-old woman with a history of pituitary tumor is found to have persistently high prolactin despite maximum dopamine agonist therapy. What is the next best step?

A. Repeat prolactin after fasting

B. Transsphenoidal surgery

C. Start corticosteroids

D. Refer for radiotherapy

E. Stop all medications

53- Which of the following hormones directly inhibits prolactin secretion?

A. TRH

B. Estrogen

C. Dopamine

D. Oxytocin

E. Progesterone

54- Which of the following is NOT a symptom of hyperprolactinemia?

A. Galactorrhea

B. Amenorrhea

C. Gynecomastia

D. Polyuria

E. Infertility

55- Which of the following is first-line treatment for a prolactinoma?

A. Radiotherapy

B. Surgery

C. Chemotherapy

D. Dopamine agonist

E. None of the above

56- What is the most common symptom of hyperprolactinemia in women?

A. Headache

B. Galactorrhea

C. Amenorrhea

D. Weight gain

E. Acne

57. What is the most common clinical feature of PCOS?

A. Chronic pelvic pain

B. Amenorrhea after age 40

C. Menstrual irregularities

D. Urinary incontinence

E. Obesity

58. Which hormone is typically elevated in PCOS?

A. Estrogen

B. Progesterone

C. Testosterone

D. Follicle-Stimulating Hormone (FSH)

E. TSH

59. Which of the following is part of the Rotterdam Criteria for diagnosing PCOS?

A. Elevated cortisol levels

B. Polycystic ovaries on ultrasound

C. Anemia

D. Underweight

E. AMH

60. What is the primary medication used to treat insulin resistance in PCOS patients?

A. Letrozole

B. Clomiphene

C. Albendazole

D. Fluoxetine

E. Metformin

61. Which of the following is NOT a potential complication of PCOS?

A. Infertility

B. Type 2 diabetes mellitus

C. Endometrial cancer

D. Acute liver failure

E. Cardiovascular diseases

62. Which of the following symptoms is commonly associated with hyperandrogenism in PCOS?

A. Hot flashes

B. Hirsutism

C. Vaginal dryness

D. Osteoporosis

E. Galactorrhea

63. Which lifestyle intervention is most effective in managing PCOS symptoms?

A. High-fat diet

B. Weight loss and exercise

C. High-protein supplements

D. Intermittent fasting alone

E. Vitamin D

64. Which of the following is considered first-line for ovulation induction in women with PCOS who desire pregnancy?

A. Clomiphene citrate

B. Finasteride

C. Letrozole

D. Oral contraceptives

E. Danazol

65. If Letrozole fails to induce ovulation in PCOS patients, what is the next step?

A. Add Metformin

B. Use Gonadotropins

C. Start Spironolactone

D. Prescribe Dexamethasone

E. Weight reduction

66. Which of the following statements regarding Clomiphene citrate is TRUE in the context of PCOS?

A. It enhances endometrial receptivity

B. It is safe for indefinite long-term use

C. It has anti-estrogenic effects on cervical mucus and endometrium

D. It is preferred over Letrozole as first-line ovulation induction agent

E. It decrease the risk of OHSS

67. Which of the following medications used in PCOS is classified as a selective estrogen receptor modulator (SERM)?

A. Letrozole

B. Spironolactone

C. Clomiphene citrate

D. Metformin

E. Myo-inositol

68. What is the primary reason Letrozole is considered superior to Clomiphene citrate in ovulation induction for PCOS?

A. Higher pregnancy rates and fewer side effects

B. Longer half-life and better tolerance

C. Stronger estrogenic stimulation

D. Direct effect on LH receptors

E. Estrogen receptor antagonism at the hypothalamus (SERM action)

69. A woman with PCOS and BMI = 34 fails lifestyle modification. She refuses ovulation induction. What is the most appropriate pharmacologic intervention to reduce long-term cardiovascular risk?

A. Oral contraceptives

B. Anti-androgens

C. Metformin

D. Statins

E. GLP-1 receptor agonists (e.g. liraglutide)

70. In which of the following patients is Clomiphene citrate least effective for ovulation induction?

A. PCOS with normal BMI and no insulin resistance

B. PCOS with obesity and hyperinsulinemia

C. PCOS with mild hirsutism

D. PCOS with normal androgen levels

E. PCOS with markedly elevated LH:FSH ratio

71. A PCOS patient undergoing ovulation induction with gonadotropins develops > 5 follicles > 12 mm by day 8. What is the most appropriate next step?

A. Administer hCG and proceed with timed intercourse

B. Continue same dose of gonadotropins

C. Cancel the cycle to prevent OHSS

D) Convert the cycle to IVF

72. What is the most important strategy to reduce the risk of OHSS in PCOS patients undergoing gonadotropin therapy?

A. Using GnRH agonist for ovulation trigger

B. Administering Clomiphene citrate beforehand

C. Using high-dose FSH stimulation from the start

D. Co-administering Metformin only

73. Which protocol is most preferred when using gonadotropins for ovulation induction in PCOS patients to minimize risks?

A. Step-down protocol

B. Constant dose protocol

C. Low-dose Step-up protocol

D. Flare protocol

74. In PCOS, why is the step-up low-dose gonadotropin protocol preferred over conventional ones?

A. It increases mono-follicular ovulation rates

B. It accelerates follicular recruitment

C. It eliminates the need for hCG trigger

D. It shortens stimulation duration

75. Which of the following is the best indicator to withhold hCG trigger in a PCOS patient on gonadotropins?

A. LH > 10 IU/L

B. E2 > 1700 pg/mL

C. Progesterone > 1.5 ng/mL

D. Endometrial thickness < 7 mm

76. Which gonadotropin-related complication is more severe in PCOS patients compared to non-PCOS women undergoing ovulation induction?

A. Luteal phase defect

B. Ovarian torsion

C. Ovarian hyperstimulation syndrome (OHSS)

D. Thin endometrium

77. Which of the following is a common clinical feature of PCOS in adolescents?

A. Early menopause

B. Amenorrhea or oligomenorrhea

C. Hot flashes

D. Increased height velocity

78. What is the first-line treatment for menstrual irregularities in adolescent PCOS with no desire for fertility?

A. Clomiphene citrate

B. Metformin

C. Combined oral contraceptives

D. GnRH analogs

79. The pathophysiology of PCOS in adolescents commonly includes:

A. Estrogen deficiency

B. Autoimmune ovarian failure

C. Insulin resistance

D. Prolactin excess

80. Which of the following metabolic risks is associated with adolescent PCOS?

A. Hypoglycemia

B. Type 2 diabetes mellitus

C. Addison's disease

D. Cushing's disease

81. Hirsutism in adolescent PCOS is caused by:

A. Estrogen excess

B. Elevated cortisol

C. Increased androgen levels

D. Hypothyroidism

82. Lifestyle modification in adolescent PCOS is aimed primarily at:

A. Reducing insulin resistance and improving symptoms

B. Improving fertility

C. Weight gain

D. Avoiding surgical treatment

83. In adolescent PCOS, which androgen is considered most reliable for biochemical hyperandrogenism diagnosis?

A. Total testosterone

B. Free testosterone

C. DHEAS

D. Androstenedione

84. The recommended approach to ovarian ultrasound in diagnosing PCOS in adolescents is:

A. Always required for diagnosis

B. Helpful if menstrual history is unavailable

C. Not recommended within 8 years of menarche

D. Used only if hormonal tests are normal

85. Metformin use in adolescent PCOS primarily targets:

A. Ovulation induction

B. Estrogen reduction

C. LH suppression

D. Insulin resistance and hyperandrogenism

86. According to international guidelines, which combination is necessary to diagnose PCOS in adolescents?

A. Oligomenorrhea + polycystic ovaries

B. Oligomenorrhea + biochemical hyperandrogenism

C. Clinical or biochemical hyperandrogenism + persistent menstrual irregularity

D. All three Rotterdam criteria must be met

87- Which of the following is the most appropriate indication for laparoscopic ovarian drilling?

A. PCOS with BMI 38

B. PCOS with hyperprolactinemia

C. PCOS with Clomiphene-resistant anovulation

D. PCOS with bilateral tubal blockage

88- A 29-year-old woman undergoes laparoscopic ovarian drilling for clomiphene-resistant PCOS. Two months later, she complains of increasing pelvic pain and worsening dysmenorrhea. Which postoperative complication is most likely?

A. Premature ovarian failure

B. Pelvic adhesions

C. Tubo-ovarian abscess

D. Endometrial hyperplasia

89- During laparoscopic ovarian drilling, excessive thermal energy is applied to the ovary. What is the most significant long-term risk of this?

A. Ovarian hyperstimulation syndrome

B. Diminished ovarian reserve

C. Increased risk of ectopic pregnancy

D. Chronic pelvic inflammatory disease

90- A woman with PCOS has tried clomiphene, letrozole, metformin, and gonadotropins without success. She is now 37 years old. What is the recommended third-line treatment?

A. IVF

B. Repeat ovarian drilling

C. Lifestyle intervention only

E. IUI alone

91. What is the hallmark feature of LUF syndrome?

A. Complete absence of follicular development

B. Ovulation without luteinization

C. Luteinization of a follicle without rupture

D. Formation of multiple cysts in the ovary

92. LUF syndrome is most commonly associated with which of the following conditions?

A. POI

B. Endometriosis

C. Turner syndrome

D. Polycystic ovarian syndrome (PCOS)

93. Which of the following is the best diagnostic tool for confirming LUF syndrome?

A. Blood progesterone level only

B. Basal body temperature charting

C. Serial transvaginal ultrasound

D. Urinary LH testing alone

94. Which medication might increase the risk of developing LUF syndrome?

A. Clomiphene citrate

B. Letrozole

C. Gonadotropins

D. Progesterone supplements

95. Which of the following is an appropriate treatment option for LUF syndrome in women undergoing ovulation induction?

A. Low-dose aspirin

B. Triggering ovulation with hCG

C. Oral contraceptives

D. Metformin alone

96. Which of the following diagnostic criteria is most specific for LUF in serial ultrasound monitoring?

A. Dominant follicle >18 mm followed by fluid in the pouch of Douglas

B. Persistent unruptured follicle >24 hours after LH surge with progesterone elevation

C. Multiple small follicles without a dominant follicle

D. Endometrial thickness <6 mm with no corpus luteum

97. What is the most appropriate management for a functional ovarian cyst?

A. Immediate laparoscopic cystectomy

B. Oral contraceptive pills to shrink the cyst

C. Observation with repeat ultrasound in 6–8 weeks

D. Chemotherapy

98. Which statement best describes the endocrine profile in LUF syndrome?

A. No LH surge, low estradiol, and low progesterone

B. Normal LH surge, normal estradiol, and normal progesterone

C. Prolonged LH elevation with low estradiol

D. Absent LH surge but high progesterone

99. According to ASRM 2021, ovulatory dysfunction is responsible for approximately what proportion of female infertility?

A. ~10%

B. ~20%

C. ~40%

D. ~60%

100. According to the WHO classification of anovulation, which group accounts for the majority of cases?

A. WHO Group I – Hypogonadotropic hypogonadal anovulation

B. WHO Group II – Normogonadotropic normoestrogenic anovulation

C. WHO Group III – Hypergonadotropic hypogonadal anovulation

D. Hyperprolactinemic anovulation

4. TUBAL FACTOR OF INFERTILITY

101. Which imaging modality is typically used first to assess tubal patency in infertility work-up?

A. MRI pelvis

B. Transvaginal ultrasound

C. Hysterosalpingography (HSG)

D. Laparoscopy

102. What is the preferred treatment in women with bilateral hydrosalpinx planning IVF?

A. Oral antibiotics

B. Salpingectomy before IVF

C. Clomiphene citrate

D. Intrauterine insemination (IUI)

103. A 32-year-old woman has unilateral tubal blockage on HSG. Next step?

A. IVF

B. Laparoscopy

C. Salpingectomy

D. Repeat HSG in 1 week

104. Which of the following findings on hysterosalpingography (HSG) most strongly predicts poor fertility outcomes?

A. Cornual spasm

B. Delayed contrast spill

C. Beaded appearance of tubes

D. Bilateral peritubal adhesions

105. In women with unilateral hydrosalpinx undergoing IVF, what has the greatest positive impact on live birth rate?

A. Antibiotic prophylaxis before oocyte retrieval

B. Transvaginal aspiration of hydrosalpinx fluid

C. Laparoscopic Tubal disconnection prior to IVF

D. Percutaneous tubal occlusion

106. In hysterosalpingography (HSG), which finding is most suggestive of tubal blockage mimicked by a transient condition rather than true obstruction?

A. Cornual spasm

B. Bilateral peritubal adhesions

C. Beaded appearance of tubes

D. Rigid tubular outline

107. What is the typical outcome of tubal cannulation in proximal tubal obstruction due to mucus plug vs true fibrosis?

A. Equally successful

B. Higher success in mucus plug cases

C. Higher success in fibrotic cases

D. Contraindicated in both cases

108. During chromopertubation, a "loculated spill" of dye suggests:

A. Normal patent tube

B. Distal tubal occlusion

C. Peritubal adhesions

D. Cornual spasm

109. Which surgical procedure is most appropriate in a woman with isolated fimbrial phimosis and good tubal length?

A. Salpingectomy

B. Neosalpingostomy

C. Salpingopexy

D. Fimbrioplasty

110. Which of the following best describes the role of assisted reproductive technologies (ART) in tubal factor infertility?

A. Only used in unexplained infertility

B. Ineffective for tubal factor

C. IVF bypasses the need for functional fallopian tubes

D. IUI is superior to IVF

5. UTERINE FACTOR OF INFERTILITY

111. Which of the following is a congenital cause of uterine factor infertility?

A. Asherman's syndrome

B. Septate uterus

C. Genital tuberculosis

D. Submucosal fibroid

112. What is the gold standard investigation for diagnosing intrauterine adhesions?

A. Hysterosalpingography (HSG)

B. Saline infusion sonography (SIS)

C. Hysteroscopy

D. Transvaginal ultrasound

113. In Asherman's syndrome, the most common cause in developing countries is:

A. Multiple fibroids

B. Genital tuberculosis

C. Endometrial hyperplasia

D. Septate uterus

114. Which type of submucosal fibroid has no intramural component according to FIGO classification?

A. Type 0

B. Type 1

C. Type 2

D. Type 3

115. The most common symptom of uterine septum is:

A. Amenorrhea

B. Recurrent pregnancy loss

C. Dysmenorrhea

D. Heavy menstrual bleeding

116. Which congenital uterine anomaly has the best reproductive prognosis after surgical correction?

A. Septate uterus

B. Unicornuate uterus

C. Bicornuate uterus

D. T-shaped uterus

117. According to FIGO classification, a submucosal fibroid with > 50% intramural component is:

A. Type 0

B. Type 1

C. Type 2

D. Type 3

118. The main mechanism of infertility in T-shaped uterus is:

A. Reduced endometrial surface area and altered receptivity

B. Tubal blockage at the uterotubal junction

C. Excessive myometrial contractility

D. Hyperplasia of the basal layer

119. According to the FIGO classification of uterine fibroids (leiomyomas), which of the following is correct?

A. Types 0–2 → Submucosal

B. Types 3–4 → Intramural

C. Types 5–7 → Subserosal

D. Type 8 → Others/Parasitic

E. All of the above

120. All of the following are true regarding a unicornuate uterus, EXCEPT:

A. It results from failure of one Müllerian duct to develop

B. It may be associated with a rudimentary horn

C. It has a strong association with renal anomalies

D. It usually has normal fertility and pregnancy outcome

6. ENDOMETRIOSIS & ADENOMYOSIS RELATED INFERTILITY

121. In women with minimal-to-mild endometriosis undergoing laparoscopy, which treatment has shown improved spontaneous pregnancy rates?

A. Diagnostic laparoscopy only

B. Laparoscopic ablation or excision of lesions

C. Long-term GnRH agonist therapy

D. Expectant management

122. What is the estimated prevalence of endometriosis among women with infertility?

A. 5–10%

B. 10–20%

C. 25–50%

D. 60–80%

123. For advanced endometriosis in infertile women, which is often the first-line assisted reproductive technique?

A. Ovulation induction with clomiphene

B. Intrauterine insemination (IUI)

C. In vitro fertilization (IVF)

D. Tuboplasty

124. In moderate-to-severe endometriosis (Stage III–IV), surgical treatment before attempting conception is most beneficial when:

A. Pelvic anatomy is significantly distorted

B. Age is >42 years

C. IVF has already failed twice

D. CA-125 is elevated but anatomy is normal

125. Which statement is true regarding surgical management of ovarian endometriomas in infertile women?

A. Always avoid cystectomy to preserve ovarian tissue

B. Cystectomy can improve pain but may reduce ovarian reserve

C. Drainage alone offers similar fertility outcomes to cystectomy

D. Surgery has no role before IVF in large endometriomas

126. Which is true about IVF outcomes in endometriosis compared to other infertility causes?

A. Always poorer in all stages of endometriosis

B. May be reduced in severe disease but similar in minimal–mild cases

C. Improved by prolonged GnRH agonist use in all cases

D. Endometriomas >6 cm should be left untreated before IVF

127. Which factor most strongly influences whether to proceed with surgery or ART in endometriosis-related infertility?

A. Size of uterus

B. Patient's age and ovarian reserve

C. CA-125 level

D. Duration of pelvic pain

128. In recurrent endometriosis with infertility, repeated surgery should be approached cautiously because:

A. It always increases AMH

B. It may further reduce ovarian reserve

C. It eliminates the need for ART

D. It has better pregnancy rates than IVF

129. A 29-year-old woman presents with 2 years of primary infertility and moderate dysmenorrhea. Transvaginal ultrasound is normal. Diagnostic laparoscopy reveals multiple superficial peritoneal implants and mild adhesions (ASRM Stage II). Both tubes are patent. What is the next best step to improve her chances of spontaneous conception?

A. Expectant management for 1 year

B. Laparoscopic ablation or excision of lesions

C. Long-term GnRH agonist therapy

D. Proceed directly to IVF

130. Long-term medical suppression after surgical treatment in women actively trying to conceive is:

A. Recommended for 6–12 months

B. Contraindicated as it delays attempts at conception

C. Essential before IVF

D. Only used in women >40 years

131. A 31-year-old woman with Stage III endometriosis and infertility is considering medical treatment before attempting conception. She asks about hormonal suppression.

Which statement is correct?

A. GnRH agonists improve pregnancy rates if used alone for 6 months

B. Combined oral contraceptives are first-line for improving conception rates

C. Danazol is preferred before ovulation induction

D. Hormonal suppression is primarily for symptom relief, not fertility enhancement

132. A 36-year-old woman with recurrent Stage IV endometriosis underwent surgery 2 years ago. She has low AMH and 3 years of infertility. What is the most appropriate management?

A. Repeat surgery

B. Ovulation induction with clomiphene

C. IVF

D. Expectant management for 6 months

133. A 32-year-old woman with Stage III endometriosis is planning IVF. She has a 4 cm asymptomatic ovarian endometrioma. What is the best management?

A. Immediate cystectomy before IVF

B. Drainage of cyst before IVF

C. Proceed to IVF without surgery

D. GnRH agonists for 6 months, then IVF

134. Which of the following medical therapies improves pregnancy rates when used alone in endometriosis-related infertility?

A. GnRH agonists

B. Progestins

C. Combined oral contraceptives

D. None of the above

135. A 36-year-old woman presents with infertility and severe dysmenorrhea. TVUS shows heterogeneous myometrium with small myometrial cysts. Which is the most likely diagnosis?

A. Endometriosis

B. Uterine fibroid

C. Adenomyosis

D. Chronic endometritis

136. Adenomyosis impairs fertility mainly through:

A. Tubal blockage

B. Ovulation failure

C. Impaired implantation

D. Cervical stenosis

137. Which surgical option may improve fertility in women with focal adenomyosis?

A. Hysterectomy

B. Adenomyomectomy

C. Endometrial ablation

D. Myomectomy

138. Which condition most commonly coexists with adenomyosis and further reduces fertility?

A. PCOS

B. Endometriosis

C. Pelvic inflammatory disease

D. Tuberculosis

139. Women with adenomyosis and infertility are at increased risk of:

A. Multiple pregnancy

B. Miscarriage

C. Ovarian hyperstimulation

D. Cervical incompetence

140. A 35-year-old woman presents with primary infertility and heavy painful periods. The gynecologist performs a transvaginal ultrasound (TVUS) as the first-line imaging test. Which of the following findings is most characteristic of adenomyosis?

A. Ovarian cysts

B. Ill-defined endo-myometrial junction (junctional zone irregularity)

C. Endometrial hyperplasia

D. Intrauterine calcifications

7. MYOMA RELATED INFERTILITY

141. Which type of fibroid is most strongly associated with reduced fertility?

A. Subserosal fibroid

B. Intramural fibroid without cavity distortion

C. Submucosal fibroid

D. Pedunculated fibroid

142. A 34-year-old woman with unexplained infertility is found to have a 5 cm intramural fibroid that does not distort the endometrial cavity. What is the best management?

A. Immediate myomectomy

B. Hysterectomy

C. Expectant management

D. Uterine artery embolization

143. Which of the following fibroid treatments is contraindicated in women desiring future fertility?

A. Hysteroscopic myomectomy

B. Laparoscopic myomectomy

C. Uterine artery embolization (UAE)

D. Open myomectomy

144. Which investigation best defines the relationship between fibroids and the endometrial cavity in the context of infertility?

A. Hysterosalpingography (HSG)

B. 2D & 3D TVUS

C. MRI

D. Ultrasound (transabdominal)

145. The recurrence rate of fibroids after myomectomy is approximately:

A. <5%

B. 10–15%

C. 20–25%

D. >50%

146. A submucosal fibroid with >50% of its volume within the endometrium is classified as:

A. Type 0

B. Type 1

C. Type 2

D. Type 3

147. Which type of fibroid is completely intramural and abuts the endometrium?

A. Type 2

B. Type 3

C. Type 4

D. Type 5

148. Which fibroid type is most likely to affect fertility by directly distorting the endometrial cavity?

A. Type 0–2

B. Type 8

C. Type 4

D. Type 6–7

149. After hysteroscopic myomectomy for submucosal fibroids, what is the minimum recommended time before attempting pregnancy?

A. One week

B. Four to six weeks

C. Three months

D. Six months

150. Which statement about intramural fibroids less than 5 cm regarding infertility is MOST accurate?

A. They have no effect on fertility outcomes

B. Surgical removal always improves pregnancy rates

C. They may negatively impact implantation but the evidence is inconclusive

D. They invariably cause recurrent miscarriage

151. After surgical treatment of fibroids in infertile women, which factor most affects subsequent pregnancy success?

A. Patient age and ovarian reserve

B. Number of fibroids removed alone

C. Presence of subserosal fibroids elsewhere

D. Use of hormone replacement therapy post-surgery

8. UNEXPLAINED INFERTILITY

152. Which of the following is least likely to be a contributing factor in unexplained infertility?

A. Gamete or embryo transport defects

B. Luteal phase defects

C. Subtle immunologic factors

D. Severe bilateral tubal blockage

153. In the initial workup for infertility, unexplained infertility is diagnosed only after:

A. Basic investigations reveal abnormal hormonal levels

B. Male factor infertility is confirmed

C. Tubal patency, ovulation, and semen analysis are normal

D. IVF is attempted and fails

154. Which first-line management strategy is often recommended for couples with unexplained infertility and a woman under 35 years old with one year of infertility?

A. Immediate IVF

B. Expectant management for up to another 12 months

C. Laparoscopic surgery

D. Donor insemination

155. Which treatment option has shown higher pregnancy rates compared to expectant management in unexplained infertility?

A. Ovulation induction with clomiphene citrate plus (IUI)

B. Progesterone supplementation only

C. Lifestyle modification alone

D. Antibiotic therapy

156. Which statement about IVF in unexplained infertility is correct?

A. IVF is generally avoided in unexplained infertility at all ages

B. IVF is often considered after failure of less invasive treatments such as IUI

C. IVF is more successful in women over 45 with unexplained infertility

D. IVF has no better success rates than expectant management

157. In couples with unexplained infertility, which of the following interventions has the strongest evidence for improving pregnancy rates after expectant management fails?

A. Laparoscopic ovarian drilling

B. Intrauterine insemination with controlled ovarian stimulation

C. Prolonged luteal phase progesterone therapy

D. Empirical antibiotic therapy

158. Which of the following is first-line active management in young couples after a period of expectant management fails?

A. In vitro fertilization (IVF) directly

B. Ovulation induction + intrauterine insemination (IUI)

C. Empirical laparoscopy

D. Donor egg IVF

159. Which statement about unexplained infertility is correct?

A. It accounts for less than 5% of infertility cases

B. Luteal phase defect is never involved

C. It cannot occur if the woman has regular cycles

D. Subtle sperm dysfunction may be a contributing factor

160. Which of the following may slightly improve live birth rates before IVF in women with unexplained infertility?

A. Short-term GnRH agonist

B. Surgical removal of corpus luteum

C. Lifestyle optimization (BMI, smoking cessation)

D. Empirical antibiotic therapy

161. A 36-year-old woman with unexplained infertility for 1 year has diminished ovarian reserve (AMH 0.8 ng/mL). What is the best management strategy?

A. Continue expectant management for 6 more months

B. OI + IUI for 6 cycles

C. Proceed to IVF

D. GnRH agonist for 3 months then IUI

162. A 30-year-old woman with unexplained infertility has undergone 3 unsuccessful cycles of clomiphene citrate + IUI. What is the next step?

A. Continue IUI for 3 more cycles

B. Switch to gonadotropin-stimulated IUI

C. Laparoscopy for diagnosis of subtle endometriosis

D. Proceed to IVF

163. Which of the following is the primary indication for IUI?

A. Severe tubal damage

B. Severe oligospermia

C. Unexplained infertility

D. Premature ovarian failure

164. After how many unsuccessful cycles of IUI should IVF be considered in a patient 27 years?

A. 2 cycles

B. 3–4 cycles

C. 6 cycles

D. 12 cycles

165. Which factor is associated with the highest success rates for IUI?

A. Woman age <35 years and infertility <3 years

B. Severe male factor infertility

C. Bilateral tubal blockage

D. Woman age >40 years

166. Which complication is most strongly associated with gonadotropin-stimulated IUI?

A. Ectopic pregnancy

B. Multiple pregnancy

C. Cervical stenosis

D. Uterine rupture

167. In IUI, sperm preparation ("washing") is performed to:

A. Increase DNA fragmentation

B. Concentrate motile sperm and remove prostaglandins

C. Induce acrosome reaction

D. Reduce sperm motility

168. Which of the following is NOT an indication for IUI?

A. Cervical mucus hostility

B. Mild male factor infertility

C. Anovulation not responsive to medical therapy

D. Donor sperm insemination

169. In a stimulated IUI cycle, the insemination is usually timed:

A. 12 hours after LH surge detection

B. 36 hours after hCG trigger injection

C. 5 days after follicle rupture

D. Any day in luteal phase

170. Which of the following semen parameters is most predictive of IUI success?

A. Morphology >4% normal forms

B. Post-wash total motile sperm count (TMSC)

C. Sperm head defects

D. Semen viscosity

171. What is the approximate live birth rate per IUI cycle in unexplained infertility with ovarian stimulation?

A. 2–3%

B. 5–10%

C. 10–15%

D. >25%

172. A 39-year-old woman with unexplained infertility is starting IUI. Which factor will most negatively affect success rates?

A. Infertility duration 2 years

B. BMI 24

C. Woman age 39 years

D. Mild asthenospermia

173. Which of the following is a contraindication to IUI?

A. Bilateral tubal blockage

B. Mild oligospermia

C. Anovulation responsive to clomiphene

D. Cervical stenosis

174. A 30-year-old woman presents with a 2-year history of infertility. She has regular ovulatory cycles, normal ovarian reserve tests, a normal semen analysis for her partner, and a normal transvaginal ultrasound. A (HSG) shows bilateral tubal patency. She meets the criteria for unexplained infertility. She asks whether she should undergo diagnostic laparoscopy and hysteroscopy before starting treatment. According to ESHRE guidelines, which of the following is the MOST appropriate recommendation regarding the use of laparoscopy and hysteroscopy in this patient?

A. Perform routine laparoscopy and hysteroscopy for all cases of unexplained infertility

B. Offer laparoscopy only to improve natural conception rates before assisted reproduction

C. Offer diagnostic laparoscopy only if symptoms or signs suggest pelvic pathology such as endometriosis

D. Replace HSG with laparoscopy as the first-line test of tubal patency in unexplained infertility

E. Perform hysteroscopy routinely before initiating any fertility treatment

175. Which of the following best describes the risk of multiple pregnancy with stimulated IUI?

A. Rare (<1%)

B. About 5–10%

C. Always >20%

D. Same as IVF

9. HIRSUTISM

176. The most common cause of hirsutism in reproductive-aged women is:

A. Androgen-secreting tumor

B. Cushing's syndrome

C. Polycystic ovary syndrome (PCOS)

D. Non-classical congenital adrenal hyperplasia (CAH)

177. Which of the following hormones is primarily responsible for hirsutism?

A. Estradiol

B. Testosterone and dihydrotestosterone (DHT)

C. Progesterone

D. Cortisol

178. A 24-year-old woman presents with hirsutism, irregular cycles, and obesity. The most likely diagnosis is:

A. PCOS

B. Cushing's disease

C. Androgen-secreting tumor

D. Non-classical CAH

179. Which scoring system is commonly used to grade hirsutism severity?

A. Apgar score

B. Ferriman–Gallwey score

C. Bishop score

D. Glasgow coma scale

180. A woman presents with rapidly progressive hirsutism and clitoromegaly. What is the next best step?

A. Reassure and start cosmetic therapy

B. Measure serum total testosterone and DHEAS

C. Start combined oral contraceptives

D. Begin spironolactone

181. Which of the following is the first-line pharmacological therapy for hirsutism in PCOS?

A. Spironolactone

B. Combined oral contraceptive pill (COCP)

C. Finasteride

D. Flutamide

182. Which drug is an anti-androgen acting as a 5α-reductase inhibitor?

A. Finasteride

B. Spironolactone

C. Flutamide

D. Metformin

183. A 26-year-old woman with PCOS and hirsutism is not planning pregnancy. Best initial management?

A. Lifestyle modification + COCP

B. Immediate IVF

C. Clomiphene citrate

D. Laparoscopic ovarian drilling

184. Which of the following androgens is exclusively adrenal in origin?

A. Testosterone

B. Androstenedione

C. DHEAS

D. DHT

185. Which enzyme defect causes non-classical congenital adrenal hyperplasia (CAH) presenting as hirsutism?

A. 11β-hydroxylase deficiency

B. 17α-hydroxylase deficiency

C. 21-hydroxylase deficiency

D. 3β-HSD deficiency

186. Main mechanism of infertility in PCOS with hirsutism is:

A. Tubal factor

B. Anovulation due to hyperandrogenemia and insulin resistance

C. Cervical mucus hostility

D. Luteal phase defect

187. Which of the following androgens, if elevated, suggests adrenal cause of hirsutism with infertility?

A. Testosterone

B. Androstenedione

C. DHEAS

D. DHT

188. In non-classical CAH (21-hydroxylase deficiency), hirsutism with infertility is due to:

A. Low cortisol

B. High LH

C. Excess adrenal androgens

D. High prolactin

189. Which is true regarding laparoscopic ovarian drilling in PCOS?

A. First-line for all women with PCOS-related infertility

B. Reserved for women resistant to clomiphene/letrozole

C. Contraindicated if hirsutism is present

D. Replaces IVF

190. Which of the following improves both hirsutism and infertility in PCOS?

A. COCP alone

B. Weight loss (lifestyle modification)

C. Spironolactone alone

D. Cosmetic hair removal

191. In which condition is glucocorticoid therapy indicated for hirsutism and infertility?

A. PCOS

B. Cushing's syndrome

C. Non-classical congenital adrenal hyperplasia (21-hydroxylase deficiency)

D. Androgen-secreting ovarian tumor

192. Mechanism of corticosteroid therapy in CAH-related hirsutism is:

A. Direct inhibition of 5α-reductase

B. Suppression of ACTH to reduce adrenal androgen production

C. Increase in SHBG

D. Blocking androgen receptors

193. A 22-year-old woman with hirsutism, irregular cycles, and infertility. Labs: Elevated 17-hydroxyprogesterone, elevated DHEAS, mildly low cortisol. Most likely diagnosis:

A. PCOS

B. Non-classical CAH

C. Androgen-secreting tumor

D. Cushing's disease

194. Which lab test is most useful to confirm non-classical CAH in a hirsute woman?

A. Serum LH/FSH ratio

B. Early morning 17-hydroxyprogesterone

C. Cortisol suppression test

D. Serum prolactin

195. A hirsute woman with infertility due to non-classical CAH is treated with glucocorticoids. Expected outcome is:

A. Restoration of ovulation and fertility

B. Immediate cosmetic resolution of hair

C. Complete cure of CAH

D. Suppression of ovarian androgen production

196. The most common enzyme deficiency causing CAH is:

A. 11β-hydroxylase deficiency

B. 21-hydroxylase deficiency

C. 17α-hydroxylase deficiency

D. 3β-hydroxysteroid dehydrogenase deficiency

197. A newborn presents with ambiguous genitalia and salt-wasting crisis. The most likely enzyme deficiency is:

A. 21-hydroxylase deficiency (salt-wasting form)

B. 11β-hydroxylase deficiency

C. 17α-hydroxylase deficiency

D. Aromatase deficiency

198. Which type of CAH is associated with hypertension and virilization?

A. 21-hydroxylase deficiency

B. 11β-hydroxylase deficiency

C. 17α-hydroxylase deficiency

D. 3β-HSD deficiency

199. Which type of CAH is associated with hypertension, hypokalemia, and sexual infantilism (under virilization in males, lack of secondary sex in females)?

A. 21-hydroxylase deficiency

B. 11β-hydroxylase deficiency

C. 17α-hydroxylase deficiency

D. 3β-HSD deficiency

200. In non-classical CAH (late-onset 21-hydroxylase deficiency), a woman may present with:

A. Ambiguous genitalia at birth

B. Salt-wasting crisis

C. Hirsutism, irregular cycles, infertility

D. Hypertension

201. Best screening test for CAH in neonates:

A. Serum cortisol

B. 17-hydroxyprogesterone

C. Plasma renin activity

D. DHEAS

202. In a hirsute infertile woman with suspected non-classical CAH, the confirmatory test is:

A. Serum testosterone

B. ACTH stimulation test (measuring 17-OHP)

C. Dexamethasone suppression test

D. GnRH stimulation test

203. The mainstay of treatment for CAH is:

A. Anti-androgens

B. Surgery only

C. Mineralocorticoid antagonists

D. Corticosteroid replacement

204. In salt-wasting CAH, what drug must be added to glucocorticoid therapy?

A. Anti-androgen

B. Mineralocorticoid (fludrocortisone)

C. Spironolactone

D. GnRH analog

205. A newborn presents with ambiguous genitalia, hyponatremia, hyperkalemia, and dehydration in the first weeks of life. The most likely cause is:

A. 21-hydroxylase deficiency (classic salt-wasting CAH)

B. 11β-hydroxylase deficiency

C. 17α-hydroxylase deficiency

D. Aromatase deficiency

10. AMENORRHEA

206. A 16-year-old girl presents with primary amenorrhea, normal breast development, but absent pubic and axillary hair. On exam, she has a blind vaginal pouch. Most likely diagnosis is:

A. Turner syndrome

B. Mayer-Rokitansky-Küster-Hauser (MRKH) syndrome

C. Complete androgen insensitivity syndrome

D. Hypogonadotropic hypogonadism

207. A 17-year-old girl with primary amenorrhea, normal secondary sexual characteristics, normal ovaries, but absent uterus on ultrasound. Most likely diagnosis:

A. MRKH syndrome

B. Turner syndrome

C. Hypothalamic amenorrhea

D. Complete androgen insensitivity

208. All are causes of primary amenorrhea with normal secondary sexual characteristics EXCEPT:

A. MRKH syndrome

B. Transverse vaginal septum

C. Imperforate hymen

D. Gonadal dysgenesis

209. All of the following are associated with high FSH/LH in primary amenorrhea EXCEPT:

A. Turner syndrome

B. Gonadal dysgenesis

C. Kallmann syndrome

D. Pure gonadal failure

210. All of the following are features of androgen insensitivity syndrome presenting with primary amenorrhea EXCEPT:

A. 46,XY karyotype

B. Normal breast development

C. Presence of uterus

D. Absent pubic and axillary hair

211. Secondary amenorrhea following dilatation & curettage for postpartum hemorrhage is most likely due to:

A. PCOS

B. Asherman's syndrome

C. Premature ovarian failure

D. Pituitary adenoma

212. All of the following are common causes of secondary amenorrhea EXCEPT:

A. PCOS

B. Asherman's syndrome

C. Hyperprolactinemia

D. Complete androgen insensitivity syndrome

213. All of the following can cause secondary amenorrhea with normal estrogen levels EXCEPT:

A. PCOS

B. Outflow tract obstruction (Asherman's)

C. Hypothalamic amenorrhea

D. Hyperprolactinemia

214. Secondary amenorrhea due to uterine causes includes all EXCEPT:

A. Asherman's syndrome

B. Uterine synechiae post-infection

C. Transverse vaginal septum

D. Endometrial tuberculosis

215. A 14-year-old girl presents with primary amenorrhea, cyclic lower abdominal pain, and a pelvic mass. On examination, there is a bulging bluish membrane at the vaginal introitus. Most likely diagnosis is:

A. Transverse vaginal septum

B. Imperforate hymen

C. MRKH syndrome

D. Androgen insensitivity syndrome

11. PUBERTY

216. Thelarche (breast budding) is the first sign of puberty in most girls. Which of the following, if present first, suggests abnormal puberty?

A. Thelarche at 10 years

B. Pubarche at 9 years before thelarche

C. Menarche at 12 years

D. Growth spurt at 11 years

217. Which of the following best indicates the onset of central (true) puberty in girls?

A. Thelarche

B. Menarche

C. Pubarche

D. Peak height velocity

218. Which of the following is the last event in normal female puberty?

A. Growth spurt

B. Thelarche

C. Pubarche

D. Menarche

219. Tanner stage 3 breast development corresponds to:

A. Only papilla elevated

B. Areola and breast in one mound, further enlargement

C. Secondary mound of areola and papilla

D. Mature breast, areola recessed

220. Precocious puberty in girls is defined as:

A. Breast development before age 10

B. Pubic hair before age 8

C. Breast development before age 8

D. Menarche before age 11

221. Which hormone primarily drives the pubertal growth spurt in girls?

A. Growth hormone alone

B. Estrogen

C. Progesterone

D. Cortisol

222. Delayed puberty in girls is defined as:

A. No thelarche by age 10

B. No menarche by age 14

C. No thelarche by age 13 or no menarche by 15

D. No menarche by 16 regardless of secondary sexual development

223. A girl develops secondary sexual characteristics in proper sequence but at a much earlier age than normal. Best term is:

A. Isosexual true precocious puberty

B. Pseudo-precocious puberty

C. Heterosexual precocious puberty

D. Premature thelarche

224. A 12-year-old girl with breast development but no pubic hair. Likely diagnosis:

A. Constitutional delay

B. Turner syndrome

C. Androgen insensitivity syndrome

D. Kallmann syndrome

225. Menarche typically occurs how many years after thelarche?

A. 1 year

B. 2–3 years

C. 4–5 years

D. At the same time

12. MALE FACTOR INFETILITY

226. The most common cause of male infertility is:

A. Hypogonadotropic hypogonadism

B. Varicocele

C. Obstructive azoospermia

D. Genetic abnormalities

227. Which of the following is a genetic cause of male infertility?

A. Klinefelter syndrome

B. Turner syndrome

C. Androgen insensitivity

D. Fragile X premutation

228. A 30-year-old man with infertility and anosmia most likely has:

A. Klinefelter syndrome

B. Kallmann syndrome

C. Sertoli cell-only syndrome

D. Prader-Willi syndrome

229. Cryptorchidism increases infertility risk because of:

A. Low LH

B. Low FSH

C. Increased testicular temperature

D. Defective Leydig cells

230. Which infection is classically associated with obstructive azoospermia?

A. Chlamydia

B. Mumps orchitis

C. Gonorrhea

D. Syphilis

231. First-line investigation for male infertility is:

A. Testicular biopsy

B. Serum testosterone

C. Scrotal ultrasound

D. Semen analysis

232. Normal semen analysis should be repeated after:

A. 1 week

B. 2 weeks

C. 3 months

D. 6 months

233. According to WHO, normal sperm concentration is:

A. >5 million/mL

B. >10 million/mL

C. >15 million/mL

D. >20 million/Ml

234. Normal sperm motility (progressive) is:

A. ≥32%

B. ≥20%

C. ≥40%

D. ≥50%

235. Normal sperm morphology (strict Kruger criteria) is:

A. ≥2%

B. ≥4%

C. ≥10%

D. ≥20%

236. Azoospermia with low FSH, low LH, low testosterone suggests:

A. Primary testicular failure

B. Pituitary or hypothalamic dysfunction

C. Klinefelter syndrome

D. Sertoli-cell only syndrome

237. Azoospermia with high FSH, high LH, low testosterone indicates:

A. Hypogonadotropic hypogonadism

B. Hypergonadotropic hypogonadism

C. Normal spermatogenesis

D. Obstructive azoospermia

238. Which hormone is secreted by Sertoli cells and reflects spermatogenesis?

A. Testosterone

B. AMH

C. DHT

D. Inhibin B

239. Varicocele is most common on:

A. Right side

B. Left side

C. Bilateral equally

D. Depends on age

240. Mechanism of infertility in varicocele is:

A. Testicular ischemia

B. Obstruction of spermatic ducts

C. Defective Sertoli cell proliferation

D. Increased scrotal temperature & oxidative stress

241. Gold standard test for varicocele diagnosis:

A. Physical exam (standing, Valsalva)

B. Scrotal ultrasound with Doppler

C. MRI pelvis

D. Venography

242. Testicular biopsy is indicated in:

A. Suspected varicocele

B. Obstructive azoospermia

C. Non-obstructive azoospermia

D. Oligospermia

243. Epididymal obstruction is most commonly due to:

A. Trauma

B. Infections

C. Tumors

D. Drugs

244. Retrograde ejaculation is diagnosed by finding sperm in:

A. Prostatic fluid

B. Post-ejaculatory urine

C. Rectal swab

D. Seminal vesicle aspirate

245. Smoking causes infertility mainly by:

A. DNA fragmentation & oxidative stress

B. Reduced FSH

C. Reduced Leydig cell function

D. Lowering libido

246. Indication for ICSI (Intracytoplasmic Sperm Injection) is:

A. Severe oligospermia

B. Normal sperm count

C. Anovulation in female

D. Tubal blockage

247. Best option for men with obstructive azoospermia but normal spermatogenesis:

A. IVF

B. IUI

C. ICSI with sperm retrieval

D. Testicular transplant

248. TESE (testicular sperm extraction) is used in:

A. Non-obstructive azoospermia

B. Oligospermia

C. Erectile dysfunction

D. Varicocele

249. A man with infertility has normal semen volume, azoospermia, normal testes, and palpable vas deferens. Likely diagnosis?

A. Obstructive azoospermia

B. Hypogonadism

C. Sertoli cell-only syndrome

D. Genetic mutation

250. In idiopathic male infertility, which empiric therapy is often tried?

A. Corticosteroids

B. Antioxidants

C. Chemotherapy

D. Testosterone replacement

ANSWERS

1	B	41	A	81	C
2	E	42	C	82	A
3	D	43	D	83	B
4	C	44	C	84	C
5	B	45	B	85	D
6	C	46	C	86	C
7	D	47	D	87	C
8	D	48	C	88	B
9	C	49	A	89	B
10	C	50	B	90	A
11	E	51	D	91	C
12	C	52	B	92	B
13	B	53	C	93	C
14	D	54	D	94	A
15	B	55	D	95	B
16	C	56	C	96	B
17	D	57	C	97	C
18	D	58	C	98	B
19	C	59	B	99	C
20	B	60	E	100	B
21	C	61	D	101	C
22	A	62	B	102	B
23	C	63	B	103	B
24	A	64	C	104	C
25	C	65	B	105	C
26	E	66	C	106	A
27	D	67	C	107	B
28	E	68	A	108	C
29	D	69	C	109	D
30	A	70	B	110	C
31	C	71	C	111	B
32	B	72	A	112	C
33	B	73	C	113	B
34	C	74	A	114	A
35	C	75	B	115	B
36	D	76	C	116	A
37	C	77	B	117	C
38	B	78	C	118	A
39	D	79	C	119	E
40	A	80	B	120	D

121	B
122	C
123	C
124	A
125	B
126	B
127	B
128	B
129	B
130	B
131	D
132	C
133	C
134	D
135	C
136	C
137	B
138	B
139	B
140	B
141	C
142	C
143	C
144	B
145	C
146	B
147	B
148	A
149	C
150	C
151	A
152	D
153	C
154	B
155	A
156	B
157	B
158	B
159	D
160	C

161	C
162	A
163	C
164	C
165	A
166	B
167	B
168	C
169	B
170	B
171	C
172	C
173	A
174	C
175	B
176	C
177	B
178	A
179	B
180	B
181	B
182	A
183	A
184	C
185	C
186	B
187	C
188	C
189	B
190	B
191	C
192	B
193	B
194	B
195	A
196	B
197	A
198	B
199	C
200	C

201	B
202	B
203	D
204	B
205	A
206	C
207	A
208	D
209	C
210	C
211	B
212	D
213	C
214	C
215	B
216	B
217	A
218	D
219	B
220	C
221	B
222	C
223	A
224	C
225	B
226	B
227	A
228	B
229	C
230	B
231	D
232	C
233	C
234	A
235	B
236	B
237	B
238	D
239	B
240	D

241	242	243	244	245	246	247	248	249	250
B	C	B	B	A	A	C	A	A	B

PART 2

TRUE/FALSE QUESTIONS IN INFERTILITY

1. In relation to ovulatory disorders:

A. Hypothalamic amenorrhea is classified as WHO Group I anovulation ( )

B. PCOS is the most common cause of WHO Group II anovulation ( )

C. Premature ovarian insufficiency belongs to WHO Group IV anovulation ( )

D. Hyperprolactinemia is categorized under WHO Group III ( )

E. Weight loss in obese women with PCOS may restore ovulation ( )

2. Concerning tubal and pelvic factors in infertility:

A. PID has significant role in the etiology of tubal infertility ( )

B. Bilateral hydrosalpinx has no impact on natural conception rates ( )

C. HSG is a useful method for initial assessment of tubal patency ( )

D. Genital tuberculosis can lead to tubo-ovarian adhesions ( )

E. Uterine fibroids have no role in infertility ( )

3. With respect to unexplained infertility:

A. Accounts for about 25% of infertility cases ( )

B. Subtle sperm dysfunction may contribute to diagnosis ( )

C. Female age has no significant impact as a prognostic factor in infertility ( )

D. Always requires immediate assisted reproduction ( )

E. Spontaneous conception may occur in some couples ( )

4. Regarding endometriosis and infertility:

A. Medical suppression of endometriosis improves fertility rates significantly ( )

B. Laparoscopy with histology has no longer the gold standard for diagnosis ()

C. Severe endometriosis may distort pelvic anatomy ( )

D. Endometriosis always presents with pelvic pain ( )

E. Adenomyosis may coexist with endometriosis and reduce fertility ( )

5. In relation to premature ovarian insufficiency:

A. Defined as loss of ovarian function before age 40 ( )

B. Diagnosis is confirmed with high FSH on two occasions 4 weeks apart ( )

C. Autoimmune disorders may contribute to the condition ( )

D. Women with POI can never conceive spontaneously ( )

E. Family history may increase the risk ( )

6. Concerning general definitions of infertility:

A. Infertility is defined as failure to conceive after 12 months of unprotected intercourse ( )

B. Secondary infertility means difficulty conceiving after a previous pregnancy ( )

C. Subfertility is often used interchangeably with infertility ( )

D. Primary infertility means no prior conception ( )

E. The global prevalence of infertility is estimated at 30–40% ( )

7. With respect to female infertility investigations:

A. FSH can be used to confirm ovulation ( )

B. Serum prolactin measurement is not part of infertility workup ( )

C. Hysterosalpingography (HSG) is a method to assess Tubal factor only ( )

D. Laparoscopy is considered the gold standard for tubal disease ( )

E. Thyroid dysfunction can contribute to infertility ( )

8. Regarding male infertility investigations:

A. Semen analysis is the first-line investigation ( )

B. Normal semen parameters guarantee fertility ( )

C. Elevated FSH is typical in obstructive azoospermia ( )

D. Testicular biopsy differentiates obstructive from non-obstructive azoospermia ( )

E. Scrotal ultrasound can identify varicocele ( )

9. In relation to lifestyle factors and infertility:

A. Obesity has no effect on ovulation ( )

B. Excessive exercise can improve ovulation ( )

C. Smoking increases infertility risk in men and women ( )

D. Alcohol intake has no impact on fertility ( )

E. Advanced maternal age reduces both oocyte quantity and quality ( )

10. Concerning hormonal influences on infertility:

A. Hyperprolactinemia can lead to anovulation ( )

B. Hypothyroidism may impair fertility ( )

C. High FSH & LH levels are seen in hypothalamic amenorrhea ( )

D. AMH is a marker of ovarian reserve ( )

E. Low FSH levels are diagnostic of PCOS ( )

11. With respect to genetic causes of infertility:

A. Klinefelter syndrome has a 47,XXY karyotype ( )

B. Turner syndrome is not associated with ovarian failure ( )

C. Y chromosome microdeletions are a genetic cause of azoospermia ( )

D. Cystic fibrosis mutations not a cause of congenital absence of the vas deferens ( )

E. Fragile X premutation may be linked to premature ovarian insufficiency ( )

12. Regarding the "FSH threshold" concept in follicular development:

A. A minimal level of FSH is required for follicular recruitment ( )

B. Once follicles are recruited, continued high FSH is essential for growth ( )

C. The dominant follicle becomes less dependent on FSH ( )

D. The threshold concept explains why few follicles keep growing ( )

E. Exogenous FSH in ovarian stimulation aims to exceed the threshold for multiple follicle growth ( )

13. In relation to epidemiology of infertility:

A. Global prevalence is about 10–15% ( )

B. Primary infertility is more common in developed countries ( )

C. Tubal disease is the leading cause of infertility in developing countries ( )

D. Male factor contributes to 10–15% of cases ( )

E. Unexplained infertility accounts for fewer than 5% of cases ( )

14. Concerning reproductive physiology and infertility:

A. The luteal phase normally lasts around 10 days ( )

B. The LH surge precedes ovulation by about 10 hours ( )

C. The follicular phase is constant in all women ( )

D. The corpus luteum produces progesterone ( )

E. Endometrial receptivity peaks in the mid-luteal phase ( )

15. Regarding hypothalamic causes of infertility:

A. Stress can suppress GnRH secretion ( )

B. Excessive exercise may cause hypothalamic amenorrhea ( )

C. High BMI is a risk factor ( )

D. High prolactin is typical of hypothalamic dysfunction ( )

E. Anorexia Nervosa may cause hypothalamic amenorrhea ( )

16. In relation to hyperprolactinemia:

A. It may cause galactorrhea and infertility ( )

B. Prolactin inhibits GnRH secretion ( )

C. Prolactinomas are always malignant ( )

D. Dopamine agonists are the mainstay of treatment ( )

E. Hypothyroidism may cause secondary hyperprolactinemia ( )

17. Concerning ovarian reserve markers:

A. AMH reflects the pool of antral follicles ( )

B. Antral follicle count is done by ultrasound ( )

C. Day-3 FSH >10 IU/L suggests low reserve ( )

D. AMH is cycle-dependent ( )

E. Ovarian reserve constant with increasing age ( )

18. With respect to semen analysis:

A. Volume >1.5 ml is abnormal ( )

B. Progressive motility >32% is considered normal ( )

C. Normal morphology >4% (strict criteria) is acceptable ( )

D. Sperm concentration >15 million/ml is abnormal ( )

E. One sample is always sufficient for diagnosis ( )

19. Regarding varicocele and infertility:

A. More common on the left side ( )

B. Associated with increased scrotal temperature ( )

C. May impair sperm motility ( )

D. Surgical correction always restores fertility ( )

E. Clinical examination is more sensitive than Doppler ultrasound ( )

20. In relation to genital tuberculosis:

A. Common cause of infertility in developing countries ( )

B. Fallopian tubes are most frequently affected ( )

C. Endometrial involvement may impair implantation ( )

D. Diagnosis is usually by endometrial biopsy ( )

E. HSG is the gold standard for diagnosis ( )

21. Concerning PCOS and infertility:

A. Associated with hyperandrogenism ( )

B. Oligo/anovulation is not common ( )

C. Polycystic ovaries on ultrasound are diagnostic alone ( )

D. Insulin resistance is often present ( )

E. First-line management includes lifestyle modification ( )

22. With respect to endometrial factors:

A. Polyps may reduce fertility ( )

B. Submucous fibroids can impair implantation ( )

C. Asherman's syndrome involves intrauterine adhesions ( )

D. Hysteroscopy is not the gold standard for diagnosis ( )

E. Endometrial thickness always predicts fertility ( )

23. Regarding endocrine disorders and infertility:

A. Hypothyroidism can cause anovulation ( )

B. Hyperthyroidism may cause menstrual irregularities ( )

C. Diabetes mellitus has no effect on fertility ( )

D. Cushing's syndrome can impair ovulation ( )

E. Late-onset CAH may mimic PCOS ( )

24. With respect to endometriomas:

A. May not reduce ovarian reserve ( )

B. Can distort pelvic anatomy ( )

C. Surgical removal always improves fertility ( )

D. Associated with chronic pelvic pain ( )

E. Found only in postmenopausal women ( )

25. Regarding congenital uterine anomalies:

A. Septate uterus is associated with recurrent pregnancy loss ( )

B. Bicornuate uterus results from incomplete fusion of Müllerian ducts ( )

C. Uterus didelphys involves two separate cavities ( )

D. Arcuate uterus has great impact on fertility ( )

E. Hysterosalpingography can differentiate all anomalies ( )

26. In relation to male endocrine causes of infertility:

A. Kallmann syndrome involves GnRH deficiency ( )

B. Elevated FSH suggests testicular failure ( )

C. Low LH and low testosterone indicate secondary hypogonadism ( )

D. Hyperprolactinemia may impair spermatogenesis ( )

E. Androgen insensitivity syndrome presents with azoospermia ( )

27. Concerning ovarian aging:

A. Oocyte quality declines with age ( )

B. Aneuploidy risk decrease with maternal age ( )

C. Fertility potential drops significantly after age 35 ( )

D. Menstrual cycle length shortens with ovarian aging ( )

E. Ovarian reserve markers remain constant with age ( )

28. With respect to cervical mucus and fertility:

A. Estrogen increases mucus spinnbarkeit ( )

B. Progesterone makes mucus thin and permeable ( )

C. Abnormal mucus may hinder sperm transport ( )

D. Infection may not alter mucus quality ( )

E. Cervical factor infertility is very common ( )

29. Regarding testicular causes of infertility:

A. Cryptorchidism is a risk factor for infertility ( )

B. Orchitis may damage spermatogenesis ( )

C. Testicular torsion has no long-term effect on fertility ( )

D. Trauma may impair testicular function ( )

E. Sertoli-cell only syndrome is a cause of azoospermia ( )

30. In relation to pelvic inflammatory disease:

A. Chlamydia trachomatis is not a common cause ( )

B. Repeated episodes increase infertility risk ( )

C. Tubal occlusion is a possible outcome ( )

D. Early antibiotic treatment prevents all sequelae ( )

E. Adhesions may form even without symptoms ( )

31. Concerning semen abnormalities:

A. Asthenozoospermia refers to low motility ( )

B. Teratozoospermia refers to abnormal morphology ( )

C. Oligozoospermia means low concentration ( )

D. Azoospermia indicates absence of sperm ( )

E. Normozoospermia excludes male infertility ( )

32. With respect to reproductive hormones in the female:

A. FSH stimulates follicular growth ( )

B. LH surge triggers ovulation ( )

C. Progesterone is secreted by granulosa cell ( )

D. Estradiol is mainly produced by granulosa cells ( )

E. Inhibin A increases in follicular phase ( )

33. Regarding the menstrual cycle and fertility:

A. Follicular phase length varies between women ( )

B. Luteal phase length is relatively constant ( )

C. Ovulation occurs around day 10 in all women ( )

D. Cervical mucus is minimal at ovulation ( )

E. Basal body temperature rises after ovulation ( )

34. In relation to sperm transport:

A. Sperm reach the fallopian tube within minutes ( )

B. Cervical mucus acts as a reservoir ( )

C. Capacitation occurs in the female tract ( )

D. Acrosome reaction is necessary for fertilization ( )

E. Uterine contractions assist sperm movement ( )

35. Concerning luteal phase defects:

A. Short luteal phase may impair implantation ( )

B. Inadequate progesterone is a feature ( )

C. Endometrial biopsy is routinely used for diagnosis ( )

D. Recurrent pregnancy loss may be linked ( )

E. Luteal support is the standard treatment ( )

36. With respect to ovarian tumors and infertility:

A. Benign cystadenomas commonly cause infertility ( )

B. Endometriomas may reduce ovarian reserve ( )

C. Surgery for ovarian tumors may damage ovarian tissue ( )

D. Malignant ovarian tumors are frequent in infertility ( )

E. Dermoid cysts have no effect on fertility ( )

37. Regarding lifestyle and male fertility:

A. Smoking increases DNA fragmentation in sperm ( )

B. Alcohol abuse may increase testosterone ( )

C. Obesity is linked to lower sperm motility ( )

D. Anabolic steroids may cause testicular atrophy ( )

E. Stress has no effect on male fertility ( )

38. In relation to age and female fertility:

A. Fertility peaks in early 20s ( )

B. Declines gradually after 25 ( )

C. Declines steeply after 37 ( )

D. Menopause occurs on average at 39 ( )

E. Oocyte number remains constant after puberty ( )

39. Concerning environmental factors:

A. Radiation has no effect on gametes ( )

B. Pesticides are linked to reduced fertility ( )

C. Heavy metals may impair spermatogenesis ( )

D. Heat exposure has no effect on sperm counts ( )

E. Mobile phones have no possible effect ( )

40. With respect to thyroid disorders:

A. Hypothyroidism can cause menstrual irregularities ( )

B. Hyperthyroidism has no effect on fertility ( )

C. TSH is the best screening test ( )

D. Thyroid antibodies may be linked to miscarriage ( )

E. Subclinical hypothyroidism has no impact ( )

41. Regarding androgen disorders:

A. Late-onset CAH may mimic PCOS ( )

B. Androgen-secreting tumors cause rapid virilization ( )

C. Hirsutism always indicates infertility ( )

D. High testosterone is common in PCOS ( )

E. DHEAS originates mainly from the adrenal gland ( )

42. In relation to metabolic factors:

A. Obesity may impair ovulation ( )

B. Insulin resistance is common in PCOS ( )

C. Metformin may restore ovulation in all women ( )

D. Hyperlipidemia has no impact on fertility ( )

E. Weight loss improves fertility outcomes ( )

43. Concerning stress and infertility:

A. Chronic stress can disrupt GnRH secretion ( )

B. Stress is a proven cause of infertility in all cases ( )

C. Psychological support may improve outcomes ( )

D. Cortisol excess impairs reproduction ( )

E. Relaxation therapy is first-line treatment ( )

44. With respect to reproductive tract infections:

A. Chlamydia is the most common cause of tubal factor infertility ( )

B. Gonorrhea can cause PID ( )

C. Viral infections commonly damage the tubes ( )

D. PID risk increases with multiple partners ( )

E. Screening and treatment reduce infertility risk ( )

45. Regarding ovarian surgery:

A. Cystectomy for endometrioma may reduce AMH ( )

B. Ovarian drilling is used for all PCOS patients ( )

C. Surgery always improves ovarian reserve ( )

D. Oophorectomy causes immediate menopause ( )

E. Laparoscopy is preferred over laparotomy ( )

46. In relation to male accessory glands:

A. Seminal vesicles contribute majority of semen volume ( )

B. Prostate secretes alkaline fluid ( )

C. Bulbourethral glands produce pre-ejaculate ( )

D. Absence of seminal vesicles always causes infertility ( )

E. Prostatic infection may impair fertility ( )

47. Regarding treatment of endometriosis-related infertility:

A. Laparoscopic excision or ablation of minimal–mild disease may improve spontaneous pregnancy rates ( )

B. Surgical removal of endometriomas always guarantees improved fertility ( )

C. Ovarian reserve may decline after cystectomy for large endometriomas ( )

D. Medical suppression with GnRH agonists improves live birth rates in infertile women ( )

E. IVF is considered an effective option in moderate to severe disease ( )

48. Regarding pharmacological treatment of PCOS in infertility:

A. Clomiphene citrate is a first-line ovulation induction agent ( )

B. Letrozole has been shown to be more effective than clomiphene ( )

C. Metformin may improve ovulation, especially in women with insulin resistance ( )

D. Combined oral contraceptives are used primarily to induce ovulation ( )

E. Gonadotropins can be used when oral agents fail ( )

49. Regarding intrauterine insemination (IUI) in Unexplained infertility:

A. IUI is commonly offered as first-line treatment when no cause of infertility is found ( )

B. Success rates are highest when combined with ovarian stimulation ( )

C. More than 6 unsuccessful IUI cycles are recommended before IVF ( )

D. Female age is an important predictor of IUI success ( )

E. The risk of multiple pregnancy increases when IUI is combined with stimulation ( )

50. Regarding Amenorrhea:

A. Primary amenorrhea = no menstruation by age 15 with normal puberty ( )

B. Pregnancy is the most common cause of secondary amenorrhea ( )

C. Thyroid disease is unrelated to amenorrhea ( )

D. Excessive exercise or weight loss may cause amenorrhea ( )

E. PCOS can cause secondary amenorrhea ( )

ANSWERS

Q	A	B	C	D	E
1	T	T	F	F	T
2	T	F	T	T	F
3	T	T	F	F	T
4	F	T	T	F	T
5	T	T	T	F	T
6	T	T	T	T	F
7	F	F	F	T	T
8	T	F	F	T	T
9	F	F	T	F	T
10	T	T	F	T	F
11	T	F	T	F	T
12	T	F	T	T	T
13	T	F	T	F	F
14	F	F	F	T	T
15	T	T	F	F	T
16	T	T	F	T	T
17	T	T	T	F	F
18	F	T	T	F	F
19	T	T	T	F	F
20	T	T	T	T	E
21	T	F	F	T	T
22	T	T	T	F	F
23	T	T	F	T	T
24	F	T	F	T	F
25	T	T	T	F	F
26	T	T	T	T	T
27	T	F	T	T	F
28	T	F	T	F	F
29	T	T	F	T	T
30	F	T	T	F	T
31	T	T	T	T	F
32	T	T	F	T	F
33	T	T	F	F	T
34	T	T	T	T	T
35	T	T	F	T	T

Q	A	B	C	D	E
36	F	T	T	F	F
37	T	F	T	T	F
38	T	T	T	F	F
39	F	T	T	F	F
40	T	F	T	T	F
41	T	T	F	T	T
42	T	T	F	F	T
43	T	F	T	T	F
44	T	T	F	T	T
45	T	F	F	T	T
46	T	F	T	F	T
47	T	F	T	F	T
48	F	T	T	F	T
49	T	T	F	T	T
50	T	T	F	T	T

PART 3

EXTENDED MATCHING QUESTIONS (EMQs) IN INFERTILITY

EMQ 1

Options:

A. Hysterosalpingography (HSG)
B. Hysteroscopy
C. Laparoscopy with chromopertubation
D. Semen analysis
E. Mid-luteal serum progesterone
F. Day 2–3 FSH and LH
G. Serum prolactin
H. Serum AMH

Scenarios:

1. A 28-year-old woman with irregular cycles. The doctor wants to confirm if ovulation is occurring.
2. A 35-year-old man with primary infertility for one-year, normal physical exam.
3. A 30-year-old woman with abnormal uterine bleeding and suspicion of intrauterine polyp.
4. A 32-year-old woman being evaluated for ovarian reserve prior to IVF.
5. A 27-year-old woman with primary infertility, requires initial assessment of tubal patency with minimal invasiveness.

EMQ 2:

Options:

A. Polycystic ovary syndrome (PCOS)
B. Hyperprolactinemia
C. Endometriosis
D. Tubal blockage (post-pelvic infection)
E. Premature ovarian insufficiency
F. Asherman's syndrome
G. Hypothalamic amenorrhea
H. Turner syndrome

Scenarios:

1. A 23-year-old woman with history of pelvic inflammatory disease. HSG shows.
2. A 29-year-old woman with secondary amenorrhea after repeated dilatation and curettage.
3. An 18-year-old girl, short stature, primary amenorrhea, absent secondary sexual characteristics.
4. A 34-year-old woman with chronic pelvic pain, dysmenorrhea, and infertility.
5. A 26-year-old obese woman with oligomenorrhea, acne, and hirsutism.

EMQ 3

Options:

A. Clomiphene citrate
B. Letrozole
C. IVF with ICSI
D. Laparoscopic ovarian drilling
E. Bromocriptine
F. Weight reduction and lifestyle modification
G. Donor oocyte IVF
H. Expectant management

Scenarios:

1. A 24-year-old woman with PCOS, irregular cycles, infertile for 1 year.
2. A couple with severe male factor infertility (oligoasthenozoospermia). Female evaluation is normal.
3. A 37-year-old woman with premature ovarian failure, undetectable ovarian reserve.
4. A 30-year-old woman with hyperprolactinemia and headaches.
5. A young couple, married for only 6 months, both healthy with no risk factors.

EMQ 4

Options:

A. Varicocele
B. Hypogonadotropic hypogonadism
C. Klinefelter syndrome
D. Obstructive azoospermia
E. Testicular torsion (past history)
F. Retrograde ejaculation
G. Y chromosome microdeletion

Scenarios:

1. Man, 35, gynecomastia, small testes, azoospermia, high FSH.
2. Man, 32, infertility, low testosterone and low gonadotropins.
3. Man, 28, infertility, semen analysis shows azoospermia but normal FSH/LH, history of vasectomy.

EMQ 5

Options:

A. HSG
B. Hysterosalpingo-contrast sonography (HyCoSy)
C. Laparoscopy with dye test
D. Hysteroscopy
E. MRI pelvis

Scenarios:

1. 27-year-old, needs outpatient minimally invasive test for tubal patency.
2. 31-year-old, infertility + severe dysmenorrhea, requires tubal evaluation and assessment for endometriosis.
3. 29-year-old, suspected intrauterine adhesions.
4. 35-year-old, requires non-radiation alternative to HSG.

EMQ 6

Options:
A. PID
B. Genital tuberculosis
C. Endometriosis
D. Salpingectomy after ectopic
E. Adhesions after abdominal surgery
F. Congenital absence of tubes

Scenarios:

1. 26-year-old, infertility, history of chlamydia infection.
2. 33-year-old, infertility after open appendectomy.
3. 25-year-old, history of ectopic pregnancy, unilateral tube removed.
4. 28-year-old, chronic pelvic pain, severe dysmenorrhea, infertility.

EMQ 7

Options:
A. Submucous fibroid
B. Asherman's syndrome
C. Chronic Endometritis
D. Endometrial polyp
E. Adenomyosis
F. Bicornuate uterus

Scenarios:

1. 29-year-old, secondary amenorrhea after repeated D&C.
2. 32-year-old, heavy periods, dysmenorrhea, bulky uterus.
3. 27-year-old, recurrent miscarriage, congenital anomaly suspected.
4. 31-year-old, menorrhagia, ultrasound shows submucosal lesion.

EMQ 8

Options:

A. Hysteroscopy
B. HSG
C. Saline infusion sonography
D. MRI
E. Pelvic ultrasound

Scenarios:

1. 28-year-old, suspected endometrial polyp.
2. 29-year-old, infertility, need to differentiate septate vs bicornuate uterus.
3. 30-year-old, recurrent miscarriage, outpatient test for uterine cavity.
4. 32-year-old, heavy bleeding, suspected fibroid.

EMQ 9

Options:

A. Dysmenorrhea
B. Deep dyspareunia
C. Infertility
D. Chronic pelvic pain
E. Adenomyosis
F. Rectovaginal nodule

Scenarios:

1. 34-year-old, infertility, severe menstrual pain.
2. 30-year-old, heavy painful periods, boggy uterus.
3. 29-year-old, painful intercourse, pelvic nodule on exam.
4. 32-year-old, persistent dull pelvic pain.

EMQ 10

Options:
A. Transvaginal ultrasound
B. MRI pelvis
C. Imaging Studies
D. Hysteroscopy
E. CA-125

Scenarios:

1. 31-year-old, suspected ovarian endometrioma.
2. 33-year-old, suspected Endometriosis, test for diagnosis.
3. 29-year-old, suspected deep infiltrating endometriosis.
4. 27-year-old, non-specific marker, raised in moderate–severe disease.

EMQ 11

Options:
A. NSAIDs
B. Combined OCPs
C. Progestins
D. GnRH agonists
E. Laparoscopic excision
F. Hysterectomy

Scenarios:

1. 24-year-old, Endometriosis, mild symptoms, not seeking pregnancy.
2. 32-year-old, Endometriosis, severe pain, wants to conceive.
3. 29-year-old, adenomyosis, not responding to medical therapy, family complete.
4. 27-year-old, pelvic pain, medical therapy contraindicated.

EMQ 12

Options:
A. Semen analysis
B. Mid-luteal progesterone
C. HSG
D. Laparoscopy
E. Thyroid function
F. AMH

Scenarios:

1. 29-year-old, initial tests all normal, unexplained infertility suspected.
2. 32-year-old, ovulation confirmed, patent tubes.
3. 27-year-old, further invasive test to exclude endometriosis.
4. 31-year-old, needs ovarian reserve checked despite normal routine workup.

EMQ 13

Options:
A. Lifestyle modification
B. Expectant management
C. Stimulated IUI
D. Tuboplasty
E. Surgery for endometriosis
F. Counseling

Scenarios:

1. 25-year-old couple, infertile for 6 months, both normal, no risk factors.
2. 28-year-old couple, 2 years unexplained infertility, both normal.
3. 31-year-old, unexplained infertility, mild endometriosis at laparoscopy.
4. 33-year-old, unexplained infertility, smoker and underweight.

EMQ 14

Options:

A. PCOS
B. Late-onset congenital adrenal hyperplasia
C. Cushing's syndrome
D. Androgen-secreting tumor
E. Idiopathic hirsutism
F. Hypothyroidism

Scenarios:

1. 25-year-old, irregular cycles, obesity, acne, hirsutism.
2. 20-year-old, rapid-onset hirsutism, clitoromegaly.
3. 27-year-old, progressive hirsutism since puberty, regular cycles, normal hormones.
4. 30-year-old, hirsutism, central obesity, purple striae.

EMQ 15

Options:

A. Serum total testosterone
B. Serum DHEAS
C. 17-hydroxyprogesterone
D. Dexamethasone suppression test
E. Pelvic ultrasound
F. TSH

Scenarios:

1. 22-year-old, hirsutism, virilization, need to exclude androgen-secreting tumor.
2. 23-year-old, hirsutism, irregular periods, suspected PCOS.
3. 24-year-old, hirsutism + hypertension, suspect CAH.
4. 29-year-old, hirsutism, obesity, purple striae.

EMQ 16

Options:

A. Laparoscopy
B. Severe male factor infertility
C. Anovulation
D. Unexplained infertility
E. Mild oligospermia
F. Ejaculatory dysfunction

Scenarios:

1. 29-year-old, infertility, HSG shows both tubes blocked.
2. 31-year-old, severe azoospermia.
3. 25-year-old, anovulatory infertility, untreated.
4. 33-year-old, infertility, retrograde ejaculation.

EMQ 17

Options:

A. Retrograde menstruation
B. Coelomic metaplasia
C. Stem cell theory
D. Lymphatic spread
E. Immune dysfunction
F. Genetic predisposition

Scenarios:

1. Theory suggesting menstrual debris implantation into peritoneal cavity.
2. Endometriosis occurring at distant sites via vascular/lymphatic spread.
3. Undifferentiated progenitor cells transforming into endometrial-like tissue.
4. Explains higher prevalence in first-degree relatives of affected women.

EMQ 18

Options:
A. Subtle endometriosis
B. Luteal phase defect
C. Cervical hostility
D. Immunological infertility
E. Mild tubal damage undetected
F. Genetic causes

Scenarios:

1. A 30-year-old, all tests normal, but laparoscopy reveals superficial implants.
2. A 29-year-old, infertility, mid-luteal progesterone consistently low.
3. A 31-year-old, infertility, abnormal post-coital test.
4. A 32-year-old, unexplained infertility, family history of recurrent miscarriage.

EMQ 19

Options:
A. Oligospermia
B. Asthenospermia
C. Teratospermia
D. Azoospermia
E. Oligoasthenoteratospermia (OAT)
F. Normozoospermia

Scenarios:

1. 33-year-old man, sperm concentration <15 million/ml.
2. 30-year-old, semen analysis shows absent sperm in ejaculate.
3. 34-year-old, low motility, poor morphology, and reduced count.
4. 29-year-old, infertility, semen report: all normal.

EMQ 20

Options:
A. Androgen insensitivity syndrome
B. Hypothalamic amenorrhea
C. Premature ovarian insufficiency
D. PCOS
E. Hyperprolactinemia
F. Late-onset congenital adrenal hyperplasia

Scenarios:

1. A 16-year-old girl with primary amenorrhea, tall stature, normal breast development, but absent pubic and axillary hair.
2. A 30-year-old woman with secondary amenorrhea, hot flushes, and high FSH.
3. A 24-year-old athlete with very low BMI, stress, and secondary amenorrhea.
4. A 26-year-old woman with irregular cycles, acne, hirsutism, and obesity.

EMQ 21

Options:
A. Lifestyle modification
B. Expectant management
C. Ovulation induction
D. Tuboplasty
E. Laparoscopic adhesiolysis
F. Counseling

Scenarios:

1. 24-year-old couple, infertile 6 months, no risk factors.
2. 28-year-old woman, BMI 34, oligomenorrhea, PCOS.
3. 29-year-old, infertility, laparoscopy reveals pelvic adhesions.
4. 31-year-old, anxious couple with unexplained infertility for 1 year, both normal.

EMQ 22

Options:
A. Galactorrhea
B. Infertility
C. Headache and visual field defect
D. Serum prolactin level
E. MRI pituitary
F. Bromocriptine
G. Cabergoline
H. Transsphenoidal surgery
I. Dopamine antagonist drugs

Scenarios:

1. A 29-year-old woman presents with secondary amenorrhea, hyperprolactinemia and difficulty conceiving.
2. A 32-year-old woman complains of bilateral milky nipple discharge and irregular cycles.
3. A 35-year-old woman with infertility has significant raised serum prolactin; the doctor requests a confirmatory imaging test.
4. A 28-year-old woman has hyperprolactinemia due to pituitary microadenoma; best first-line pharmacological treatment.
5. A 30-year-old woman developed hyperprolactinemia after starting antipsychotic therapy.
6. A 34-year-old woman with macroadenoma presents with headaches and bitemporal hemianopia.

EMQ 23

Options:
A. Low FSH, LH & E2
B. Low estradiol
C. POI
D. Functional hypothalamic amenorrhea
E. Kallmann syndrome
F. Pituitary tumor

G. GnRH pulsatile therapy
H. Gonadotropin injections (FSH + LH)
I. IVF directly

Scenarios:

1. A 22-year-old athlete with amenorrhea after excessive training and significant weight loss.
2. A 19-year-old girl with primary amenorrhea, absent sense of smell, low gonadotropins.
3. A 27-year-old woman with secondary amenorrhea after pituitary surgery.
4. A 28-year-old woman with infertility due to hypo-hypo anovulation; she wants pregnancy – best first-line treatment.
5. A 24-year-old woman with hypogonadotropic hypogonadism not responding to lifestyle changes; next step in ovulation induction.
6. A 30-year-old woman with hot flushes, high FSH, low estradiol.

EMQ 24
Options:
A. Hirsutism
B. Obesity
C. Polycystic ovaries on ultrasound
D. Insulin resistance
E. Increased LH:FSH ratio
F. Lifestyle modification (weight reduction)
G. Letrozole
H. Clomiphene citrate
I. Metformin

Scenarios:

1. A 26-year-old woman with infertility, irregular cycles every 2–3 months, and acne.
2. A 24-year-old woman with BMI 34, acanthosis nigricans, and oligomenorrhea.

3. A 22-year-old woman with infertility; labs show elevated LH:FSH ratio and androgen excess.
4. A 29-year-old woman with PCOS planning pregnancy; best first-line drug for ovulation induction.
5. A 27-year-old woman with PCOS and BMI 35; most effective initial management before drug therapy.
6. A 25-year-old woman with PCOS and metabolic syndrome; adjuvant drug to improve insulin sensitivity and cycles.

EMQ 25

Options:

A. Amenorrhea before age 40
B. Hot flushes & night sweats
C. High FSH, low estradiol
D. Fragile X premutation
E. Turner syndrome
F. Autoimmune thyroid disease
G. Hormone replacement therapy (HRT)
H. Donor oocyte IVF
I. Bone density loss
J. Normal FSH, normal estradiol

Scenarios:

1. A 32-year-old woman presents with 6 months of amenorrhea and menopausal symptoms.
2. A 19-year-old girl with primary amenorrhea, short stature, webbed neck, streak ovaries.
3. A 28-year-old woman with secondary amenorrhea, strong family history of Fragile X syndrome.
4. A 34-year-old woman with POI; counseling includes risk of autoimmune comorbidity.

5. A 30-year-old woman with POI; complains of hot flushes and urogenital atrophy; best symptomatic treatment.
6. A 29-year-old woman with POI; wishes to conceive.

EMQ 26

Options:
A. Dysmenorrhea
B. Menorrhagia
C. Dyspareunia
D. Enlarged boggy uterus
E. MRI pelvis
F. Transvaginal ultrasound
G. Adenomyosis
H. LNG-IUS (Mirena)
I. Hysterectomy
J. GnRH agonists

Scenarios:

1. A 34-year-old woman with heavy, painful periods and primary infertility.
2. A 38-year-old woman with adenomyosis; uterus enlarged, soft and tender on bimanual exam.
3. A 30-year-old woman with adenomyosis; best non-invasive imaging modality.
4. A 33-year-old woman with severe dysmenorrhea, not planning pregnancy; medical option that reduces bleeding and pain.
5. A 42-year-old woman, family complete, adenomyosis resistant to medical therapy.
6. A 29-year-old woman with adenomyosis-related pain; medical option acting by down-regulating pituitary-ovarian axis.

EMQ 27

Options:

A. Adenomyosis
B. Endometrioma
C. Transvaginal ultrasound
D. MRI pelvis
E. Ovarian reserve reduction
F. Medical suppression (OCPs, progestins, GnRH agonists)
G. Expectant management

Scenarios:

1. A 29-year-old woman with chronic pelvic pain, infertility, and ultrasound showing a unilocular cyst with ground-glass echogenicity.
2. A 30-year-old woman with endometrioma confirmed by imaging, not planning pregnancy, needs pain control.
3. A 27-year-old woman with endometrioma after laparoscopic excision, concern is decline in this ovarian function marker.
4. A 33-year-old woman with asymptomatic endometrioma, size <4 cm, not currently seeking pregnancy.

EMQ 28

Options:

A. Dysmenorrhea
B. Deep dyspareunia
C. Chronic pelvic pain
D. Infertility
E. Ovarian endometrioma
F. Rectovaginal nodule
G. Laparoscopy
H. Transvaginal ultrasound
I. NSAIDs and hormonal suppression
J. Laparoscopic excision/ablation

Scenarios:

1. A 29-year-old woman presents with severe cyclical pelvic pain and painful intercourse. On exam, a tender nodule is felt in the posterior vaginal fornix.
2. A 26-year-old woman with chronic pelvic pain and dysmenorrhea not relieved by simple analgesics; diagnostic test.
3. A 28-year-old woman with endometriosis, mild symptoms, not currently trying to conceive; best first-line management.
4. A 30-year-old woman with minimal to mild endometriosis and infertility; she desires pregnancy — best surgical approach.

EMQ 29

Options:

A. Oligomenorrhea more than 2 years after menarche
B. Clinical hyperandrogenism (hirsutism, acne)
C. Biochemical hyperandrogenism (↑ testosterone, ↑ DHEAS)
D. Polycystic ovarian morphology on ultrasound
E. Exclude other causes (CAH, Cushing's, androgen-secreting tumor)
F. Lifestyle modification (weight loss, exercise)
G. Combined oral contraceptives
H. Metformin
I. Irregular cycles within 1 year of menarche (normal variant)
J. Risk of metabolic syndrome

Scenarios:

1. A 17-year-old girl, 4 years post-menarche, presents with regular cycles but has coarse facial hair and moderate acne.
2. A 15-year-old girl, 8 months after menarche, irregular cycles — reassurance given as this is physiological.
3. A 17-year-old overweight girl with oligomenorrhea and hirsutism; lab shows elevated total testosterone.

4. A 16-year-old with PCOS, BMI 32; first-line non-pharmacological intervention.
5. A 17-year-old with PCOS, no desire for fertility, wants treatment for acne and cycle regulation.
6. A 16-year-old girl with PCOS; counseling includes long-term risk of diabetes and cardiovascular disease.

EMQ 30

Options:

A. Anovulatory infertility
B. Normal follicular growth without rupture
C. Mid-luteal serum progesterone
D. Ultrasound follicle tracking
E. Endometrial biopsy
F. NSAID use as a precipitating factor
G. Ovulation induction with clomiphene/letrozole
H. hCG trigger for follicle rupture

Scenarios:

1. A 28-year-old woman with infertility; endometrial biopsy was previously used to diagnose this condition but is now obsolete.
2. A 27-year-old woman with suspected LUF; best non-invasive method to detect follicle growth without rupture.
3. A 29-year-old woman using NSAIDs chronically for dysmenorrhea develops LUF-related infertility.
4. A 32-year-old woman with LUF; ovulation induction is initiated.

EMQ 31

Options

A. Thelarche (breast development)
B. Pubarche (appearance of pubic/axillary hair)
C. Menarche (onset of menstruation)

D. GnRH pulsatility from hypothalamus
E. Tanner staging
F. Delayed puberty
G. Precocious puberty
H. Turner syndrome
I. Constitutional delay of puberty
J. Estrogen effect on endometrium

Scenarios

1. A 10-year-old girl presents with breast budding, considered the first physical sign of puberty in females.
2. A 12-year-old girl comes with first menstrual bleeding, marking the end-stage of pubertal development.
3. A 14-year-old girl has not developed secondary sexual characteristics; bone age is delayed, family history similar.
4. A 7-year-old girl presents with pubic hair and breast enlargement earlier than expected for her age.
5. A 16-year-old girl has short stature, streak ovaries, and primary amenorrhea; karyotype shows 45,XO.
6. A 12-year-old girl's puberty is assessed by breast size and pubic hair distribution using this clinical tool.
7. Cyclical release of this hormone from the hypothalamus triggers puberty onset.
8. A 13-year-old girl shows endometrial proliferation on ultrasound, explained by this hormone's effect.

EMQ 32

Options

A. Turner syndrome (45,XO)
B. Polycystic ovary syndrome (PCOS)
C. Hypothalamic amenorrhea (stress/exercise/weight loss)
D. Hyperprolactinemia

E. Asherman's syndrome
F. Premature ovarian insufficiency (POI)
G. Thyroid dysfunction
H. Progesterone challenge test
I. Estrogen + progesterone challenge test
J. Pregnancy

Scenarios

1. A 28-year-old woman presents with secondary amenorrhea, galactorrhea, and high prolactin levels.
2. A 17-year-old girl presents with primary amenorrhea, short stature, webbed neck, and streak ovaries.
3. A 22-year-old athlete with very low BMI develops amenorrhea after intensive training.
4. A 30-year-old woman with irregular menses, hirsutism, obesity, and polycystic ovaries on ultrasound.
5. A 36-year-old woman with secondary amenorrhea, hot flushes, and FSH in menopausal range.
6. A 25-year-old woman with secondary amenorrhea and abnormal TSH levels.
7. A 27-year-old woman with amenorrhea; after giving oral progesterone she has withdrawal bleeding.
8. A 29-year-old woman with amenorrhea does not bleed after progesterone test but does bleed after combined estrogen + progesterone test.

ANSWERS

EMQ	1	2	3	4	5	6	7	8
1	E	D	B	H	A	-	-	-
2	D	F	H	C	A	-	-	-
3	B	C	G	E	H	-	-	-
4	C	B	D	-	-	-	-	-
5	A	C	D	B	-	-	-	-
6	A	E	D	C	-	-	-	-
7	B	E	F	A	-	-	-	-
8	A	D	C	E	-	-	-	-
9	A	E	F	D	-	-	-	-
10	A	C	B	E	-	-	-	-
11	A	E	F	E	-	-	-	-
12	E	A	D	F	-	-	-	-
13	B	C	E	A	-	-	-	-
14	A	D	E	C	-	-	-	-
15	A	E	C	D	-	-	-	-
16	A	B	C	F	-	-	-	-
17	A	D	C	F	-	-	-	-
18	A	B	C	F	-	-	-	-
19	A	D	E	F	-	-	-	-
20	A	C	B	D	-	-	-	-
21	B	A	E	F	-	-	-	-
22	B	A	E	G	I	H	-	-
23	D	E	A	G	H	C	-	-
24	C	D	E	G	F	I	-	-
25	C	E	D	F	G	H	-	-
26	G	D	F	H	I	J	-	-
27	B	F	E	G	-	-	-	-
28	F	G	I	J	-	-	-	-
29	B	I	C	F	G	J	-	-
30	E	D	F	H	-	-	-	-
31	A	C	I	G	H	E	D	J
32	D	A	C	B	F	G	H	I

PART 4

CASE-BASED & SHORT ESSAY QUESTIONS IN INFERTILITY

CASE NO. (1) INFERTILITY WORKUP

A 29-year-old Woman presents with Infertility, her husband is healthy, with no previous children.

1. Define infertility. How do you differentiate primary vs secondary infertility?
2. What is the normal fecundability per cycle and cumulative pregnancy rate per year in healthy couples?
3. When should infertility evaluation start in: women <35 years, women ≥35 years, women ≥40 years?
4. What is the difference between sterility and subfertility?
5. Define fecundability and fecundity.
6. What is the prevalence of infertility worldwide?
7. What are the main risk factors for female infertility?
8. How does age affect fertility in females?
9. How does BMI (obesity or underweight) affect fertility?
10. What key points should be covered in the history of an infertile couple?
11. What are the important points in the male partner's history?
12. What general examination findings may suggest infertility causes?
13. What gynecological examination findings may be relevant in infertility assessment?
14. What are the first-line investigations for an infertile couple?
15. What hormonal tests are usually done for the female partner?
16. What imaging is used to assess uterine cavity and tubal patency?
17. What is the role of semen analysis in male infertility evaluation?

18. When would you request genetic testing (karyotype, Y-chromosome microdeletion, CFTR mutation)?
19. Outline the general management steps of an infertile couple.
20. What are the roles of lifestyle modification in infertility treatment?
21. What are the measures to optimize natural fertility?
22. When should you refer to assisted reproductive technologies (ART)?
23. What are the ethical considerations in infertility management?
24. How do you counsel a couple about prognosis in infertility?

CASE NO. (2) ASSESEMENT OF OVULATION

A 27-year-old woman presents with 18 months of primary infertility. She reports irregular cycles ranging from 30–60 days. She is otherwise healthy. Husband's semen analysis is normal. She wants to know if she is ovulating regularly.

1. What are the clinical features suggesting ovulation in a normal cycle?
2. How can basal body temperature (BBT) be used in assessment of ovulation? What are its limitations?
3. What is the role of mid-luteal serum progesterone in confirming ovulation? What cut-off value is considered diagnostic?
4. How can ultrasound folliculometry be used to monitor ovulation?
5. What are the sonographic signs of ovulation?
6. What is the role of serum LH monitoring in prediction of ovulation?
7. What is the role of cervical mucus assessment (Spinnbarkeit, ferning) in ovulation monitoring?
8. How can endometrial biopsy be used to confirm ovulation? Is it still commonly used?

9. What are the advantages and disadvantages of each method of ovulation assessment?
10. What is the role of ultrasound in infertility workup?

CASE NO. (3) OPTIMIZING NATURAL FERTILITY

A 29-year-old woman and her 32-year-old husband present with 10 months of infertility. Both are healthy, non-smokers, and have no significant medical history. Her cycles are regular every 28–30 days. Husband's semen analysis is normal. They ask what they can do to maximize their chance of natural conception.

1. What advice would you give a couple regarding timing and frequency of intercourse to maximize chances of conception?
2. What is the fertile window in the menstrual cycle?
3. How can couples identify the fertile window (e.g., cervical mucus changes, LH kits, cycle tracking)?
4. What lifestyle factors can negatively impact natural fertility in both men and women?
5. How does female age affect natural fertility?
6. What is the effect of obesity or being underweight on fertility?
7. How does smoking, alcohol, and caffeine intake influence fertility?
8. What is the role of stress and sleep in natural conception chances?
9. What preconception supplements are recommended to optimize fertility (e.g., folic acid, vitamin D)?
10. How long should a couple try to conceive naturally before seeking medical advice?

11. What advice is given regarding the use of lubricants during intercourse and their effect on sperm motility?
12. How can management of chronic conditions (thyroid disease, diabetes, PCOS) improve natural fertility outcomes?

CASE NO. (4) HYPOGONADOTROPIC HYPOESTROGENIC ANOVULATION

A 32-year-old woman with a history of severe postpartum hemorrhage presents with secondary amenorrhea for 12 months and seek for pregnancy. She also reports failure of lactation.

1. What is the most likely diagnosis?
2. What are the common causes of Hypogonadotropic Hypoestrogenic Anovulation?
3. How does Hypo hypo lead to infertility?
4. How is it diagnosed?
5. What are the typical clinical features?
6. How is it managed?
7. Which types of gonadotropins and trigger injections would you use?
8. Define anovulation. What is the difference between anovulation and oligo-ovulation?
9. What are the most common causes of anovulation?
10. What is the difference between the WHO and FIGO classification systems for anovulation?
11. Give examples of WHO group III hypergonadotropic hypoestrogenic anovulation.
12. How would you investigate a woman with suspected anovulation?
13. What is the role of mid-luteal progesterone in diagnosing anovulation?

14. How do you use ultrasound folliculometry in evaluating anovulatory patients?
15. What is the role of lifestyle modification in management of anovulatory infertility?

CASE NO. (5) POLYCYSTIC OVARY SYNDROME (PCOS)

A 24-year-old woman presents with primary infertility and irregular cycles. She has acne, hirsutism, and BMI of 34. Ultrasound shows polycystic ovarian morphology. Labs: AMH 8 ng/mL, LH/FSH ratio 2:1, testosterone mildly elevated, prolactin and TSH normal.

1. What is the definition of PCOS?
2. What are the Rotterdam diagnostic criteria for PCOS?
3. What are the steps for diagnosis of PCOS according to international evidence-based guidelines for PCOS, 2023?
4. What are the main clinical features of PCOS?
5. How do you investigate a woman suspected of PCOS?
6. What ultrasound features are typical of polycystic ovaries?
7. What are the main endocrine abnormalities found in PCOS?
8. How does PCOS lead to infertility?
9. What is the role of lifestyle modification in PCOS management?
10. What pharmacological options are available for ovulation induction in PCOS?
11. Compare clomiphene citrate and letrozole for ovulation induction in PCOS.
12. What is the role of gonadotropins in treatment of PCOS infertility?

13. What is ovarian drilling and when is it considered?
14. What are the long-term health risks associated with PCOS?
15. How do you counsel a PCOS patient regarding metabolic syndrome and cardiovascular risk?
16. What is the risk of endometrial hyperplasia/carcinoma in PCOS and why?
17. How do you manage hirsutism in PCOS?
18. What is the role of metformin in PCOS management?
19. What is the recommended gonadotropins protocol for induction of ovulation by gonadotropins?
20. What are indications of IVF/ICSI in cases of PCOS?

CASE NO. (6) ADOLESCENT PCOS

A 16-year-old girl presents with irregular cycles since menarche (intervals of 2–3 months). She complains of acne and increased facial hair. BMI is 30. Labs: LH mildly elevated, testosterone mildly increased.

1. What is the definition of PCOS in adolescents?
2. Why is diagnosing PCOS more challenging in adolescents compared to adults?
3. What are the limitations of applying the Rotterdam criteria in adolescents?
4. What are the most reliable diagnostic criteria for PCOS in adolescence?
5. What are the typical clinical features of adolescent PCOS?

6. How do menstrual irregularities differ between normal puberty and PCOS?
7. What is the role of biochemical testing (androgens, LH/FSH) in diagnosis?
8. What are the ultrasound features of adolescent ovaries, and are they reliable for PCOS diagnosis?
9. What conditions should be excluded before diagnosing PCOS in adolescents?
10. What are the first-line management strategies for adolescent PCOS?
11. What is the role of lifestyle modification and weight reduction in management?
12. What is the role of combined oral contraceptives in adolescent PCOS?
13. When is metformin indicated in adolescents with PCOS?
14. How do you manage hirsutism and acne in adolescent PCOS?
15. What are the long-term health risks if PCOS starts in adolescence?

CASE NO. (7) PREMATURE OVARIAN INSUFFICIENCY (POI)

A 29-year-old woman presents with secondary amenorrhea for 7 months and hot flushes. She is married for 3 years and trying to conceive. Hormonal profile shows: FSH 42 IU/L, LH 28 IU/L, estradiol 10 pg/ml, AMH undetectable. Transvaginal ultrasound shows small ovaries with very few antral follicles.

1. What is the definition of premature ovarian insufficiency (POI)?
2. What is the difference between POI and premature menopause?
3. What are the diagnostic criteria of POI?
4. What are the common causes of POI?

5. How would you differentiate between Primary Ovarian Insufficiency (POI), Turner's syndrome, and Resistant Ovary Syndrome?
6. What genetic disorders are associated with POI (e.g., Turner syndrome, Fragile X premutation)?
7. What iatrogenic factors can lead to POI?
8. What are the typical clinical features of POI?
9. How do you investigate a woman suspected of POI?
10. What are the characteristic hormone profile findings in POI?
11. How do you differentiate POI from hypothalamic amenorrhea?
12. What is the natural course and variability of ovarian function in POI?
13. What are the fertility implications of POI?
14. What fertility options are available for women with POI?
15. What is the role of hormone replacement therapy (HRT) in POI?
16. What are the risks of untreated POI?
17. How do you counsel a patient with POI regarding fertility preservation or future pregnancy?
18. What is the psychosocial impact of POI and how can it be addressed?

CASE NO. (8) HYPERPROLACTINEMIA

A 29-year-old woman presents with 18 months of primary infertility and amenorrhea for 6 months. She reports galactorrhea. Pregnancy test is negative. Labs: Prolactin 120 ng/mL, TSH normal, FSH and LH low. MRI of pituitary shows a 4 mm microadenoma.

1. What is hyperprolactinemia? What is the normal serum prolactin range?
2. What are the physiological causes of hyperprolactinemia?

3. What are the pathological causes of hyperprolactinemia?
4. What are the drug-induced hyperprolactinemia?
5. How does hyperprolactinemia lead to infertility?
6. What are the common symptoms in women with hyperprolactinemia?
7. What is the management of prolactinoma during pregnancy?
8. How do you confirm the diagnosis of hyperprolactinemia?
9. What are the prolactin levels in micro- and macroprolactinemia??
10. What is the role of thyroid function tests in evaluation of hyperprolactinemia?
11. What imaging is indicated for suspected pituitary adenoma?
12. What are the first-line treatments for hyperprolactinemia?
13. Compare bromocriptine and cabergoline in the management of hyperprolactinemia.
14. When is surgery indicated in hyperprolactinemia?
15. What is the impact of hyperprolactinemia on ovulation and menstrual cycle?
16. How do you monitor treatment response in hyperprolactinemia?
17. What is galactorrhea, incidence, common causes and management?
18. What is the difference between hyperprolactinemia and galactorrhea?

CASE NO. (9) TUBAL FACTOR OF INFERTILITY

A 30-year-old woman presents with 3 years of primary infertility. She has a history of pelvic inflammatory disease at age 22 and was treated for chlamydia. Her cycles are regular, hormonal profile normal, and her partner's semen analysis is normal. Hysterosalpingogram (HSG) shows bilateral tubal blockage.

1. What is the contribution of tubal factor to female infertility (percentage)?
2. What are the common causes of tubal infertility?
3. How does pelvic inflammatory disease (PID) lead to tubal factor infertility?
4. What is the role of genital tuberculosis in tubal infertility?
5. What are the risk factors for hydrosalpinx?
6. How does hydrosalpinx affect IVF outcomes?
7. What are the methods to assess tubal patency?
8. What are the advantages and disadvantages of hysterosalpingography (HSG)?
9. What are the advantages and disadvantages of sonohysterography / HyCoSy?
10. What is the role of laparoscopy with chromopertubation in tubal assessment?
11. How do you manage unilateral tubal block?
12. How do you manage bilateral tubal block?
13. What are the indications for salpingectomy before IVF?
14. What is the role of tuboplasty or reconstructive surgery in tubal infertility?
15. How does endometriosis contribute to tubal factor infertility?
16. What preventive measures can reduce the incidence of tubal infertility?
17. What are the indications for IVF/ICSI in tubal factor infertility?

CASE NO. (10) UTERINE FACTOR OF INFERTILITY

A 26-year-old woman presents with infertility and two recurrent first-trimester miscarriages. She has regular menses and no history of pelvic infection or surgery. Imaging (3D ultrasound, HSG, MRI) shows a normal external uterine contour with a fibrous septum dividing the uterine cavity. Ovaries and tubes are normal.

1. What is the contribution of uterine factor to female infertility (percentage)?
2. What are the causes of uterine factor infertility?
3. How do congenital uterine anomalies cause infertility?
4. Differentiate between septate, bicornuate, unicornuate, and didelphys uterus in terms of fertility outcome.
5. What imaging modalities are used to diagnose congenital uterine anomalies?
6. What is the role of 3D ultrasound and MRI in uterine anomaly assessment?
7. How do acquired uterine pathologies (fibroids, polyps, adhesions) affect fertility?
8. Which types of fibroids are most likely to impair implantation and pregnancy?
9. How do submucous fibroids affect IVF/ICSI outcome?
10. What are the treatment options for submucous fibroids?
11. What is Asherman's syndrome and how does it cause infertility?
12. How is intrauterine adhesion diagnosed?
13. What is the role of hysteroscopy in diagnosis and management of uterine factor infertility?
14. What are the indications for hysteroscopic polypectomy in infertility?

15. How do endometrial pathologies (thin endometrium, endometritis) affect implantation?

16. What preventive or pre-IVF measures can be taken to optimize the uterine environment?

CASE NO. (11) ENDOMETRIOSIS RELATED INFERTILITY

A 32-year-old woman presents with 4 years of infertility and severe progressive dysmenorrhea. She also reports deep dyspareunia and chronic pelvic pain that worsens during menstruation. Her menstrual cycles are regular. Pelvic examination reveals tenderness in the posterior fornix

1. What is endometriosis and what are the common sites of implantation?
2. What is the relationship between endometriosis and infertility?
3. What are the possible mechanisms by which endometriosis reduces fertility?
4. How does endometrioma affect ovarian reserve and oocyte quality?
5. What are the clinical features of endometriosis in women presenting with infertility?
6. How is endometriosis staged/classified (e.g., rASRM classification)?
7. How is endometriosis diagnosed? What is the role of laparoscopy?
8. What is the role of ultrasound and MRI in the diagnosis of endometriosis?
9. How does endometriosis affect IVF/ICSI outcomes?
10. What is the management of minimal to mild endometriosis in infertility?
11. What is the role of surgical treatment (laparoscopic ablation/excision) in endometriosis-related infertility?

12. What is the management of moderate to severe endometriosis related infertility?
13. What are the risks of surgical removal of endometrioma on ovarian reserve?
14. What is the role of medical treatment (GnRH agonists, progestins) in endometriosis-related infertility?
15. What is the role of pretreatment with GnRH agonists before IVF in women with endometriosis?
16. How do adenomyosis and endometriosis differ in their impact on fertility?
17. How do you counsel a woman with endometriosis about natural conception, surgery, and ART options?

CASE NO. (12) ENDOMETRIMA

A 30-year-old woman presents with primary infertility for 3 years. She has regular cycles but complains of pelvic pain that worsens around menstruation. Ultrasound shows a 5 cm left ovarian cyst with homogeneous "ground glass" appearance.

1. What is the most likely diagnosis in this patient?
2. How does an endometrioma typically appear on ultrasound?
3. What is the relationship between endometrioma and infertility?
4. What are the differential diagnoses of an ovarian cyst in a reproductive-age woman?
5. What investigations are useful to confirm the diagnosis and exclude malignancy?

6. How do you differentiate a functional cyst from a pathological cyst on ultrasound?
7. What is the gold standard for diagnosing endometriosis?
8. How should you manage a 5 cm endometrioma in a woman desiring fertility and when should be removed before IVF?
9. What medical options exist for endometrioma?
10. When is IVF indicated in women with endometrioma and infertility?
11. What are the risks of ovarian cystectomy in infertility management?

CASE NO. (13) ADENOMYOSIS

A 37-year-old woman presents with 3 years of secondary infertility. She reports progressively worsening dysmenorrhea and menorrhagia. Ultrasound shows a globular enlarged uterus with heterogeneous myometrium and multiple myometrial cysts, suggestive of adenomyosis. Ovarian reserve is normal; partner's semen analysis is normal.

1. What is adenomyosis and how does it differ from endometriosis?
2. What are the common clinical features of adenomyosis?
3. How does adenomyosis contribute to infertility?
4. What is the role of ultrasound in the diagnosis of adenomyosis?
5. What are the typical MRI findings of adenomyosis?
6. What is the relationship between adenomyosis and recurrent implantation failure (RIF)?
7. How do you differentiate adenomyosis from fibroids on imaging?
8. What is the role of GnRH agonist therapy before IVF in women with adenomyosis?

9. What is the role of progestins or LNG-IUS in adenomyosis management?
10. When is surgical management (adenomyomectomy) indicated in adenomyosis?
11. What is the role of high-intensity focused ultrasound (HIFU) or uterine artery embolization in adenomyosis and fertility?
12. How do you counsel a woman with adenomyosis regarding her fertility and IVF success chances?

CASE NO. (14) FIBROIDS

A 35-year-old woman presents with 2 years of secondary infertility and heavy menstrual bleeding. Transvaginal ultrasound shows a 4 cm submucosal fibroid distorting the uterine cavity and a 6 cm intramural fibroid not distorting the endometrium. Ovarian reserve and partner's semen analysis are normal.

1. What are uterine fibroids (leiomyomas) and what types exist according to location?
2. Which types of fibroids are most strongly associated with infertility?
3. How do submucous fibroids impair fertility?
4. What is the effect of large intramural fibroids on implantation and IVF outcome?
5. Do subserosal fibroids usually affect fertility?
6. How are fibroids diagnosed on ultrasound?
7. What is the role of saline infusion sonohysterography (SIS) and hysteroscopy in diagnosing fibroids?
8. What is the role of MRI in fibroid assessment before IVF/ICSI?

9. How do fibroids increase the risk of miscarriage and adverse obstetric outcomes?
10. What are the indications for myomectomy in infertile women?
11. What are the routes of myomectomy (hysteroscopic, laparoscopic, open) and when is each indicated?
12. What is the impact of myomectomy on future fertility and pregnancy outcomes?
13. How long should a patient wait before attempting conception after myomectomy?
14. What is the role of medical treatment (GnRH agonists, SPRMs) in fibroids and fertility?
15. What is the effect of fibroids on IVF/ICSI success rates?
16. How do you counsel a woman with fibroids who is planning IVF?

CASE NO. (15) UNEXPLAINED INFERTILITY

A 29-year-old woman with 2 years of primary infertility. Her cycles are regular, mid-luteal progesterone confirms ovulation, HSG shows bilateral patent tubes, husband's semen analysis is normal. Both partners are otherwise healthy.

1. What is the definition of unexplained infertility?
2. What baseline investigations should be normal before labeling a couple as unexplained infertility?
3. What is the approximate prevalence of unexplained infertility among infertile couples?

4. What are the possible underlying mechanisms of unexplained infertility?
5. How long should a couple try to conceive naturally before starting treatment if diagnosed with unexplained infertility?
6. What is the role of expectant management in unexplained infertility?
7. What are the indications for ovulation induction with timed intercourse and IVF in unexplained infertility?
8. What is the role of IUI in unexplained infertility?
9. What is the role of IVF/ICSI in unexplained infertility?
10. What are the prognostic factors affecting spontaneous pregnancy rates in unexplained infertility?
11. What is the impact of female age on prognosis in unexplained infertility?
12. How many IUI cycles are usually recommended before moving to IVF?
13. What is the evidence for using clomiphene citrate or letrozole in unexplained infertility?
14. What is the role of gonadotropins with IUI in unexplained infertility?
15. How do guidelines (e.g., ESHRE, ASRM) recommend managing unexplained infertility?
16. What is the risk of multiple pregnancy in treatment of unexplained infertility with ovulation induction?
17. How do you counsel a couple with unexplained infertility regarding prognosis and treatment options?

CASE NO. (16) HIRSUTISM

A 23-year-old woman presents with excessive hair growth on the face and chest for 3 years. She also reports irregular cycles. BMI is 31. Examination shows terminal hair on chin and upper lip (Ferriman-Gallwey score 14). No clitoromegaly or deep voice.

1. What is the definition of hirsutism? How is it different from hypertrichosis?
2. What is the role of androgens in the pathophysiology of hirsutism?
3. What is the most common cause of hirsutism in women of reproductive age?
4. What endocrine disorders can present with hirsutism?
5. What are the clinical features that suggest androgen-secreting tumors?
6. How do you assess the severity of hirsutism clinically?
7. What is the Ferriman–Gallwey score?
8. What baseline investigations are indicated in a woman presenting with hirsutism?
9. What is the role of serum testosterone and DHEAS in evaluation?
10. When should you suspect late-onset congenital adrenal hyperplasia?
11. What is the role of imaging (pelvic US, adrenal CT/MRI) in evaluation of hirsutism?
12. How do you manage hirsutism in PCOS patients?
13. What is the role of combined oral contraceptives in treatment?
14. What is the role of antiandrogens (spironolactone, cyproterone acetate, finasteride)?
15. Why must antiandrogens always be combined with contraception?

16. What is the role of insulin sensitizers (metformin) in managing hirsutism in PCOS?
17. What cosmetic treatments are available for hirsutism?
18. How do you counsel a patient with hirsutism about prognosis and long-term management?

CASE NO. (17) CONGENITAL ADRENAL HYPERPLASIA

A 22-year-old woman presents with irregular cycles, infertility, and hirsutism. On examination she has acne, increased body hair, and mild clitoromegaly. Hormonal profile: 17-hydroxyprogesterone markedly elevated, testosterone mildly elevated, prolactin and TSH normal.

1. What is congenital adrenal hyperplasia (CAH)?
2. What is the most common enzyme deficiency causing CAH?
3. What is the difference between classical and non-classical CAH?
4. How does classical CAH usually present in females?
5. How does non-classical CAH present in adolescence and adulthood?
6. How does CAH cause infertility in women?
7. What are the typical hormonal findings in CAH (17-hydroxyprogesterone, androgens, cortisol)?
8. What is the role of ACTH stimulation test in diagnosing CAH?
9. What are the main differential diagnoses of hyperandrogenism in women?
10. How does CAH differ from PCOS clinically and biochemically?
11. What are the reproductive implications of CAH in men?
12. What is the role of glucocorticoid therapy in CAH management?

13. How does glucocorticoid treatment improve fertility in women with CAH?
14. What is the role of mineralocorticoid replacement in CAH?
15. What fertility treatment options are available for women with CAH who fail to conceive naturally?
16. What are the risks of pregnancy in women with CAH, and how is management adapted?
17. How do you counsel a couple regarding genetic risk and inheritance of CAH?

CASE NO. (18) INTRAUTERINE INSEMINATION (IUI)

A 32-year-old woman presents with 3 years of primary infertility. Her cycles are regular, ovulation is confirmed, HSG shows bilateral patent tubes. Husband's semen analysis shows mild oligoasthenozoospermia (15 million/mL, progressive motility 30%). The couple asks if they are candidates for IUI.

1. What is intrauterine insemination (IUI) and how does it differ from intracervical insemination?
2. What are the main indications for IUI?
3. What are the contraindications for IUI?
4. What are the prerequisites before offering IUI?
5. How is the semen sample prepared for IUI?
6. What is the rationale behind semen washing before insemination?
7. What is the role of ovulation induction in IUI cycles?
8. Which drugs are commonly used for ovarian stimulation in IUI?

9. What is the optimal timing of IUI in relation to ovulation trigger?
10. How many IUI cycles are generally recommended before moving to IVF?
11. What are the success rates of IUI compared to natural conception and IVF?
12. What factors influence the success rate of IUI?
13. What are the possible complications of IUI?
14. What is the risk of multiple pregnancy in IUI with stimulation?
15. How does IUI success differ in cases of unexplained infertility, mild male factor, and cervical factor?
16. What is the role of luteal phase support in IUI cycles?
17. How do international guidelines (ESHRE/ASRM) recommend using IUI in infertility management?

CASE NO. (19) PUBERTY

A 12-year-old girl is brought by her mother because she has started breast development but has not yet started menstruating. Mother is worried about whether this is normal.

1. What is the average age of onset of puberty in girls?
2. What is the normal sequence of pubertal events in females?
3. What are the Tanner stages of breast development?
4. What are the Tanner stages of pubic hair development?
5. What is the average age of menarche?
6. What hormonal changes initiate puberty in girls?
7. What is the role of GnRH pulsatility in female puberty?

8. What is the role of FSH and LH in follicular development during puberty?
9. What are the signs of adrenarche in girls?
10. What is precocious puberty in girls? Define the age cut-off.
11. Differentiate between central (gonadotropin-dependent) and peripheral (gonadotropin-independent) precocious puberty.
12. What are the common causes of central precocious puberty in girls?
13. What are the common causes of peripheral precocious puberty in girls?
14. What is delayed puberty in girls? Define the age cut-off.
15. What are the common causes of delayed puberty in girls?
16. What is the role of bone age assessment in evaluating delayed or precocious puberty?
17. What is the role of pelvic ultrasound in the evaluation of female puberty disorders?
18. When is karyotyping indicated in girls with delayed puberty?
19. How is central precocious puberty managed in girls?
20. How is delayed puberty managed in girls (constitutional vs pathological)?

CASE NO. (20) AMENORRHEA

A 16-year-old girl presents with no menstruation since puberty. She has normal breast development and pubic hair. Her BMI is normal. On examination, external genitalia appear normal, but the vagina ends in a blind pouch. Pelvic ultrasound shows absent uterus and normal ovaries.

1. What is the definition of primary amenorrhea?

2. What is the definition of secondary amenorrhea?
3. What is the commonest cause of secondary amenorrhea?
4. What is the most important first step in evaluating secondary amenorrhea?
5. What are the common causes of primary amenorrhea with normal secondary sexual characteristics?
6. What are the common causes of primary amenorrhea with absent secondary sexual characteristics?
7. How do you differentiate between outflow tract obstruction and ovarian causes of amenorrhea?
8. What is Asherman's syndrome and how does it present?
9. What is the role of the progesterone challenge test in evaluating amenorrhea?
10. How do you interpret a positive vs negative progesterone withdrawal test?
11. What is the role of the estrogen–progesterone challenge test?
12. How do you use serum FSH and LH levels to differentiate causes of amenorrhea?
13. What are the typical hormone findings in hypothalamic amenorrhea?
14. What are the typical hormone findings in premature ovarian insufficiency?
15. How does hyperprolactinemia cause amenorrhea?
16. What is the role of thyroid dysfunction in amenorrhea?
17. How do you evaluate amenorrhea in a woman with suspected androgen excess?
18. What imaging is useful in primary amenorrhea?
19. How is primary amenorrhea due to Mullerian agenesis managed?
20. How is secondary amenorrhea due to hypothalamic dysfunction managed?

CASE NO. (21) MALE FACTOR INFERTILITY

A 34-year-old man presents with 2 years of infertility. His wife has a normal evaluation. Semen analysis shows: volume 2 mL, concentration 8 million/mL, motility 20%, morphology 2% normal forms. He has no history of mumps orchitis, surgery, or systemic illness. Examination reveals normal secondary sexual characteristics and bilateral testes 15 mL each.

1. What is the contribution of male factor to overall infertility cases (percentage)?
2. What are the main causes of male infertility?
3. What is the difference between obstructive and non-obstructive azoospermia?
4. How is semen analysis performed and what parameters are evaluated according to WHO criteria?
5. What are the normal reference values for sperm concentration, motility, and morphology?
6. What is oligospermia, asthenospermia, teratospermia, and oligoasthenoteratospermia (OAT)?
7. What are the common lifestyle and environmental risk factors affecting male fertility?
8. How do varicoceles affect male fertility?
9. What is the role of hormonal evaluation in male infertility?
10. How do you differentiate between primary testicular failure and secondary hypogonadism in male infertility?
11. What is the role of genetic testing (karyotype, Y chromosome microdeletion, CFTR mutation) in male infertility?

12. What is the role of testicular biopsy in male infertility evaluation?
13. How does infection (orchitis, prostatitis, STDs) contribute to male infertility?
14. What is the role of antioxidant therapy in male infertility?
15. What are the options for sperm retrieval in azoospermic men (PESA, TESA, micro-TESE)?
16. What is the role of ICSI in severe male factor infertility?
17. How does advanced paternal age affect fertility and ART outcomes?
18. What is the clinical significance of sperm DNA fragmentation tests in male infertility?
19. How do endocrine disorders (thyroid, prolactin, diabetes) affect male fertility?
20. How do you counsel a man with severe male factor infertility about fertility options?

VOLUME 2

IVF/ICSI

PART 1

SINGLE BEST ANSWERS (SBAs) & MULTIPLE CHOICE QUESTIONS (MCQs) IN IVF/ICSI

PREPARATION OF THE PATIENT BEFORE IVF/ICSI

1- Which lifestyle modification is most evidence-based for improving IVF/ICSI outcomes before treatment?

A. Switching from coffee to green tea

B. Achieving BMI within the normal range and stopping smoking

C. Using herbal fertility supplements

D. Reducing screen time before sleep

2-Which of the following thyroid profiles is considered acceptable before starting IVF stimulation?

A. TSH < 5.0 mIU/L regardless of thyroid antibodies

B. TSH < 10.0 mIU/L if asymptomatic

C. Any TSH level as long as free T4 is normal

D. TSH levels are not relevant for IVF outcomes

E. TSH < 2.5 mIU/L in women planning pregnancy

3- In women with recurrent implantation failure planning IVF, which test is most relevant before starting stimulation?

A. Endometrial scratching

B. Semen culture

C. Hysteroscopy

D. Ovarian biopsy

E. Karyotyping of embryos before transfer

4- A 30-year-old woman is preparing for IVF. Which ovarian reserve test is most predictive of ovarian response to stimulation?

A. Serum FSH on day 3

B. Serum AMH (Anti-Müllerian Hormone)

C. Serum Estradiol (E2) on day 3

D. Serum Progesterone in luteal phase

E. Mid-cycle LH surge

5- Which uterine assessment is most useful before starting IVF?

A. CT scan of the pelvis

B. Hysterosalpingography (HSG) only

C. TVUS

D. MRI of the uterus in all patients

E. No uterine assessment is required

6- Which male partner test is routinely required before IVF/ICSI?

A. Karyotyping

B. Semen analysis

C. Testicular biopsy

D. Scrotal MRI

E. Y-chromosome microdeletion test

7- Which of the following endocrine tests is routinely recommended before IVF in women?

A. DHEA-S, Cortisol, Testosterone

B. LH surge test kits

C. Growth hormone assay

D. FSH, LH, E2, AMH, TSH, Prolactin

E. ACTH stimulation test

8- A 34-year-old woman is preparing for IVF. Which of the following baseline investigations is NOT routinely recommended?

A. CBC and blood group

B. Viral markers (HIV, HBV, HCV, syphilis)

C. Chest X-ray

D. AMH and AFC

E. TSH and prolactin

9-Which factor has the strongest impact on ICSI success rates?

A. Number of oocytes retrieved

B. Maternal age and Embryo quality

C. Sperm morphology alone

D. Duration of infertility

E. Type of culture media used

10- What is the approximate live birth rate per embryo transfer with ICSI in women aged 40–42?

A. ~5–10%

B. ~15–20%

C. ~30–35%

D. ~40–50%

E. Same as women <35 years

11- Which of the following has been shown to decrease ICSI success rates significantly?

A. Endometrial thickness > 8 mm at transfer

B. Use of blastocyst transfer

C. Use of frozen embryo transfer (FET)

D. Antagonist stimulation protocol

E. Maternal age > 38 years

12- What is the approximate cumulative pregnancy rate after 3–4 ICSI cycles in women < 35 years?

A. 10–20%

B. 30–40%

C. 50–60%

D. 70–80%

E. >90%

13- Which of the following uterine factors is most strongly linked to reduced ICSI success?

A. Adenomyosis

B. Retroverted uterus

C. Thin endometrium (< 7 mm)

D. Fibroid < 2 cm not distorting cavity

E. Cervical ectropion

14- Which laboratory factor has the greatest influence on embryo implantation rates in ICSI?

A. Embryologist's technique in injection

B. Incubator culture conditions

C. Sperm preparation method

D. Type of catheter used for transfer

E. Use of ICSI instead of conventional IVF

15- Which of the following is considered the most reliable predictor of ovarian response to stimulation in IVF?

A. Day 3 FSH

B. Antral Follicle Count (AFC)

C. Serum Estradiol (E2) on day 3

D. Serum LH on day 3

E. Mid-cycle progesterone

16- What is the typical threshold of AMH (Anti-Müllerian Hormone) that suggests a poor ovarian response to stimulation?

A. < 1.1 ng/ml

B. < 2.5 ng/ml

C. < 3.5 ng/ml

D. < 5 ng/ml

E. < 10 ng/ml

17- A 36-year-old woman has AMH = 4.0 ng/ml and AFC = 22 Which response is most likely during stimulation?

A. Low response

B. Normal response

C. High response

D. No oocyte retrieval possible

E. Premature ovarian failure

18- What is the expected ovarian response in a woman with AMH 2.5 ng/ml and AFC 12?

A. Poor responder

B. Normal responder

C. Hyper-responder

D. Premature ovarian failure

E. Unpredictable response

19- A woman with AMH 0.5 ng/ml and AFC 3 is likely to:

A. Have a high risk of OHSS

B. Be a poor responder with low oocyte yield

C. Respond normally to 150 IU stimulation

D. Have >50% chance of live birth per cycle

E. Not require gonadotropin stimulation

20- When counselling a 32-year-old woman with normal ovarian reserve and her partner with severe male factor infertility about ICSI, which of the following statements is most accurate?

A. The chance of pregnancy per cycle is >70% regardless of age or embryo quality.

B. The average clinical pregnancy rate per cycle is around 30–40% in women under 35.

C. Fertilization rates with ICSI are usually lower than conventional IVF.

D. Cumulative live birth rates after 3 cycles remain below 40%.

E. Maternal age has little effect on ICSI success rates compared to male factor.

21- Which of the following is a well-established indication for ICSI rather than conventional IVF?

A. Unexplained infertility with normal semen parameters

B. Young female with high ovarian reserve undergoing elective egg freezing

C. Tubal factor infertility with normal semen analysis

D. Mild endometriosis with normal sperm count

E. Severe oligospermia or azoospermia requiring surgical sperm retrieval

22- Which of the following scenarios is NOT a standard indication for IVF/ICSI?

A. Severe oligospermia with total motile sperm count <5 million

B. Bilateral tubal obstruction confirmed by laparoscopy

C. Failure of intrauterine insemination (IUI) after 6 cycles in unexplained infertility

D. Primary ovarian insufficiency with FSH persistently >40 IU/L

E. Endometriosis stage IV with distorted pelvic anatomy

AGONISTS PROTCOLS

23- What is the main mechanism of GnRH agonist long protocol in ovarian stimulation?

A. Direct stimulation of LH surge for ovulation

B. Pituitary down-regulation after initial flare effect

C. Suppression of ovarian estrogen receptors

D. Direct stimulation of FSH release

E. Inhibition of progesterone production by corpus luteum

24- When is GnRH agonist typically started in the long protocol?

A. Mid-luteal phase of the preceding cycle

B. Day 1 of stimulation

C. Mid-cycle after LH surge

D. After triggering ovulation

E. Only in the luteal support phase

25- Which of the following is an advantage of the long GnRH agonist protocol compared to antagonist protocol?

A. Shorter duration of stimulation

B. Reduced risk of OHSS

C. More synchronized follicular cohort

D. No risk of cyst formation

E. Lower gonadotropin dose required

26- The flare protocol (short agonist protocol) is most commonly used in:

A. High responders at risk of OHSS

B. Low responders / diminished ovarian reserve

C. Women with PCOS and high AMH

D. Women requiring PPOS stimulation

E. Patients with recurrent implantation failure

27- What is the main rationale for using the short GnRH agonist protocol?

A. To suppress ovarian activity before stimulation

B. To take advantage of the initial FSH/LH flare up effect

C. To reduce risk of OHSS in high responders

D. To prevent follicular synchronization

E. To shorten luteal phase support duration

28- What is the usual clinical marker used to confirm down-regulation before starting stimulation in long protocol?

A. Serum progesterone >5 ng/ml

B. AMH <1 ng/ml

C. Peak estradiol level >250 pg/ml

D. Follicle size >14 mm on ultrasound

E. Serum estradiol <50 pg/ml with suppressed LH, FSH and thin endometrium

29- Which of the following is a disadvantage of long protocol?

A. Risk of premature LH surge

B. Longer duration of treatment and higher gonadotropin dose

C. Poor synchronization of follicle growth

D. Inability to suppress pituitary gonadotropins

E. Lack of down-regulation

30- Which finding suggests that an ovarian cyst is functionally active and may interfere with stimulation?

A. Diameter <3 cm, estradiol <40 pg/ml

B. Thin-walled, unilocular cyst with no vascularity

C. Persistent but stable size over 2 cycles

D. Diameter >5 cm, estradiol >50 pg/ml

E. Hemorrhagic appearance but low estradiol

31- What is the management option for ovarian cyst with high E2, before stimulation in a long protocol?

A. Ignore and proceed with stimulation

B. High-dose gonadotropin stimulation

C. Immediate hCG trigger

D. Switch to clomiphene induction

E. Cyst aspiration under ultrasound guidance

32- Which of the following complications is more likely with long agonist protocol compared to antagonist?

A. OHSS (Ovarian Hyperstimulation Syndrome)

B. Poor ovarian response

C. Thin endometrium

D. Luteal phase defect

E. Increased miscarriage rate

33- The ultrashort GnRH agonist protocol is characterized by:

A. Continuous use until oocyte retrieval

B. Administration of the agonist for only 2–3 days, starting on day 1 of the menstrual cycle, to take advantage of the initial flare-up effect

C. Use only in luteal phase for luteal support

D. Combination with letrozole for PCOS patients

E. Higher pregnancy rates in all women

34- What is the main purpose of pituitary down-regulation in the long protocol?

A. To increase progesterone levels in luteal phase

B. To decrease FSH sensitivity of ovaries

C. To stimulate endometrial proliferation

D. To prevent premature LH surge and spontaneous ovulation

E. To improve sperm penetration of zona pellucida

35- Which of the following best describes the sequence in the long protocol?

A. Start gonadotropins → later add agonist → trigger ovulation

B. Start agonist → achieve down-regulation → add gonadotropins → hCG trigger → oocyte retrieval

C. Start gonadotropins and agonist together → continue till trigger

D. Start antagonist in luteal phase → switch to agonist

E. Begin luteal support before starting stimulation

36- A known side effect during the down-regulation phase of the long protocol is:

A. Hot flushes and hypoestrogenic symptoms

B. Premature ovulation

C. Increased endometrial receptivity

D. Rapid follicular recruitment

E. Increased progesterone secretion

37- What is the typical endometrial appearance that indicates adequate pituitary suppression before gonadotropin stimulation in a long protocol?

A. Thick, trilaminar endometrium >10 mm

B. Thin endometrium < 6 mm

C. Echogenic endometrium ≥12 mm

D. Irregular endometrium with cystic changes

E. Absent endometrium

ANTAGONIST PROTOCOL

38- What is the main mechanism of GnRH antagonists in ovarian stimulation?

A. Initial flare of gonadotropins followed by suppression

B. Stimulation of LH surge to induce ovulation

C. Direct competitive blockade of GnRH receptors → immediate LH/FSH suppression

D. Down-regulation of pituitary over several weeks

E. Direct inhibition of ovarian estrogen receptors

39- In the antagonist protocol, when are GnRH antagonists usually introduced?

A. Mid-luteal phase of the previous cycle

B. Day 1 of stimulation

C. Once the leading follicle reaches ~12–14 mm

D. Only after ovulation trigger

E. During the luteal support phase

40- Which of the following is a major advantage of antagonist protocol compared to agonist long protocol?

A. Higher pregnancy rates in all age groups

B. Lower risk of OHSS and shorter treatment duration

C. More synchronized follicular cohort

D. Better endometrial receptivity

E. Lower gonadotropin consumption in all patients

41- Which ovulation trigger is most useful in antagonist cycles to reduce OHSS risk?

A. hCG trigger only

B. Dual trigger (hCG + GnRH agonist)

C. GnRH agonist trigger

D. Natural LH surge

E. No trigger required

42- Which patient population benefits most from the antagonist protocol?

A. Poor responders with low AMH

B. Women with recurrent implantation failure

C. Patients requiring frozen oocyte preservation

D. Women with endometriosis

E. Women at high risk of OHSS (e.g., PCOS, high AMH)

43- Which of the following is a disadvantage of the antagonist protocol compared to the long agonist protocol?

A. Higher gonadotropin dose requirement

B. Increased risk of OHSS

C. Asynchronization of follicles

D. Longer duration of stimulation

E. Lower Pregnancy rate

44- Why is the GnRH antagonist protocol often preferred in fertility preservation (oncology patients)?

A. It enhances oocyte quality

B. It eliminates the need for gonadotropins

C. It allows simultaneous endometrial receptivity testing

D. It avoids the need for oocyte vitrification

E. It reduces stimulation duration, allowing faster treatment

45- Which of the following is true regarding LH surge suppression in antagonist protocol?

A. Antagonists completely eliminate risk of LH surge

B. Antagonists require 2–3 weeks before suppression is achieved

C. Antagonists act immediately without initial flare

D. LH surge is more frequent with antagonists than agonists

E. Antagonists increase endogenous FSH release

46- Which of the following is not a routine indication for using the antagonist protocol?

A. PCOS patients

B. Patients with high AMH

C. Poor responders needing flare effect

D. Patients undergoing fertility preservation

E. High-risk OHSS candidates

47- In terms of patient experience, antagonist protocol is preferred because:

A. It requires fewer injections and shorter duration of treatment

B. It eliminates the need for gonadotropins

C. It guarantees higher pregnancy rates

D. It avoids monitoring during stimulation

E. It reduces cost in all patients

48- What is the first step in a GnRH antagonist stimulation cycle?

A. Start GnRH antagonist in the luteal phase

B. Begin controlled ovarian stimulation with gonadotropins on day 2–3 of cycle

C. Give GnRH agonist for down-regulation before stimulation

D. Start luteal progesterone support immediately

E. Perform oocyte retrieval on day 3 of stimulation

49- When is Fixed GnRH antagonist usually started during stimulation?

A. Day 1 of stimulation

B. After triggering ovulation

C. During luteal support phase

D. Day 6 of Stimulation

E. One week before stimulation

50- What is the main purpose of adding GnRH antagonist during stimulation?

A. To synchronize follicle growth

B. To prevent premature LH surge and ovulation

C. To improve endometrial receptivity

D. To increase oocyte yield

E. To enhance sperm penetration

51- What strategy can improve synchronization of follicles in antagonist cycles?

A. Using a mid-luteal agonist pretreatment

B. Starting stimulation without any pretreatment

C. Stopping gonadotropins for the first 5 days

D. Using a dual trigger on day 1

E. Avoiding estradiol pretreatment

52- Which of the following best describes the clinical pregnancy and live birth rates when comparing GnRH antagonist protocol to the long agonist protocol in IVF?

A. Antagonist protocol has consistently higher live birth rates.

B. Long agonist protocol has consistently higher live birth rates.

C. Recent studies show comparable pregnancy and live birth rates between the two protocols.

D. Antagonist protocol is inferior in poor responders but superior in high responders.

E. Live birth rates are significantly lower with antagonist due to poor endometrial receptivity.

PROGESTIN-PRIMED OVARIAN STIMULATION PROTOCOL

53- What is the main mechanism of Progestin-Primed Ovarian Stimulation (PPOS)?

A. Suppression of follicle recruitment in the luteal phase

B. Progesterone administration in follicular phase prevents premature LH surge

C. Stimulation of endogenous FSH secretion

D. Down-regulation of GnRH receptors over 2 weeks

E. Direct stimulation of granulosa cell proliferation

54- Which of the following is a mandatory step after PPOS stimulation?

A. Fresh embryo transfer in the same cycle

B. Routine ovarian drilling before retrieval

C. Freeze-all embryos for later transfer (FET)

D. Luteal support with estrogen and progesterone during same cycle

E. Use of GnRH agonist trigger only

55- Which patients benefit most from PPOS protocol?

A. Women with PCOS at risk of OHSS

B. Women needing fertility preservation (e.g., oncology)

C. Oocyte donors

D. Patients requiring freeze-all strategy for any reason

E. All of the above

56- Which of the following is an advantage of PPOS compared to antagonist protocol?

A. Allows fresh embryo transfer with improved implantation

B. Oral administration is simpler and cheaper than antagonists

C. Reduces need for luteal support after transfer

D. Eliminates risk of OHSS completely

E. Provides higher live birth rates in all groups

57- Which statement is true regarding limitations of PPOS?

A. It cannot effectively prevent premature LH surge

B. It requires embryo cryopreservation

C. It causes ovarian cyst formation more often than agonist protocols

D. It is contraindicated in PCOS patients

E. It gives lower fertilization rates compared to ICSI

58- Why is fresh embryo transfer not performed in PPOS cycles?

A. Because progesterone causes premature luteal phase defect

B. Because oocyte quality is reduced in PPOS

C. Because progestins directly damage embryos

D. Because endometrium becomes non-receptive due to early progesterone exposure

E. Because gonadotropins are ineffective with progestins

59- Which type of progestin is commonly used in PPOS protocols?

A. Letrozole

B. Medroxyprogesterone acetate or dydrogesterone

C. GnRH antagonist tablets

D. Clomiphene citrate

E. Tamoxifen

60- In PPOS, when is progestin typically started?

A. Luteal phase of the previous cycle

B. After hCG trigger

C. After oocyte retrieval

D. Only during luteal support

E. Day 2 of ovarian stimulation together with gonadotropins

61- A 30-year-old woman with diminished ovarian reserve (AMH 0.8 ng/ml) is scheduled for IVF. Doctor considers PPOS protocol. Which statement is correct?

A. PPOS improves ovarian reserve and increases AMH

B. PPOS prevents premature LH surge but does not improve oocyte number in low responders

C. PPOS guarantees higher pregnancy rates compared to antagonist

D. PPOS allows fresh transfer safely

E. PPOS should never be used in poor responders

62- A 29-year-old woman with PCOS is stimulated using PPOS. She develops >20 follicles >17 mm. Which trigger and next step are most appropriate?

A. hCG trigger followed by fresh transfer

B. Dual trigger (hCG + agonist) and fresh transfer

C. GnRH agonist trigger followed by freeze-all strategy

D. No trigger and cancel cycle

E. Progesterone trigger with immediate fresh transfer

DOUBLE STIMULATION PROTOCOL

63- What is the main rationale for Double Stimulation protocol in IVF?

A. To reduce gonadotropin requirement

B. To take advantage of follicular recruitment in both follicular and luteal phases

C. To avoid embryo freezing

D. To improve endometrial receptivity

E. To prevent OHSS

64- Which patient population benefits most from DuoStim?

A. High responders with PCOS

B. Low responders or women with poor ovarian reserve

C. Women with tubal factor infertility

D. Normal responders

E. Women undergoing fresh transfer cycles

65- When is the second stimulation started in DuoStim?

A. Immediately after ovulation trigger

B. After menstruation in next cycle

C. After luteal support is completed

D. Anytime in mid-cycle

E. In luteal phase, 3–5 days after oocyte retrieval

66- What is usually required in DuoStim after both stimulations?

A. Fresh embryo transfer

B. Endometrial scratching

C. Freeze-all embryos strategy

D. Natural conception attempt

E. Use of clomiphene only

67- What is the main advantage of DuoStim in oncofertility patients?

A. Reduces need for GnRH antagonist

B. Allows rapid accumulation of oocytes in a short time before chemotherapy

C. Improves endometrial receptivity for fresh transfer

D. Increases fertilization rates independent of ovarian reserve

E. Avoids need for oocyte vitrification

68- Which of the following is true about follicular waves in humans that support DuoStim?

A. Only one wave of follicular recruitment per cycle exists

B. Multiple follicular waves occur, including in luteal phase

C. Follicular recruitment is absent in luteal phase

D. Luteal follicles cannot respond to gonadotropins

E. Oocyte competence is lower in luteal phase than follicular phase

69- What is the expected oocyte competence in luteal phase stimulation compared to follicular phase stimulation?

A. Always inferior

B. Always superior

C. Comparable when culture and freezing are optimized

D. Non-viable oocytes are retrieved in luteal phase

E. No oocytes are retrieved in luteal phase

70- Which of the following is a limitation of DuoStim protocol?

A. Requires freeze-all strategy, no fresh transfer possible

B. Lower oocyte yield compared to single stimulation

C. Cannot be used in poor responders

D. Contraindicated in fertility preservation

E. Associated with lower fertilization rates

71- Which ovarian stimulation drugs are used in both follicular and luteal stimulations of DuoStim?

A. Only clomiphene citrate

B. Only GnRH agonist

C. Progesterone alone

D. Gonadotropins with GnRH antagonist co-treatment

E. hCG alone

72- Which trigger is used at the end of each stimulation phase in DuoStim cycles to induce final oocyte maturation?

A. Recombinant LH trigger

B. GnRH agonist trigger - hCG trigger

C. Kisspeptin Trigger

D. Progesterone trigger

E. No trigger is required in DuoStim

MODIFIED NATURAL CYCLE STIMULATION

73- Which patient population benefits most from modified natural cycle IVF?

A. Women with very high ovarian reserve (AMH >7 ng/ml)

B. Low responders with very low ovarian reserve

C. Patients with normal ovarian reserve undergoing first IVF

D. Women seeking elective egg freezing

E. All patients equally

74- What is a major limitation of modified natural cycle IVF?

A. High gonadotropin cost

B. Increased OHSS risk

C. Lower embryo quality in all cases

D. Increased luteal support requirement

E. Low oocyte yield and higher risk of cycle cancellation

75- In terms of cumulative live birth rates, how does mild stimulation compare to conventional stimulation after several cycles?

A. Always inferior regardless of patient group

B. Comparable if multiple cycles are performed (similar cumulative success)

C. Always superior due to better oocyte quality

D. Inferior because no embryos can be frozen

E. Cannot be compared scientifically

GONADOTROPINS

76- What is the typical starting gonadotropin dose in a standard conventional IVF stimulation protocol for a normal responder?

A. 75–150 IU/day

B. 150–225 IU/day

C. 300–450 IU/day

D. 50 IU/day

E. >600 IU/day

77- What is the maximum dose of gonadotropin is appropriate for low responders?

A. 75 IU/day

B. 100–150 IU/day

C. 300 IU/day

D. 450–600 IU/day

E. No gonadotropins required

78- In high responders, what is the minimum starting dose?

A. 75 IU/day

B. 150 IU/day

C. 300 IU/day

D. 450 IU/day

E. > 450 IU/day

79- Which of the following factors is most important in determining the starting gonadotropin dose?

A. Endometrial thickness alone

B. Day 21 progesterone level

C. Tubal patency

D. Number of previous pregnancies

E. Maternal age, AMH, antral follicle count and BMI

80- Why is adjustment of gonadotropin dose in the mid-stimulation phase generally not recommended?

A. The ovary does not respond to gonadotropins at all

B. Follicular cohort is already recruited, and further dose changes do not significantly affect outcome

C. It increases the chance of multiple pregnancy

D. It always improves oocyte quality but reduces embryo number

E. It is prohibited by IVF regulations

81- What is the main purpose of monitoring during controlled ovarian stimulation in ICSI cycles?

A. To confirm ovulation has occurred

B. To adjust luteal support dose

C. To track follicular growth and prevent premature LH surge or OHSS

D. To assess endometrial receptivity after transfer

E. To monitor embryo development directly inside the ovary

82- Which hormone is most useful for monitoring the risk of OHSS during ovarian stimulation?

A. FSH

B. Progesterone

C. AMH

D. Estradiol (E2)

E. Inhibin B

83- When is progesterone measurement during stimulation most clinically relevant?

A. Day 2 of cycle

B. Mid-stimulation (day 5–6)

C. On trigger day, to rule out premature luteinization

D. After embryo transfer

E. After luteal support

84- What is the typical follicle size on ultrasound considered adequate to give ovulation trigger in ICSI cycles?

A. 10–12 mm

B. 12–14 mm

C. 18–20 mm

D. 8–10 mm

E. >25 mm

85- What is the most appropriate frequency of monitoring in the mid to late stimulation phase of an ICSI cycle?

A. Daily ultrasound and hormones from day 2

B. Every 2–3 days until follicles reach ~16 mm, then more frequent if needed

C. Only one ultrasound before trigger

D. Monitoring is unnecessary with antagonist protocol

E. Weekly monitoring

86- Which of the following findings suggests premature LH surge during ICSI monitoring?

A. Low estradiol with small follicles

B. Follicles 12 mm with estradiol <100 pg/ml

C. Endometrium 4 mm on day 10

D. AMH <1 ng/ml

E. Elevated progesterone >1.5 ng/ml before trigger

87- What is the significance of endometrial thickness monitoring during ICSI stimulation?

A. Thin endometrium (<8 mm) may be associated with poor implantation

B. Thick endometrium (>12 mm) always guarantees pregnancy

C. Endometrial measurement determines gonadotropin dose

D. Endometrium is irrelevant in ICSI cycles

E. Endometrial thickness should not be measured

88- On day 10 of stimulation, a 30-year-old woman has 12 follicles ≥18 mm, estradiol = 2800 pg/ml, and progesterone = 0.9 ng/ml. What is the next best step?

A. Continue stimulation for 2 more days

B. Give ovulation trigger and schedule oocyte retrieval

C. Cancel the cycle

D. Add antagonist to prevent LH surge

E. Start luteal support immediately

89- A 32-year-old woman on antagonist protocol is monitored on day 8. She has 8 follicles 15–17 mm, estradiol = 2200 pg/ml, and progesterone = 2.1 ng/ml. What is the interpretation?

A. Normal response, ready for trigger

B. Premature luteinization; consider freeze-all strategy

C. Poor ovarian response

D. High risk of OHSS, cancel cycle immediately

E. Inadequate stimulation, increase gonadotropins

90- On day 9, a 36-year-old woman shows only 2 follicles (14–15 mm) and estradiol = 150 pg/ml despite 300 IU/day gonadotropins. What does this indicate?

A. High responder, risk of OHSS

B. Premature LH surge

C. Normal stimulation, continue as planned

D. Poor ovarian response, consider cycle cancellation

E. Endometrial pathology

91- A 29-year-old woman on long protocol shows endometrium 5 mm on day 11 despite good follicular growth (7 follicles ≥18 mm, estradiol = 2400 pg/ml). What is the concern?

A. Thin endometrium may reduce implantation, consider freeze-all

B. Risk of premature ovulation

C. High risk of OHSS

D. Poor ovarian response

E. Multiple pregnancy risk

92- A 27-year-old woman with PCOS is undergoing ovarian stimulation for ICSI. On day 11, ultrasound shows 18 follicles ≥17 mm. Serum estradiol is 3800 pg/ml, progesterone = 1.0 ng/ml. What is the best next step?

A. Proceed with hCG trigger and fresh embryo transfer

B. Proceed with GnRH agonist trigger & freeze-all strategy

C. Cancel the cycle to avoid complications

D. Continue stimulation for 2–3 more days

E. Reduce gonadotropin dose and delay trigger

93- A 30-year-old woman has follicles 12–14 mm with E2 = 800 pg/ml on day 9. What should be the next step?

A. Trigger ovulation now

B. Continue stimulation and re-monitor after 2 days

C. Cancel the cycle

D. Switch to natural cycle

E. Give luteal support

94- Which patient group may benefit from adding recombinant LH to stimulation?

A. PCOS patients with high LH

B. Women with tubal factor infertility

C. Women with hypogonadotropic hypogonadism & Low Responder

D. Women with high AMH

E. All normal responders

95- What is the main advantage of recombinant FSH over urinary-derived FSH?

A. Higher OHSS risk

B. Higher purity and batch-to-batch consistency

C. Contains LH activity

D. Lower cost

E. Better implantation rates in all patients

96- A 32-year-old woman with hypogonadotropic hypogonadism is planned for IVF. Which stimulation regimen is most appropriate?

A. rFSH alone

B. Recombinant LH alone

C. hCG only

D. Clomiphene citrate only

E. hMG (contains both FSH and LH activity)

97- According to ESHRE guidelines, how do recombinant and urinary gonadotropins compare in terms of live birth outcomes?

A. Recombinant is clearly superior

B. Urinary is clearly superior

C. Both show comparable efficacy in terms of live birth rates

D. Recombinant is inferior in poor responders

E. Urinary products are no longer recommended

98- Which factor is most important when choosing between urinary and recombinant gonadotropins in daily practice (as per ESHRE)?

A. Patient preference, cost, and availability

B. Superiority of recombinant in all outcomes

C. LH contamination in urinary products

D. Mandatory use of recombinant in high responders

E. Prohibition of urinary use in Europe

TRIGGERING OF OVULATION

99- A 27-year-old woman with PCOS undergoing ovarian stimulation has 22 follicles ≥17 mm and estradiol 4500 pg/ml. What is the safest trigger?

A. hCG trigger only

B. GnRH agonist trigger

C. Dual trigger (hCG + agonist)

D. No trigger, cancel cycle

E. Recombinant LH trigger

100- A 36-year-old Low responder with AMH 0.5 ng/ml shows 4 follicles 16–18 mm on day 11 of stimulation. In her previous cycle, most retrieved oocytes were immature. Which trigger is most appropriate?

A. hCG trigger only

B. GnRH agonist trigger

C. Dual trigger (hCG + GnRH agonist)

D. No trigger, wait longer

E. Recombinant LH trigger

101- Why can GnRH agonist trigger not be used in long agonist protocol cycles?

A. It causes excessive OHSS

B. Pituitary is desensitized and cannot release endogenous LH

C. It leads to multiple pregnancies

D. It increases risk of premature luteinization

E. It reduces oocyte quality

102- What is the typical timing of oocyte retrieval after ovulation trigger?

A. 12–18 hours

B. 24 hours

C. 34–36 hours

D. 48–60 hours

E. 72 hours

103- A 30-year-old woman on a long GnRH agonist protocol is ready for oocyte retrieval. Which trigger option is possible in her cycle?

A. GnRH agonist trigger

B. hCG trigger

C. Dual trigger (agonist + hCG)

D. Recombinant LH

E. Both A and B

104- A 29-year-old antagonist cycle patient has 10 follicles 17–19 mm and estradiol 2500 pg/ml. She is not at high risk of OHSS. Which trigger is most appropriate?

A. hCG trigger

B. GnRH agonist trigger

C. Dual trigger

D. Cancel cycle

E. Progesterone trigger

105- Why does hCG trigger carry a higher risk of OHSS compared to GnRH agonist trigger?

A. Because hCG is less effective at binding LH receptors

B. Because hCG has a longer half-life, prolonging luteotropic stimulation

C. Because hCG fails to induce luteinization

D. Because hCG suppresses estradiol levels

E. Because hCG causes poor oocyte maturation

106- Which step in oocyte development is completed after hCG trigger?

A. Transition from metaphase I to metaphase II

B. Initiation of follicle recruitment

C. Germ cell migration

D. Formation of primary follicles

E. Completion of zygote cleavage

107- Which source is urinary hCG derived from?

A. Recombinant DNA technology

B. Human menopausal urine

C. Placental tissue culture

D. Synthetic peptide

E. Pituitary extracts

108- A 34-year-old woman on conventional IVF protocol receives urinary hCG 10,000 IU. What is the main mechanism by which hCG induces final oocyte maturation?

A. Binding FSH receptors on granulosa cells

B. Binding LH receptors and resuming meiosis in the oocyte

C. Increasing AMH production in granulosa cells

D. Directly stimulating progesterone receptors

E. Inhibiting estradiol secretion

109- A 29-year-old woman with PCOS (antagonist protocol) has 20 follicles ≥18 mm, estradiol = 4000 pg/ml. The clinician is considering ovulation trigger. What is the main mechanistic difference between using hCG vs GnRH agonist in this case?

A. hCG directly increases FSH secretion, while GnRH agonist increases AMH

B. hCG works through estrogen receptors, while GnRH agonist works through progesterone receptors

C. hCG prevents cumulus expansion, while GnRH agonist enhances it

D. hCG shortens luteal phase, while GnRH agonist prolongs it

E. hCG acts directly on granulosa LH receptors to mimic LH surge, while GnRH agonist induces an endogenous LH surge from the pituitary

110- Which source is recombinant hCG produced from?

A. Chinese Hamster Ovary (CHO) cells using recombinant DNA technology

B. Human menopausal urine

C. Synthetic LH analogues

D. Pituitary extracts

E. Placental tissue

111- Which hCG preparation has higher purity and batch-to-batch consistency?

A. Urinary hCG

B. Recombinant hCG

C. Both equal

D. Neither

E. Depends on patient age

112- What is the standard dose of urinary hCG trigger for final oocyte maturation?

A. 250 μg

B. 10,000 IU

C. 75–150 IU

D. 1,500 IU

E. 50 μg

113- What is the standard dose of recombinant (rhCG) trigger?

A. 5,000 IU

B. 10,000 IU

C. 150 μg subcutaneous

D. 1,500 IU

E. 500 μg

114- What is the range of GnRH agonist dose (triptorelin) used as ovulation trigger in antagonist cycles?

A. 0.1- 0.4 mg subcutaneous

B. 1 mg subcutaneous

C. 5,000 IU intramuscular

D. 250 μg subcutaneous

E. 3.75 mg depot

115- Which combination is typically used in dual trigger?

A. rFSH + GnRH agonist

B. Low-dose hCG (1,500 IU- 5000) + GnRH agonist (0.1–0.2 mg)

C. Full-dose hCG (10,000 IU) + rLH

D. Progesterone + GnRH agonist

E. rFSH + hCG

116- In which patient scenario is dual trigger most useful?

A. High responders with very high OHSS risk

B. Women with recurrent cycles of immature oocytes despite hCG trigger

C. Women with hypogonadotropic hypogonadism

D. Patients on long agonist protocol

E. Patients with tubal factor infertility

117- What is the main advantage of dual trigger compared with hCG trigger alone?

A. It reduces gonadotropin cost

B. It eliminates the need for monitoring

C. It provides both endogenous LH/FSH surge and exogenous hCG support

D. It allows natural conception during stimulation

E. It reduces embryo cryopreservation rates

118- Which of the following is NOT true about dual trigger?

A. It may improve maturity of retrieved oocytes

B. It may improve fertilization and pregnancy rates in some patients

C. It completely eliminates OHSS risk in high responders

D. It combines agonist + low-dose hCG

E. It is often used in antagonist cycles

119- What is the main difference between dual trigger and double trigger?

A. Dual trigger uses hCG only, while double trigger uses agonist only

B. Dual trigger gives agonist + hCG together, while double trigger separates timing (agonist ~40h, hCG ~34h before retrieval)

C. Dual trigger is used in poor responders, double trigger in PCOS

D. Double trigger eliminates luteal support need

E. There is no difference

120- A 37-year-old woman on 300 IU rFSH daily shows no follicular growth and E2 <100 pg/ml on day 10 of stimulation. What is the best step?

A. Continue stimulation 3 more days

B. Increase dose to 450 IU

C. Add clomiphene citrate

D. Cancel the cycle

E. Trigger ovulation

121- A 29-year-old woman with PCOS on Long protocol has 30 follicles >16 mm and E2 = 6,000 pg/ml on day 11. What is the best decision?

A. Proceed with hCG trigger

B. Proceed with agonist trigger

C. Cancel the cycle to avoid OHSS

D. Add cabergoline and continue

E. Continue stimulation

122- A 27-year-old PCOS patient on Long agonist protocol develops very high estradiol (E2 = 4500 pg/ml) with >30 follicles on day 8. What is the best rescue strategy to prevent OHSS?

A. Proceed with hCG 10,000 IU trigger

B. Continue long agonist protocol and cancel the cycle

C. Switch to antagonist protocol to allow agonist trigger later

D. Give dual trigger (hCG + agonist)

E. Reduce gonadotropins and continue same protocol

123- Which of the following is TRUE about kisspeptin trigger?

A. It completely replaces hCG in all IVF centers

B. It induces an endogenous LH surge with lower OHSS risk

C. It is contraindicated in PCOS patients

D. It acts as a luteal phase support

E. It directly induces cumulus expansion

124- What is the current status of kisspeptin trigger in IVF practice?

A. Standard of care worldwide

B. Still considered investigational with ongoing clinical trials

C. Only approved for poor responders

D. Mandatory for all antagonist cycles

E. Banned due to side effects

125- A patient with 1 mature follicle, E2 200 pg/ml is upset about continuing IVF. What is the best counselling point?

A. Cycle must be cancelled

B. It is better to freeze all embryos

C. IVF will not work without at least 10 oocytes

D. Increasing gonadotropins now will improve outcome

E. Even a single good-quality oocyte can result in pregnancy

OOCYTE RETRIEVAL

126- Which needle size is most commonly used for oocyte retrieval?

A. 18–20 gauge

B. 10–14 gauge

C. 25–30 gauge

D. 8–12 gauge

E. 30–35 gauge

127- Which complication is most directly related to oocyte retrieval procedure?

A. Tubal blockage

B. Ovarian hyperstimulation syndrome

C. Pelvic infection or bleeding

D. Cervical incompetence

E. Premature luteinization

128- Which of the following is TRUE about oocyte retrieval?

A. It is performed 12 hours after trigger

B. It requires full bladder preparation

C. It always requires general anesthesia

D. It is done without any anesthesia

E. It is performed under transvaginal ultrasound guidance

129- What is the usual flushing medium used during oocyte retrieval?

A. Normal saline

B. Phosphate-buffered saline

C. Culture media with heparin

D. Pure distilled water

E. No medium is required

130- What is the expected oocyte recovery rate from aspirated follicles?

A. 10–20%

B. 30–40%

C. 50–60%

D. 70–80%

E. 100%

131- What is the most important step immediately after retrieving oocytes?

A. Freeze all oocytes directly

B. Transfer oocytes into culture medium at 37°C

C. Inject sperm immediately into all oocytes

D. Wash oocytes with distilled water

E. Add hCG to oocytes

132- Which of the following is a relative contraindication for oocyte retrieval?

A. Uncorrected coagulopathy

B. Tubal factor infertility

C. Male factor infertility

D. Low AMH

E. Endometriosis

133- A 29-year-old woman undergoes oocyte retrieval 20 hours after hCG trigger. No oocytes are found. What is the most likely reason?

A. Empty follicle syndrome

B. Premature ovulation

C. Early retrieval before maturation

D. Ovarian torsion

E. Infection

134- A 32-year-old woman undergoes oocyte retrieval 40 hours after trigger. Most follicles are collapsed, and no oocytes are recovered. What is the most likely cause?

A. Delayed retrieval after ovulation

B. Empty follicle syndrome

C. Poor ovarian response

D. Technical error in aspiration

E. Endometriosis

135- A patient undergoing oocyte retrieval complains of severe abdominal pain and hypotension during the procedure. What is the most likely complication?

A. OHSS

B. Bowel injury

C. Hemoperitoneum due to vascular injury

D. Pelvic infection

E. Cyst rupture

136- A 34-year-old woman develops fever, pelvic pain, and foul discharge 3 days after oocyte retrieval. What is the most likely diagnosis?

A. Ovarian hyperstimulation syndrome

B. Pelvic infection

C. Ectopic pregnancy

D. Endometrial polyp

E. Luteal cyst

137- A 28-year-old PCOS patient has 25 follicles aspirated but only 5 oocytes retrieved. What is the most likely explanation?

A. Empty follicle syndrome

B. OHSS

C. Premature luteinization

D. Low recovery rate due to technical issues

E. Poor egg quality

138- A 30-year-old patient undergoes oocyte retrieval under transvaginal ultrasound. Suddenly, bright echogenic fluid appears in the pouch of Douglas. What is the most likely cause?

A. Ovarian cyst rupture

B. Pelvic infection

C. Bleeding from punctured vessel

D. Endometrioma leakage

E. Ascites due to OHSS

139- A 40-year-old Low responder undergoes retrieval with 3 follicles > 18 mm, but no oocytes are obtained despite proper aspiration. What is the diagnosis?

A. Empty follicle syndrome

B. Premature ovulation

C. Ovulatory dysfunction

D. Technical error

E. OHSS

140- A 27-year-old woman complains of shoulder pain and abdominal distension after oocyte retrieval. What is the most likely cause?

A. OHSS ascites

B. Hemoperitoneum

C. Bowel injury

D. Pneumoperitoneum

E. Infection

141- During oocyte retrieval, the patient suddenly develops bradycardia and hypotension. What is the immediate step?

A. Continue aspiration quickly

B. Stop procedure, give IV fluids, and manage anesthesia complication

C. Increase sedation dose

D. Convert to laparoscopy

E. Proceed with hCG injection

142- A patient has retrieval of 12 mature follicles, but only 3 oocytes are obtained. What is the most appropriate next cycle modification?

A. Increase gonadotropin dose

B. Change aspiration needle or technique

C. Switch to IUI

D. Cancel future IVF attempts

E. Use clomiphene citrate only

143- Which of the following is the most accurate predictor of oocyte yield at retrieval?

A. Serum progesterone level on trigger day

B. Serum estradiol concentration on trigger day

C. Antral follicle count (AFC) at baseline

D. Number of follicles ≥16–18 mm on ultrasound at trigger

E. Endometrial thickness on trigger day

144- Which factor is most strongly associated with "Empty Follicle Syndrome"?

A. Low AMH

B. PCOS

C. Faulty hCG trigger administration or timing

D. High BMI

E. Premature LH surge

145- Which of the following is the most common immediate complication of oocyte retrieval?

A. Ovarian torsion

B. Bowel injury

C. Pelvic bleeding/hemoperitoneum

D. Bladder perforation

E. Sepsis

146- Which anesthesia protocol is most commonly used worldwide for oocyte retrieval?

A. General anesthesia with intubation

B. Local infiltration only

C. Conscious sedation/IV anesthesia (e.g., midazolam + propofol)

D. Spinal anesthesia

E. Epidural anesthesia

147- Which factor most influences the success rate of oocyte retrieval procedure?

A. Size of aspiration needle

B. Endometrial receptivity

C. Serum progesterone level

D. Day of embryo transfer

E. Operator experience and technique

148- What is the best strategy if no oocytes are obtained despite adequate follicular aspiration?

A. Repeat trigger and reschedule retrieval

B. Rescue ICSI

C. Repeat aspiration immediately with flushing and lab recheck for oocytes

D. Cancel cycle

E. Convert to IUI

149- Which of the following is a late complication of oocyte retrieval?

A. OHSS

B. Vaginal laceration

C. Hemoperitoneum

D. Bowel perforation

E. Anesthetic reaction

150- Which structure is punctured first during transvaginal oocyte retrieval?

A. Ovarian capsule directly

B. Endometrial cavity

C. Fallopian tube

D. Vaginal wall then ovarian capsule

E. Cervix

151- A 28-year-old woman with previous pelvic surgery has ovaries that are adherent high in the pelvis and not accessible by vaginal ultrasound. What is the best retrieval approach?

A. Cancel the cycle

B. Proceed with transvaginal retrieval despite difficulty

C. Transabdominal ultrasound-guided follicular aspiration

D. Convert to IUI

E. Blind aspiration through uterine cavity

152- A 35-year-old patient undergoing oocyte retrieval has ovarian follicles located posterior to the uterus. Which approach ensures safe retrieval?

A. Transvaginal aspiration through posterior fornix

B. Transabdominal blind aspiration

C. Hysteroscopic retrieval

D. Laparotomy

E. No retrieval possible

153- Which of the following is a relative contraindication for transvaginal oocyte retrieval at the usual site?

A. Severe pelvic abscess

B. Tubal factor infertility

C. Endometriosis

D. Previous cesarean section

E. Irregular cycles

154- What type of suction pressure is usually applied during follicular aspiration?

A. 20–50 mmHg

B. 80–120 mmHg

C. 200–250 mmHg

D. 300–400 mmHg

E. No suction is applied

155- A 34-year-old woman with known endometriosis is undergoing oocyte retrieval. On ultrasound, a left ovarian endometrioma (4 cm) is seen. What is the best approach?

A. Aspirate the endometrioma to improve follicle access

B. Avoid puncturing the endometrioma and aspirate only follicles

C. Convert to laparoscopic retrieval

D. Cancel the cycle

E. Puncture both follicles and endometrioma together

156- During oocyte retrieval, the needle accidentally punctures an endometrioma. The follicular fluid appears brownish. What is the most important next step?

A. Stop procedure and cancel cycle

B. Continue aspiration, change the needle and give prophylactic antibiotics

C. Discard the contaminated oocytes immediately

D. Flush the ovary with normal saline

E. Switch to abdominal retrieval

157- In a patient with large endometriomas (> 5 cm) obstructing follicle access during IVF retrieval, what is the best long-term management before the next cycle?

A. Expectant management only

B. Always aspirate the endometrioma during retrieval

C. Suppress with clomiphene citrate

D. Surgical cystectomy before next IVF attempt

E. High-dose gonadotropin stimulation

158- What is the most common cause of empty follicle syndrome?

A. True ovarian resistance to hCG

B. Incorrect administration or timing of hCG trigger

C. Premature LH surge

D. Poor egg quality

E. Ovarian cyst rupture

159- Which of the following is considered "true" EFS?

A. Oocytes absent due to early retrieval before 34 hours post-trigger

B. Faulty injection technique of hCG

C. hCG vial expired

D. Delay in aspiration >40 hours post-trigger

E. No oocytes retrieved despite correct hCG administration and adequate timing

160- Which patient characteristic is more commonly associated with true EFS?

A. Young age with PCOS

B. Older age with poor ovarian reserve

C. High AMH

D. Obesity

E. Hypothyroidism

161- Which laboratory test can help differentiate false from true EFS on retrieval day?

A. Serum progesterone

B. Serum estradiol

C. Serum β-hCG level

D. Serum AMH

E. Serum FSH

162- A 29-year-old PCOS patient undergoes oocyte retrieval. Only follicular fluid is obtained despite >15 large follicles on ultrasound. Serum β-hCG on retrieval day is <5 mIU/ml. What is the most likely cause?

A. True EFS

B. False EFS due to failed hCG injection

C. Poor egg quality

D. Premature luteinization

E. Low AMH

163- A 42-year-old woman with very low AMH undergoes retrieval after correct hCG. No oocytes are obtained. β-hCG is >100 mIU/ml. What is the likely cause?

A. True EFS

B. False EFS

C. Poor technique

D. Premature LH surge

E. OHSS

164- A 30-year-old woman with normal ovarian reserve undergoes oocyte retrieval 36 hrs after hCG trigger. No oocytes are obtained. Serum β-hCG on retrieval day is < 5 mIU/ml. What is the most appropriate next step?

A. Repeat retrieval immediately without any change

B. Administer a "rescue" dose of hCG (or GnRH agonist) and reschedule retrieval 36 hrs later

C. Cancel the cycle completely

D. Switch to natural cycle IVF in the same attempt

E. Start luteal support as usual

165- A 37-year-old woman with bilateral hydrosalpinges has fluid in the uterine cavity after retrieval. What is the best long-term management

before the next IVF cycle?

A. Continue same stimulation protocol

B. Salpingectomy before next cycle

C. High-dose gonadotropins next cycle

D. Use donor embryos

E. Add antibiotics in luteal phase

166- A 31-year-old woman after oocyte retrieval develops fluid in the endometrial cavity due to intrauterine infection. What is the most likely consequence if fresh transfer is done?

A. Increased implantation rate

B. Higher chance of multiple pregnancy

C. Improved endometrial receptivity

D. Reduced OHSS risk

E. Higher risk of miscarriage and implantation failure

167- A 32-year-old woman undergoing IVF is noted to have intrauterine fluid on ultrasound at the time of oocyte retrieval. Repeat scan on day 5 (embryo transfer day) shows complete resolution of the fluid. What is the best management?

A. Cancel embryo transfer and freeze all embryos

B. Proceed with fresh embryo transfer as fluid has resolved

C. Aspirate the endometrial cavity before transfer

D. Start antibiotics and postpone transfer

E. Give GnRH agonist and cancel transfer

168- A 34-year-old woman undergoing IVF shows intrauterine fluid on ultrasound at oocyte retrieval. On day 5, before planned blastocyst transfer, the fluid is still present in the endometrial cavity. What is the best management?

A. Proceed with fresh embryo transfer despite the fluid

B. Aspirate the intrauterine fluid immediately before transfer

C. Cancel fresh transfer and freeze all embryos (freeze-all strategy)

D. Give luteal support and continue transfer

E. Perform hysteroscopy at the same time as transfer

169- A 31-year-old woman undergoing transvaginal oocyte retrieval suddenly develops hematuria after the procedure. What is the most likely complication?

A. Ureteric injury

B. Bladder injury from puncture needle

C. Vaginal wall tear

D. Renal trauma

E. Uterine perforation

170- A patient develops fever, suprapubic pain, and dysuria 48 hrs after oocyte retrieval. What is the most likely diagnosis?

A. Urinary tract infection secondary to bladder injury

B. Endometritis

C. OHSS

D. Vaginal infection

E. Ovarian cyst rupture

171- During oocyte retrieval, blood-stained urine appears in the Foley catheter bag. What should be the immediate next step?

A. Abort the procedure immediately

B. Catheterize the bladder and monitor urine output

C. Perform laparotomy

D. Ignore and proceed with embryo transfer

E. Start luteal phase support

172- Which factor increases the risk of bladder injury during oocyte retrieval?

A. Small ovaries close to uterine wall

B. Bilateral endometriomas

C. High ovaries located anteriorly behind bladder

D. PCOS with multiple follicles

E. Use of GnRH antagonist

173- A 34-year-old woman with severe endometriosis undergoes oocyte retrieval. 12 hours later, she develops abdominal pain, fever, and peritonitis. What is the most likely complication?

A. OHSS

B. Vaginal bleeding

C. Bowel perforation

D. Bladder injury

E. Endometritis

174- Which patient factor increases the risk of bowel injury during oocyte retrieval?

A. PCOS with multiple follicles

B. History of pelvic surgery with adhesions

C. High ovarian reserve

D. Use of antagonist protocol

E. Young age

175- A woman develops fever, abdominal distension, and diarrhea 24 hrs after oocyte retrieval. Which investigation is most useful to confirm bowel injury?

A. Ultrasound pelvis

B. Plain abdominal X-ray

C. CT abdomen with contrast

D. Serum β-hCG

E. Hysterosalpingogram

176- What is the immediate management if bowel perforation is suspected after oocyte retrieval?

A. Start luteal support and observe

B. Broad-spectrum IV antibiotics and urgent surgical consultation

C. Oral antibiotics only

D. Cancel embryo transfer only

E. Repeat ultrasound and continue stimulation

177- A 29-year-old woman develops mild vaginal spotting after oocyte retrieval. She is hemodynamically stable. What is the best next step?

A. Immediate laparotomy

B. Vaginal packing and observation

C. Broad-spectrum antibiotics

D. Cancel embryo transfer

E. Start anticoagulants

178- A 34-year-old patient develops moderate vaginal bleeding after retrieval, but vitals are stable. Which of the following is most appropriate?

A. Vaginal wall suturing or cauterization if bleeding point visible

B. Observation only

C. Exploratory laparotomy

D. Blood transfusion immediately

E. Start luteal support

179- Which factor most predisposes to vaginal bleeding during oocyte retrieval?

A. Use of antagonist protocol

B. Puncture of vaginal wall vessels by aspiration needle

C. Thin endometrium

D. Low AMH

E. Retroverted uterus

180- A 36-year-old woman presents with heavy vaginal bleeding 1 hr after retrieval, pulse 120 bpm, BP 80/50 mmHg. What is the immediate management?

A. Observation only

B. Start oral antibiotics

C. Delay intervention until next day

D. IV fluids + blood transfusion + surgical hemostasis

E. Administer progesterone support

181- Which of the following is NOT routinely required before oocyte retrieval in IVF?

A. CBC

B. Viral screening (HIV, HBsAg, HCV, VDRL)

C. Coagulation profile

D. Chest CT scan

E. Pelvic ultrasound

182- A 38-year-old woman scheduled for oocyte retrieval is on anticoagulation. Which pre-procedure test is mandatory?

A. Serum electrolytes

B. Coagulation profile (INR, aPTT)

C. Endometrial biopsy

D. Chest X-ray

E. DEXA scan

183- Before oocyte retrieval, what is the recommended timing of serum β-hCG testing?

A. 6 hrs after trigger

B. On the morning of retrieval (to confirm adequate trigger)

C. 48 hrs before trigger

D. 1 week before retrieval

E. Not required

184- What is the minimum serum β-hCG level required on the day of oocyte retrieval to ensure adequate trigger?

A. 10 IU/L

B. 20 IU/L

C. 40 IU/L

D. 80 IU/L

E. 150 IU/L

LUTEAL PHASE SUPPORT

185- What is the main reason luteal phase support is required in IVF cycles?

A. To prevent premature ovulation

B. To increase follicular growth

C. To reduce estradiol levels

D. To induce LH surge

E. Because ovarian stimulation and oocyte retrieval impair corpus luteum function

186- Which hormone is the cornerstone of luteal phase support in IVF?

A. Estradiol

B. GnRH agonist

C. FSH

D. LH

E. Progesterone

187- A 35-year-old woman undergoes fresh embryo transfer. When should luteal phase support be started?

A. On day 1 of stimulation

B. On day of trigger

C. On the day of retrieval or within 1–2 days after retrieval

D. On the day of pregnancy test

E. After luteal progesterone drop

188- Which route of progesterone administration is most commonly used in IVF luteal support?

A. Oral

B. Transdermal

C. Vaginal or intramuscular

D. Subcutaneous FSH

E. Sublingual

189- A 29-year-old woman with recurrent implantation failure asks about adding estrogen to luteal support. Which statement is correct?

A. Estrogen is never used in luteal support

B. Estrogen may be added with progesterone in some protocols to improve endometrial receptivity

C. Estrogen replaces progesterone fully

D. Estrogen is only given to PCOS patients

E. Estrogen is contraindicated with agonist protocols

190- For how long is luteal phase support typically continued after embryo transfer?

A. Until day 7 after transfer

B. Until pregnancy test (day 14)

C. Until 8–10 weeks of gestation if pregnancy occurs

D. Until delivery

E. Only 2 days post-transfer

191- A 28-year-old PCOS patient is a high responder, 22 oocytes retrieved, at risk of OHSS. Which luteal phase support should be avoided?

A. Vaginal progesterone

B. Intramuscular progesterone

C. Low-dose hCG injections

D. Vaginal micronized progesterone + estradiol

E. Subcutaneous progesterone

192- A 30-year-old woman with OHSS risk undergoes freeze-all strategy. What luteal phase support is needed in this cycle?

A. Standard progesterone and estrogen support

B. No luteal support is required if no fresh transfer is performed

C. High-dose hCG support

D. Only oral dydrogesterone

E. GnRH agonist injection

193- A 34-year-old patient has progesterone < 8 ng/ml on day of transfer despite luteal support. What is the appropriate action?

A. Cancel transfer

B. Add additional progesterone (IM or vaginal)

C. Switch to natural cycle

D. Give GnRH antagonist

E. Stop luteal support

194- A 27-year-old woman at high risk of OHSS underwent antagonist protocol and received a GnRH agonist trigger. Fresh embryo transfer is planned. Which of the following best describes the recommended intensive luteal phase support in this setting?

A. Strong LPS by Progesterone + estradiol

B. Vaginal progesterone alone is sufficient

C. High-dose hCG every 2 days for luteal support

D. No luteal support is required after agonist trigger

E. Oral dydrogesterone alone

195- A 33-year-old IVF patient refuses vaginal progesterone for luteal support. What is the best alternative option?

A. Oral dydrogesterone

B. No luteal support is needed

C. Only estradiol tablets

D. Clomiphene citrate

E. Bromocriptine

196- What is the typical dose of progesterone and oral dydrogesterone for luteal support in IVF cycles?

A. Progesterone 50–100 mg IM daily; Dydrogesterone 10 mg twice daily

B. Progesterone 10 mg IM weekly; Dydrogesterone 5 mg once daily

C. Progesterone 400 mg IM daily; Dydrogesterone 40 mg once weekly

D. Progesterone 1000 mg IM daily; Dydrogesterone 20 mg once daily

E. Progesterone not required; Dydrogesterone 2.5 mg once daily

197- Which of the following is NOT an advantage of dydrogesterone compared to vaginal progesterone?

A. Oral route, patient-friendly

B. Better compliance

C. No local vaginal irritation

D. Always superior pregnancy rates in all patients

E. Can be combined with estradiol if needed

EMBRYO TRANSFER

198- What is the preferred route for embryo transfer?

A. Transabdominal

B. Transcervical under ultrasound guidance

C. Transmyometrial

D. Hysteroscopic transfer

E. Laparoscopic transfer

199- What is the optimal day for blastocyst transfer in IVF cycles?

A. Day 1

B. Day 2

C. Day 3

D. Day 5

E. Day 7

200- What is the Minimum endometrial thickness for embryo transfer?

A. 5 mm

B. 6 mm

C. 8 mm

D. 10 mm

E. Thickness does not matter

201- Which catheter is preferred for embryo transfer?

A. Sharp metallic catheter

B. Soft flexible catheter

C. Rigid plastic catheter

D. Foley's catheter

E. Uterine sound

202- Which is TRUE regarding embryo transfer?

A. Antibiotic prophylaxis is always required

B. Embryos should be placed 1.5 cm from fundal endometrium

C. Sharp rigid catheter increases implantation

D. Ultrasound is not necessary

E. Thick endometrium >14 mm is mandatory

203- What is the most common complication of embryo transfer?

A. OHSS

B. Infection

C. Multiple pregnancy

D. Endometrial perforation

E. Cervical trauma

204- A 32-year-old woman scheduled for embryo transfer is found to have endometrial thickness of 5 mm on the day of transfer. What is the best management?

A. Proceed with fresh transfer

B. Freeze all embryos and prepare endometrium in a subsequent cycle

C. Add hCG injection and proceed

D. Repeat endometrial scratching

E. Cancel stimulation permanently

205- During embryo transfer, the catheter repeatedly fails to pass through a stenotic cervix. What is the best strategy?

A. Cancel embryo transfer immediately

B. Use force to pass catheter through cervix

C. Perform a mock transfer or cervical dilatation before actual transfer

D. Switch to trans-myometrial transfer without attempt

E. Push catheter into fundus to ensure entry

206- A 35-year-old woman undergoing embryo transfer has intrauterine fluid noted in the cavity at the time of transfer. What is the best step?

A. Proceed with fresh embryo transfer

B. Aspirate fluid and continue transfer

C. Cancel fresh transfer and freeze all embryos

D. Administer antibiotics and transfer embryos

E. Continue luteal support and transfer as planned

207- A 28-year-old IVF patient has an embryo transfer planned. Which measure improves pregnancy rates during ET?

A. Empty bladder during procedure

B. Full bladder with ultrasound guidance

C. Transfer under general anesthesia

D. Using rigid catheter

E. Performing blind transfer

208- A 29-year-old woman undergoing her first IVF cycle with good prognosis asks how many embryos should be transferred. According to guidelines, what is the safest option?

A. 1 embryo (single ET)

B. 2 embryos

C. 3 embryos

D. 4 embryos

E. 5 embryos

209- A 40-year-old woman with multiple failed IVF attempts requests more embryos to be transferred. What is the maximum recommended number of embryos in women ≥ 40 years?

A. 1 embryo

B. 2 embryos

C. 3 embryos

D. 4 embryos

E. Unlimited

210- During embryo transfer, blood is noted on the catheter tip after withdrawal. What does this indicate?

A. Successful implantation

B. Cervical or endometrial trauma, may reduce implantation rate

C. Ovarian injury

D. Multiple gestation likelihood

E. Increased receptivity

211- A 35-year-old patient after embryo transfer develops severe abdominal distension, dyspnea, and hemoconcentration. What is the likely complication?

A. Pelvic infection

B. Ovarian hyperstimulation syndrome (OHSS)

C. Endometrial perforation

D. Bowel perforation

E. Bladder trauma

212- A 31-year-old woman undergoes ET. Two weeks later, β-hCG is 1500 but no intrauterine sac is visible on TVUS. What complication should be suspected?

A. Normal delayed implantation

B. Ectopic pregnancy

C. OHSS

D. Cervical trauma

E. Empty follicle syndrome

213- A 28-year-old woman had 3 cleavage-stage embryos transferred. She later develops triplet pregnancy. What is the main clinical concern?

A. High risk of miscarriage, prematurity, and maternal complications

B. Better success rate

C. Higher endometrial receptivity

D. Lower cost of IVF

E. Reduced implantation risk

214- Day 3 embryo transfer refers to:

A. Transfer of zygotes

B. Transfer of cleavage-stage embryos

C. Transfer of blastocysts

D. Transfer of morula

E. Transfer of gametes

215- Day 5 embryo transfer corresponds to which developmental stage?

A. Oocyte

B. Zygote

C. Cleavage embryo

D. Blastocyst

E. Morula

216- Which of the following describes "sequential embryo transfer"?

A. Transfer of gametes into fallopian tube

B. Transfer of cleavage-stage embryo followed by blastocyst in same cycle

C. Transfer of frozen embryos only

D. Transfer of zygote and gametes together

E. Two transfers in two consecutive cycles

217- Which of the following is an example of a soft embryo transfer catheter?

A. Wallace catheter

B. Tomcat catheter

C. Cook K-jet catheter

D. Both A and C

E. Foley's catheter

218- What is the main advantage of soft embryo transfer catheters compared to rigid catheters?

A. Easier to visualize under X-ray

B. Cheaper and reusable

C. Always requires cervical dilatation

D. Allows faster transfer

E. Less traumatic to endometrium and higher implantation rates

219- Which type of catheter may be used in cases of difficult embryo transfer with cervical stenosis?

A. Wallace soft catheter

B. Tomcat rigid catheter

C. Foley's catheter

D. Urinary catheter

E. Pediatric feeding tube

220- Which embryo transfer catheter is commonly described as a "two-step" system (outer sheath + inner soft catheter)?

A. Tomcat catheter

B. Frydman catheter

C. Labotect catheter

D. Wallace catheter

221- Which catheter design improves ease of negotiation through cervix but may increase trauma risk?

A. Curved rigid catheter

B. Straight rigid catheter

C. Soft flexible catheter

D. Metallic catheter

E. Balloon catheter

222- What is the recommended bladder status during embryo transfer?

A. Empty bladder

B. Overfilled bladder

C. Moderately full bladder

D. No relation to bladder filling

E. Catheterized bladder

223- When should the embryo be released from the catheter during ET?

A. Immediately after entering cervix

B. In lower uterine segment

C. At target site under US guidance with slow release

D. At external cervical os

E. Anywhere in uterine cavity, no difference

224- Which factor has the greatest impact on ET success rates?

A. Type of catheter used

B. Experience and skill of the operator

C. Embryo stage only

D. Bladder filling

E. Anesthesia used

225- What should be checked after withdrawing the catheter?

A. Presence of blood only

B. Presence of mucus only

C. Presence of retained embryos in catheter tip

D. Nothing is required

E. Endometrial thickness

226- Which of the following is NOT part of proper embryo transfer technique?

A. Use of ultrasound guidance

B. Full or moderately full bladder

C. Gentle passage of soft catheter

D. Checking catheter for retained embryos

E. Performing sharp cervical dilatation routinely

227- A 33-year-old woman undergoes embryo transfer. The catheter meets resistance at the internal os and force is applied. Later, blood is seen on the catheter tip and no pregnancy occurs. What is the most likely cause of failure?

A. Endometrial thinness

B. Traumatic transfer with bleeding

C. Poor embryo quality

D. OHSS

E. Multiple embryo transfer

228- A 29-year-old woman has an embryo transfer. Ultrasound shows embryos deposited very close (<0.5 cm) to the fundal endometrium. Pregnancy test is negative. What is the most likely cause of failed transfer?

A. Embryos expelled from cavity

B. Endometrial receptivity issue

C. Improper deposition site (too fundal, possible trauma)

D. Cervical stenosis

E. Poor luteal support

229- A 37-year-old woman with endometrium measuring 5 mm undergoes ET. Embryos fail to implant. What is the most likely cause of failed transfer?

A. Poor ovarian stimulation

B. Thin endometrium (<7 mm)

C. Operator error

D. Multiple embryo transfer

E. OHSS

230- A 31-year-old woman with history of multiple failed transfers is found to have chronic endometritis on hysteroscopy. What is the most likely cause of failure?

A. Technical difficulty in transfer

B. Poor ovarian reserve

C. High progesterone level

D. Endometrial receptivity problem due to inflammation

E. Operator inexperience

231- A 30-year-old woman with hydrosalpinx is planned for IVF. Which preventive measure improves implantation rates before embryo transfer?

A. Immediate embryo transfer without intervention

B. Salpingectomy before IVF

C. Endometrial scratching during stimulation

D. High-dose luteal progesterone only

E. Antibiotics before oocyte retrieval

232- A 36-year-old woman with recurrent implantation failure undergoes evaluation. Endometrial receptivity analysis (ERA) shows displaced window of implantation. What preventive strategy can improve outcome in next transfer?

A. Change stimulation protocol only

B. Perform personalized embryo transfer (pET) according to ERA result

C. Always transfer more embryos

D. Add low-dose aspirin

E. Routine hysteroscopy before every transfer

233- During ET, blood and mucus were repeatedly found on catheter tip in a previous failed attempt. Which preventive measure reduces this risk?

A. Avoid mock transfer

B. Gentle cervical cleaning before catheter insertion

C. Use of sharp rigid catheter

D. Immediate embryo release at cervix

E. No ultrasound guidance

234- A 40-year-old woman with recurrent failed transfers is found to have thin endometrium (5 mm). Which preventive strategy should be applied?

A. Proceed with fresh ET

B. Always transfer >3 embryos to increase chance

C. Ignore endometrial thickness if embryo quality is high

D. Use rigid catheter

E. Freeze embryos and optimize endometrium in subsequent cycle

235- What is the main advantage of Day 5 (blastocyst) transfer compared to Day 3 transfer?

A. Reduced implantation rates

B. Reduced lab culture time

C. Always eliminates multiple pregnancy

D. Lower embryo quality

E. Higher synchronization with endometrium and better selection of viable embryos

236- In which situation might Day 3 embryo transfer be considered instead of Day 5?

A. When many embryos of excellent quality are available

B. When few embryos are available and concern exists about extended culture survival

C. When OHSS risk is high

D. When endometrium is thin

E. Always in first IVF attempt

237- Which factor is most important in determining the optimal day of embryo transfer?

A. Patient age alone

B. Ovarian stimulation protocol

C. Embryo developmental stage and quality

D. Number of previous IVF attempts

E. Use of donor sperm

238- What is the advantage of Frozen Blastocyst Transfer compared to Fresh Blastocyst Transfer in high responders?

A. Lower implantation rates

B. Reduced risk of OHSS and better endometrial receptivity

C. Always requires donor uterus

D. Avoids need for luteal phase support

E. Eliminates embryo selection

239- A 30-year-old woman undergoes Day 5 blastocyst transfer. She asks whether strict bed rest after the procedure will improve her chances of pregnancy. What should she be advised?

A. Strict bed rest for 48 hours significantly increases pregnancy rates

B. 24 hours of complete bed rest is mandatory

C. Normal daily activity can be resumed; prolonged bed rest does not improve outcomes

D. Hospital admission for observation is recommended

E. Avoid all physical activity for 2 weeks

240- A 32-year-old woman undergoes embryo transfer and asks if sexual intercourse during the luteal phase improves implantation chances. What is the most appropriate advice?

A. Intercourse after ET improves implantation and is recommended routinely

B. Intercourse after ET reduces implantation rates due to uterine contractions

C. Intercourse after ET has no proven effect and is completely unrestricted

D. Intercourse should be strictly avoided for 3 months after ET

E. Intercourse is mandatory on day of transfer to improve outcome

241- A 29-year-old woman has undergone Day 5 blastocyst transfer. She asks when she can safely resume sexual intercourse. What is the most appropriate advice?

A. Immediately after embryo transfer with no restriction

B. Avoid intercourse for the entire first trimester

C. Resume only after fetal cardiac activity is confirmed

D. Intercourse is contraindicated after IVF in all cases

E. Avoid until pregnancy test result (≈ 2 weeks after ET)

242- A 31-year-old woman underwent Day 5 embryo transfer and asks if she can continue her daily gym workouts with moderate-intensity exercise. What is the most appropriate advice?

A. Strenuous exercise should be avoided; light to moderate activity is acceptable

B. Stop all exercise until delivery

C. Exercise has no effect and can be continued at any intensity

D. Exercise is contraindicated until luteal phase support is stopped

E. Exercise improves implantation and should be increased

243- A 34-year-old IVF patient had blastocyst transfer yesterday and is planning a long car trip (5 hours). What should you advise?

A. Travel is strictly contraindicated after ET

B. She may travel with normal precautions, as it does not reduce success

C. Travel is only safe after positive pregnancy test

D. She should remain on bed rest for 1 week before traveling

E. Air travel only is allowed, not car travel

244- A 30-year-old woman after embryo transfer asks about drinking coffee. What is the best advice?

A. Caffeine should be completely eliminated

B. Coffee improves implantation and should be encouraged

C. Caffeine should be stopped until luteal support is completed

D. Moderate caffeine intake (<200 mg/day, ~1–2 cups coffee) is acceptable

E. Tea is allowed but coffee is not

245- All of the following interventions are proven to improve pregnancy rates after embryo transfer EXCEPT:

A. Abdominal ultrasound guidance

B. Use of soft embryo transfer catheters

C. Removal of cervical mucus

D. Acupuncture during transfer

E. Correct placement of catheter tip 1.5–2 cm from fundus

246- Which of the following about embryo transfer is NOT true?

A. Full bladder improves visualization during ultrasound-guided transfer

B. Blood on catheter tip may reduce implantation rates

C. Embryo should be deposited at cervical os to avoid trauma

D. Operator's skill is a major determinant of success

E. Immediate ambulation after ET does not reduce pregnancy rates

247- A 32-year-old woman undergoes IVF. She asks about the expected pregnancy success rates depending on embryo transfer strategy. Which statement is most accurate?

A. Day 3 cleavage-stage transfer generally has higher success than Day 5 blastocyst transfer

B. Day 5 blastocyst transfer often shows higher implantation and live birth rates compared to Day 3 transfer

C. Fresh embryo transfer always has better success than frozen embryo transfer in all patients

D. Frozen embryo transfer may be more successful than fresh transfer in high responders or OHSS risk patients

E. Both B and D are correct

FROZEN EMBRYO TRANSFER

248- Which of the following about frozen embryo transfer is TRUE?

A. FET can only be done in stimulated cycles

B. FET is always inferior to fresh ET in live birth rates

C. FET can be performed in natural or hormonally prepared cycles

D. FET requires laparoscopic guidance

E. FET is contraindicated in high responders

249- All of the following are advantages of frozen embryo transfer EXCEPT:

A. Allows time for endometrial recovery and optimization

B. Reduces risk of OHSS by avoiding fresh transfer in high responders

C. Enables embryo banking for future attempts

D. Always guarantees higher implantation rate compared to fresh transfer

E. Permits preimplantation genetic testing before transfer

250- Which of the following is NOT true regarding the timing of FET?

A. In natural cycles, transfer is timed to spontaneous ovulation

B. In artificial cycles, endometrium is prepared with estrogen and progesterone

C. Blastocyst FET is performed 5 days after ovulation/progesterone start

D. Cleavage-stage FET is performed 7 days after progesterone start

E. Synchronization between endometrium and embryo stage is crucial

251- All of the following are FALSE regarding outcomes of frozen embryo transfer EXCEPT:

A. FET is associated with lower implantation rates in PCOS

B. FET is associated with reduced OHSS risk

C. FET cannot result in live birth if embryos are vitrified

D. FET is contraindicated after previous cesarean section

E. FET requires general anesthesia

252- Which of the following is TRUE about natural cycle frozen embryo transfer?

A. Requires exogenous estrogen and progesterone throughout

B. Relies on spontaneous ovulation and endogenous hormones

C. Not suitable for ovulatory women

D. Always superior to hormone replacement cycles in all patients

E. Requires daily GnRH agonist injections

253- In hormone replacement cycles for FET, endometrial preparation typically includes:

A. Estrogen followed by progesterone supplementation

B. FSH stimulation alone

C. GnRH agonist trigger and no hormones

D. LH injections only

E. Prolactin supplementation

254- Modified natural cycle FET differs from true natural cycle in that:

A. Requires high-dose gonadotropins

B. Uses estrogen and progesterone from day 1

C. Always needs surgical intervention

D. Embryos are transferred without regard to ovulation

E. Ovulation is triggered with hCG

255- Hormone replacement cycles for FET are particularly useful in:

A. Women with regular cycles

B. Women with anovulation or irregular cycles

C. Women with OHSS risk

D. All patients regardless of cycle status

E. Only in women >40 years

256- The most critical factor in timing frozen embryo transfer is:

A. Endometrial thickness >5 mm

B. Synchronization between progesterone exposure and embryo developmental stage

C. Number of embryos available

D. Presence of corpus luteum

E. Estradiol peak level

257- A 36-year-old professional requires flexible timing for embryo transfer due to work constraints. Which FET protocol provides the most control over scheduling?

A. Natural cycle

B. Modified natural cycle only

C. Hormone replacement cycle (HRT-FET)

D. Minimal stimulation cycle

E. Fresh transfer

258- A 28-year-old woman with short follicular phase has unpredictable premature LH surges. Which protocol minimizes this problem?

A. Natural cycle FET

B. Modified natural cycle with hCG trigger

C. No luteal support

D. Fresh embryo transfer only

E. FET without monitoring

259- A 34-year-old woman undergoing FET is found to have a thin endometrium (<6 mm) in a natural cycle. What is the best option?

A. Proceed with natural cycle transfer

B. Ignore endometrial thickness if embryo quality is good

C. Use clomiphene citrate stimulation

D. Switch to hormone replacement cycle with high-dose estrogen to optimize lining

E. Perform immediate transfer and add aspirin

260- A 27-year-old woman is a high responder with 30 oocytes retrieved. Embryos are frozen to avoid OHSS. Which FET protocol is most flexible for subsequent safe transfer?

A. Natural cycle only

B. Hormone replacement cycle

C. Modified natural cycle

D. Either natural or HRT depending on cycle pattern

E. No transfer is recommended

261- Which of the following is NOT true regarding hormone replacement cycle (HRT-FET)?

A. Endometrium is prepared with estrogen followed by progesterone

B. Useful in women with anovulation or irregular cycles

C. Provides flexibility in scheduling transfer

D. Always requires corpus luteum formation

E. Can be combined with GnRH agonist pretreatment

262- Which of the following statements about FET is FALSE?

A. Synchronization of endometrium and embryo stage is critical for success

B. HRT-FET is the method of choice for women with PCOS and irregular cycles

C. Natural cycle FET is possible in women with regular ovulation

D. Blastocyst transfer in FET is usually done 5 days after starting progesterone

E. Endometrial preparation is unnecessary in all cases

263- A 34-year-old IVF patient has serum progesterone >1.5 ng/ml on the day of trigger. Which of the following is FALSE?

A. This may reduce endometrial receptivity in a fresh transfer

B. Freeze-all strategy with subsequent FET is recommended

C. FET allows correction of endometrial asynchrony

D. Proceeding with fresh transfer improves implantation rates

E. Blastocysts can be vitrified and transferred later

264- A 29-year-old woman is undergoing HRT-FET. Which of the following is NOT true about timing?

A. Cleavage-stage embryos are usually transferred on Day 3 after progesterone start

B. Blastocysts are usually transferred on Day 5 after progesterone start

C. Synchronization of progesterone exposure with embryo stage is essential

D. Estradiol dose adjustment before progesterone start can optimize lining

E. The timing of transfer does not matter once endometrium is thick enough

265- Which of the following serum progesterone levels on the day of trigger or before embryo transfer is associated with reduced implantation rates in fresh IVF cycles?

A. <0.5 ng/mL

B. 0.5–1.0 ng/mL

C. >1.5 ng/mL

D. 2.5–3.0 ng/mL always optimal

E. Progesterone level has no impact

266- In frozen embryo transfer (HRT-FET), what is the recommended minimum serum progesterone level on the day before transfer to ensure endometrial receptivity?

A. ≥2 ng/mL

B. ≥5 ng/mL

C. ≥15 ng/ml

D. No threshold required

E. ≥8–10 ng/Ml

Preimplantation Genetic Testing (PGT) & Genetics)

267- Which of the following is the main indication for sex selection using preimplantation genetic diagnosis (PGD/PGT)?

A. To increase implantation rate in IVF

B. To prevent transmission of X-linked genetic disorders

C. To improve endometrial receptivity

D. To enhance ovarian stimulation response

E. To reduce multiple pregnancy

268- At what embryonic stage is biopsy most commonly performed for preimplantation genetic testing (PGT)?

A. Oocyte before fertilization

B. Zygote (Day 1)

C. Cleavage-stage embryo (Day 3, blastomere biopsy) or blastocyst (Day 5, trophectoderm biopsy)

D. During implantation

E. After fetal heartbeat detection

269- Sex selection for non-medical (social) reasons is generally considered:

A. Universally accepted and recommended

B. Mandatory in all IVF cycles

C. More effective than sperm sorting

D. Banned or restricted in many countries due to ethical concerns

E. Without any ethical issues

270- Which of the following is NOT a valid medical indication for preimplantation genetic diagnosis?

A. Carrier of X-linked recessive disease

B. Couples at risk of chromosomal translocations

C. Recurrent pregnancy loss due to genetic abnormality

D. Maternal age >40 without genetic disease

E. Autosomal recessive disorder risk in couple

271- All of the following are advantages of PGD/PGT EXCEPT:

A. Avoids transmission of severe genetic diseases

B. Reduces miscarriage rates in some couples

C. Allows elective single embryo transfer with euploid embryos

D. Can be combined with IVF/ICSI protocols

E. Guarantees 100% healthy live birth without need for prenatal testing

272- All of the following statements about sex selection via PGD are TRUE EXCEPT:

A. Used to prevent X-linked disease inheritance

B. Can be performed by FISH, PCR, or NGS methods

C. Social sex selection is ethically debated

D. Increases ovarian response and oocyte yield

E. Usually requires IVF/ICSI for embryo biopsy

273- A couple has a family history of Duchenne Muscular Dystrophy (X-linked recessive). They request IVF. What is the best strategy to prevent disease transmission?

A. Fresh embryo transfer without testing

B. PGD with sex selection to transfer only female embryos

C. IUI with donor sperm

D. Prenatal amniocentesis only

E. High-dose progesterone support

274- A 35-year-old woman with three consecutive miscarriages is found to have a balanced translocation. What is the role of PGD/PGT in this case?

A. No benefit, since translocations cannot be detected

B. Only sperm sorting is indicated

C. PGT-SR (structural rearrangement) to identify normal/balanced embryos before transfer

D. Fresh transfer without testing

E. Embryo freezing without biopsy

275- A 40-year-old woman undergoing IVF requests information about improving live birth rate. Which of the following is most useful?

A. PGD/PGT-A (aneuploidy screening) to select euploid embryos

B. Routine fresh transfer of all embryos

C. Acupuncture before transfer

D. Sperm DNA fragmentation test

E. Increased luteal support only

276- A couple are both carriers of β-thalassemia. What is the best reproductive option?

A. IVF with PGD/PGT-M to detect unaffected embryos

B. Fresh transfer without testing

C. Only sperm sorting

D. Prenatal diagnosis after conception

E. Adoption is the only option

277- All of the following are true regarding Preimplantation Genetic Testing for Monogenic disorders (PGT-M) EXCEPT:

A. Used for single-gene disorders such as β-thalassemia, cystic fibrosis

B. Requires family-specific genetic probe/testing

C. Can help in avoiding X-linked disorders

D. Detects embryo aneuploidy universally in all chromosomes

E. Usually performed with IVF/ICSI cycles

278- All of the following are true regarding Preimplantation Genetic Testing for Structural Rearrangements (PGT-SR) EXCEPT:

A. Used for balanced or unbalanced chromosomal translocations

B. Can reduce recurrent pregnancy loss due to chromosomal abnormalities

C. Detects gene mutations like cystic fibrosis and sickle cell anemia

D. Requires IVF/ICSI for embryo biopsy

E. Aims to select embryos with normal/balanced karyotype

279- Which of the following statements is FALSE regarding PGT?

A. PGT requires embryo biopsy at cleavage or blastocyst stage

B. IVF/ICSI is required to obtain embryos for testing

C. PGT completely eliminates the risk of affected child, so prenatal testing is unnecessary

D. Different types exist: PGT-M, PGT-A, PGT-SR

E. Can be combined with cryopreservation and FET strategies

280- All of the following are appropriate indications for PGT EXCEPT:

A. Couples carrying single-gene mutations (PGT-M)

B. Carriers of chromosomal translocations (PGT-SR)

C. Women with advanced maternal age or RIF (PGT-A)

D. Social sex selection in healthy couples with no genetic disease

E. Recurrent miscarriage due to genetic cause

281- A 28-year-old couple are both carriers of cystic fibrosis (autosomal recessive). Which PGT is most appropriate?

A. PGT-A

B. PGT-M

C. PGT-SR

D. No PGT is indicated

E. Only sperm sorting

282- A couple have a balanced translocation on karyotype. Which PGT method is indicated?

A. PGT-A

B. PGT-M

C. PGT-SR

D. No testing needed

E. Fresh transfer only

283- A 41-year-old woman with repeated IVF failures asks about improving her chance of live birth. Which type of PGT is most appropriate?

A. PGT-M

B. PGT-A

C. PGT-SR

D. None; only donor oocytes are possible

E. Social sex selection

284- All of the following scenarios are correct indications for PGT-SR EXCEPT:

A. Balanced translocation carrier

B. Inversions or structural chromosomal rearrangements

C. Robertsonian translocation

D. Single-gene mutation like sickle cell anemia

E. Recurrent miscarriage due to parental chromosomal abnormality

285- Which of the following Y-chromosome microdeletions is most commonly associated with severe oligospermia or azoospermia?

A. AZFa

B. AZFb

C. AZFc

D. SRY mutation

E. CFTR mutation

286- A 26-year-old man presents with azoospermia, small firm testes, gynecomastia, and elevated FSH. Karyotype shows 47,XXY. What is the diagnosis?

A. Kallmann syndrome

B. Klinefelter syndrome

C. Turner syndrome

D. Y-chromosome deletion

E. Androgen insensitivity

287- Which of the following female genetic abnormalities is associated with premature ovarian insufficiency (POI)?

A. 45,X (Turner syndrome)

B. FMR1 premutation (Fragile X)

C. 47,XXX

D. AZFc microdeletion

E. SRY translocation

288- A 17-year-old girl with primary amenorrhea and short stature is found to have streak ovaries. Karyotype is 45, X. What is the underlying cause of infertility?

A. Androgen insensitivity

B. Y chromosome microdeletion

C. CFTR mutation

D. Turner syndrome

E. Pituitary adenoma

289- What proportion of embryos from women ≥40 years are expected to be aneuploid?

A. ~10%

B. ~25%

C. ~50%

D. >70%

E. None

290- The main role of Preimplantation Genetic Testing for Aneuploidy (PGT-A) is to:

A. Detect single-gene disorders

B. Detect chromosomal structural rearrangements

C. Select euploid embryos to reduce miscarriage and improve implantation

D. Increase ovarian response

E. Enhance endometrial receptivity

291- All of the following are consequences of embryonic aneuploidy EXCEPT:

A. Implantation failure

B. Early miscarriage

C. Congenital malformation syndromes (e.g., Down syndrome)

D. Increased risk of OHSS

E. Reduced live birth rates

292- A 39-year-old woman has undergone multiple IVF cycles with good-quality embryos but recurrent implantation failure. Karyotyping is normal. What is the most likely cause?

A. Embryonic aneuploidy due to advanced maternal age

B. Endometrial polyp

C. Cervical stenosis

D. Technical error during transfer

E. Hydrosalpinx

293-All of the following statements about aneuploidy are TRUE EXCEPT:

A. The most common mechanism is meiotic nondisjunction

B. Aneuploidy risk increases with maternal age

C. PGT-A guarantees a healthy baby without need for prenatal testing

D. Aneuploidy is the leading cause of first-trimester miscarriage

E. Aneuploidy can occur in both oocytes and sperm

294- Which of the following is the most common chromosomal aneuploidy compatible with live birth?

A. Trisomy 13 (Patau)

B. Trisomy 18 (Edwards)

C. Trisomy 21 (Down syndrome)

D. Turner syndrome (45,X)

E. Triploidy

295- The incidence of both Down syndrome and Edwards syndrome increases with:

A. Paternal age

B. Maternal age

C. Stimulation protocol used in IVF

D. Number of embryos transferred

E. Endometrial thickness

296- Which of the following is TRUE regarding Edwards syndrome (Trisomy 18)?

A. It is more common than Down syndrome

B. Most affected fetuses die in utero or within the first year of life

C. Associated with high survival into adulthood

D. Strongly linked to paternal age only

E. It improves fertility potential in females

297- Which of the following is used for prenatal detection of trisomies like Down and Edwards?

A. Serum markers and nuchal translucency in first trimester

B. Semen analysis

C. Hysterosalpingogram

D. Laparoscopy

E. Embryo grading only

298- All of the following are TRUE regarding Down and Edwards syndromes EXCEPT:

A. Both are caused by nondisjunction events

B. Both are associated with increased maternal age

C. Down syndrome is the most common trisomy at live birth

D. Edwards syndrome has better long-term survival than Down syndrome

E. PGT-A can help in preventing transfer of affected embryos in IVF

299- Which genetic study is indicated in couples with recurrent pregnancy loss?

A. Parental karyotype to detect translocations

B. FMR1 testing

C. CFTR mutation screening

D. PGT-A only

E. Endometrial biopsy

300- All of the following genetic studies are useful in infertility EXCEPT:

A. Karyotyping in azoospermia or recurrent pregnancy loss

B. Y-chromosome microdeletion analysis in severe male factor infertility

C. CFTR mutation analysis in men with CBAVD

D. FMR1 premutation testing in women with POI

E. ABO blood group typing in recurrent implantation failure

301- All of the following are correct indications for PGT-SR EXCEPT:

A. Balanced Robertsonian translocation carrier

B. Inversions or structural chromosomal rearrangements

C. Recurrent pregnancy loss due to structural abnormality

D. Single-gene disorder like cystic fibrosis

E. Reciprocal translocation carrier

302- NGS (Next Generation Sequencing) in IVF is mainly used for:

A. Detecting sperm motility disorders

B. Comprehensive chromosome screening (PGT-A, PGT-M, PGT-SR)

C. Endometrial thickness assessment

D. Follicular growth monitoring

E. Oocyte retrieval guidance

303- A 40-year-old woman undergoing IVF requests the best method to select chromosomally normal embryos. Which genetic testing method is most appropriate?

A. FISH limited to a few chromosomes

B. Karyotyping only

C. NGS-based PGT-A

D. Hysteroscopy

E. AMH testing

304- A couple are carriers of β-thalassemia and undergo IVF. Which advanced technology can detect single-gene mutations at embryo stage?

A. NGS-based PGT-M

B. Endometrial receptivity analysis (ERA)

C. FISH

D. AMH assay

E. HSG

305- All of the following are correct about NGS in IVF EXCEPT:

A. It can detect aneuploidy across all 24 chromosomes

B. It is more comprehensive than FISH and array-CGH

C. It may be applied for PGT-M (monogenic) and PGT-SR (structural)

D. It completely eliminates the need for prenatal genetic testing

E. It can analyze multiple embryos at the same time

306- A 39-year-old woman undergoes IVF. The lab offers FISH to test embryos for aneuploidy. Which limitation should be explained?

A. FISH can only analyze a limited number of chromosomes

B. FISH is superior to NGS in detecting mosaicism

C. FISH detects all chromosomal abnormalities

D. FISH is cheaper but guarantees live birth

E. FISH is the gold standard for all PGT

307- A couple with recurrent pregnancy loss undergoes array-CGH on embryos. Which is TRUE about array-CGH compared to FISH?

A. Detects only 5–10 chromosomes like FISH

B. Detects aneuploidy across all 24 chromosomes

C. Cannot be used for embryos

D. Less accurate than ultrasound in detecting aneuploidy

E. Completely replaces NGS in modern practice

308- A 41-year-old IVF patient asks for the most comprehensive test for embryo aneuploidy and mosaicism detection. Which method is best?

A. FISH

B. Array-CGH

C. Karyotype

D. NGS

E. HSG

309- A couple with a balanced translocation is planning IVF. Which method is MOST appropriate for embryo testing today?

A. FISH only

B. Array-CGH only

C. NGS-based PGT-SR

D. ERA test

E. AMH level

ANSWERS

1	B	36	A
2	E	37	B
3	C	38	C
4	B	39	C
5	C	40	B
6	B	41	C
7	D	42	E
8	C	43	C
9	B	44	E
10	A	45	C
11	E	46	C
12	D	47	A
13	C	48	B
14	B	49	D
15	B	50	B
16	A	51	A
17	C	52	C
18	B	53	B
19	B	54	C
20	B	55	E
21	E	56	B
22	D	57	B
23	B	58	D
24	A	59	B
25	C	60	E
26	B	61	B
27	B	62	C
28	E	63	B
29	B	64	B
30	D	65	E
31	E	66	C
32	A	67	B
33	B	68	B
34	D	69	C
35	B	70	A

71	D	106	A
72	B	107	B
73	B	108	B
74	E	109	E
75	B	110	A
76	B	111	B
77	C	112	B
78	B	113	E
79	E	114	A
80	B	115	B
81	C	116	B
82	D	117	C
83	C	118	C
84	C	119	B
85	B	120	D
86	E	121	C
87	A	122	C
88	B	123	B
89	B	124	B
90	D	125	E
91	A	126	A
92	B	127	C
93	B	128	E
94	C	129	C
95	B	130	D
96	E	131	B
97	C	132	A
98	A	133	C
99	B	134	A
100	C	135	C
101	B	136	B
102	C	137	D
103	B	138	C
104	A	139	A
105	B	140	B

141	B	176	B
142	B	177	B
143	D	178	A
144	C	179	B
145	C	180	D
146	C	181	D
147	E	182	B
148	C	183	B
149	A	184	C
150	D	185	E
151	C	186	E
152	A	187	C
153	A	188	C
154	B	189	B
155	B	190	C
156	B	191	C
157	D	192	B
158	B	193	B
159	E	194	A
160	B	195	A
161	C	196	A
162	B	197	D
163	A	198	B
164	B	199	D
165	B	200	C
166	E	201	B
167	B	202	B
168	C	203	C
169	B	204	B
170	A	205	C
171	B	206	C
172	C	207	B
173	C	208	A
174	B	209	C
175	C	210	B

211	B	246	C
212	B	247	E
213	A	248	C
214	B	249	D
215	D	250	D
216	B	251	B
217	D	252	B
218	E	253	A
219	B	254	E
220	D	255	B
221	A	256	B
222	C	257	C
223	C	258	B
224	B	259	D
225	C	260	B
226	E	261	D
227	B	262	E
228	C	263	D
229	B	264	E
230	D	265	C
231	B	266	E
232	B	267	B
233	B	268	C
234	E	269	D
235	E	270	D
236	B	271	E
237	C	272	D
238	B	273	B
239	C	274	C
240	B	275	A
241	E	276	A
242	A	277	D
243	B	278	C
244	D	279	C
245	D	280	D

281	B
282	C
283	B
284	D
285	C
286	B
287	B
288	D
289	D
290	C
291	D
292	A
293	C
294	C
295	B
296	B
297	A
298	D
299	A
300	E
301	D
302	B
303	C
304	A
305	D
306	A
307	B
308	D
309	C

MALE FACTOR INFERTILITY IN IVF/ICSI

310- Which of the following is TRUE regarding male factor infertility?

A. It accounts for less than 10% of infertility cases

B. Semen analysis should be performed at least twice, 2–3 weeks apart

C. Y chromosome microdeletions have no role in azoospermia

D. Varicocele is unrelated to male infertility

E. Only female evaluation is needed initially

311- A 28-year-old man with azoospermia has small testes, high FSH, and karyotype 47,XXY. What is the diagnosis?

A. Kallmann syndrome

B. Klinefelter syndrome

C. Y-chromosome microdeletion

D. Varicocele

E. CBAVD

312- All of the following are correct about ICSI in male factor infertility EXCEPT:

A. Allows fertilization with very low sperm counts

B. Requires surgical sperm retrieval in azoospermia

C. Completely eliminates genetic risks associated with male infertility

D. Can be used in severe oligospermia

E. Is the most effective ART option in male factor infertility

313- All of the following statements about varicocele and infertility are correct EXCEPT:

A. It is the most common correctable cause of male infertility

B. Associated with impaired spermatogenesis due to testicular hyperthermia

C. Surgical correction may improve semen parameters and pregnancy rates

D. Varicocelectomy is indicated in all men regardless of fertility status

E. It is more common on the left side due to venous anatomy

314- All of the following are pre-testicular causes of male infertility EXCEPT:

A. Hypogonadotropic hypogonadism

B. Pituitary adenoma

C. Hyperprolactinemia

D. Varicocele

E. Kallmann syndrome

315- A 32-year-old man presents with azoospermia. All of the following are correct about his evaluation EXCEPT:

A. Karyotype should be considered if non-obstructive azoospermia is suspected

B. Y-chromosome microdeletion testing is indicated

C. CFTR mutation analysis is indicated if CBAVD is suspected

D. Semen analysis alone is enough to identify exact cause without further workup

E. Testicular biopsy may help differentiate obstructive vs non-obstructive

316- A 27-year-old man with azoospermia, gynecomastia, and small testes is found to have karyotype 47,XXY. All of the following are correct EXCEPT:

A. Klinefelter syndrome is associated with hypergonadotropic hypogonadism

B. Testicular biopsy may rarely yield sperm for ICSI

C. Men with Klinefelter are at increased risk of metabolic and endocrine disorders

D. Genetic counseling should be offered before ART

E. IVF with ICSI completely eliminates the risk of genetic transmission

317- A 24-year-old man presents with azoospermia, low FSH and LH, and low testosterone. All of the following are correct EXCEPT:

A. This is a pre-testicular cause of male infertility

B. May be seen in Kallmann syndrome

C. Can be treated with gonadotropin replacement to induce spermatogenesis

D. Requires orchiectomy for definitive management

E. Semen analysis may improve after hormonal therapy

318- All of the following are correct regarding semen sample collection EXCEPT:

A. Abstinence period should be 2–7 days

B. Sample should be examined within 1 hour of collection

C. Two abnormal samples are needed before confirming male factor

D. Lubricated condom can be used for collection routinely

E. Sample is usually obtained by masturbation

319- According to WHO 2010 reference values, which of the following is NOT correct?

A. Normal sperm concentration ≥15 million/ml

B. Normal morphology ≥4%

C. Normal progressive motility ≥32%

D. Semen volume ≥1.5 ml

E. Normal vitality ≥20% live sperm

320- A 30-year-old man has semen analysis showing volume 2.0 ml, sperm concentration 10 million/ml, progressive motility 40%, morphology 6%. What is the abnormality?

A. Normal semen analysis

B. Oligozoospermia

C. Asthenozoospermia

D. Teratozoospermia

E. Necrozoospermia

321- A 28-year-old man has semen analysis: concentration 30 million/ml, progressive motility 10%, morphology 6%. Diagnosis?

A. Teratozoospermia

B. Asthenozoospermia

C. Oligoasthenoteratozoospermia (OAT)

D. Normal

E. Necrozoospermia

322- Semen analysis: concentration 25 million/ml, motility 45%, morphology 2% normal forms. Which is correct?

A. Normal semen analysis

B. Oligozoospermia

C. Teratozoospermia

D. Necrozoospermia

E. Asthenozoospermia

323- Semen analysis shows sperm concentration 20 million/ml, motility 0%, and viability (eosin test) shows all sperm dead. What is this condition?

A. Azoospermia

B. Necrozoospermia

C. Asthenozoospermia

D. Teratozoospermia

E. Cryptozoospermia

324- Semen analysis: volume 1 ml, concentration 5 million/ml, motility 15%, morphology 2%. Which diagnosis applies?

A. Oligozoospermia only

B. Asthenozoospermia only

C. Teratozoospermia only

D. Oligoasthenoteratozoospermia (OAT syndrome)

E. Necrozoospermia

325- All of the following are possible causes of azoospermia EXCEPT:

A. Klinefelter syndrome

B. Y-chromosome microdeletion

C. CBAVD (obstructive)

D. Pituitary hypogonadism

E. Teratozoospermia

326- A 32-year-old man presents with infertility. Semen analysis: volume 2.5 ml, azoospermia. Physical exam: normal testes, palpable vas deferens absent bilaterally. Hormones: FSH, LH, Testosterone all normal. Question: What is the MOST likely cause?

A. Primary testicular failure

B. Klinefelter syndrome

C. CBAVD (Congenital bilateral absence of vas deferens)

D. Y chromosome microdeletion

E. Hypogonadotropic hypogonadism

327- 28-year-old man with infertility. Semen analysis: azoospermia. Testes small & firm. Hormones: FSH ↑↑, LH ↑, Testosterone ↓. Karyotype: 47,XXY. Which diagnosis fits best?

A. Hypogonadotropic hypogonadism

B. Obstructive azoospermia

C. Klinefelter syndrome → Non-obstructive azoospermia

D. CBAVD

E. Retrograde ejaculation

328- A 35-year-old man with infertility. Semen analysis: azoospermia, volume 0.3 ml. Hormones: FSH, LH, Testosterone normal. History: retrograde ejaculation after spinal surgery. Which is the next step?

A. Varicocelectomy

B. Check post-ejaculatory urine for sperm

C. Testicular biopsy immediately

D. Start gonadotropin therapy

E. Repeat semen analysis only

329- All of the following features suggest NON-obstructive azoospermia EXCEPT:

A. Elevated FSH

B. Small firm testes

C. Chromosomal abnormalities (e.g., Klinefelter)

D. CFTR mutation

E. Sertoli-cell only syndrome

330- A 32-year-old man with azoospermia has normal FSH, LH, and testosterone. Testes are normal size, but vas deferens is absent bilaterally. Which sperm retrieval method is most appropriate?

A. TESA

B. TESE

C. Micro-TESE

D. PESA

E. Electroejaculation

331- A 28-year-old man with azoospermia, small firm testes, and elevated FSH is diagnosed with Klinefelter syndrome. Which method gives the best chance of retrieving sperm?

A. PESA

B. MESA

C. Micro-TESE

D. Electroejaculation

E. Repeat semen analysis only

332- Azoospermic patient scheduled for ICSI. All of the following are valid sperm retrieval methods EXCEPT:

A. PESA

B. MESA

C. TESA

D. Micro-TESE

E. ERA test

333- A patient undergoes Micro-TESE and sperm are retrieved. Which of the following statements is FALSE?

A. Retrieved sperm can be used immediately for ICSI

B. Retrieved sperm can be cryopreserved for later cycles

C. Micro-TESE minimizes testicular damage compared to multiple biopsies

D. Sperm retrieval guarantees high fertilization and live birth rates

E. Surgical retrieval may fail in some patients

334- A 32-year-old man with obstructive azoospermia undergoes PESA, but no sperm are obtained. What is the best next step?

A. TESE from testicular tissue

B. ERA test

C. Endometrial biopsy in partner

D. Repeat semen analysis

E. AMH level testing

335- All of the following are reasonable options after failed sperm retrieval in non-obstructive azoospermia EXCEPT:

A. Donor sperm insemination

B. Adoption

C. Repeat Micro-TESE in the same sitting

D. Counseling about low chances of biological paternity

E. PGT-SR on embryos

336- All of the following statements correctly differentiate IVF from ICSI EXCEPT:

A. In IVF, multiple motile sperm are added around the oocyte, while in ICSI, a single sperm is directly injected into the oocyte cytoplasm.

B. ICSI is mainly indicated in severe male factor infertility, whereas IVF is suitable if sperm parameters are normal.

C. ICSI requires micromanipulation equipment, while IVF does not.

D. In both IVF and ICSI, embryos are cultured and transferred similarly.

E. IVF completely prevents polyspermy, while ICSI cannot.

337- A 32-year-old couple presents with infertility for 4 years. The male partner has severe oligoasthenoteratozoospermia (sperm concentration 2 million/ml, progressive motility 10%, normal morphology 2%). Which ART method is MOST appropriate?

A. Conventional IVF

B. Intrauterine insemination (IUI)

C. ICSI (Intracytoplasmic sperm injection)

D. Expectant management

E. Natural cycle monitoring only

338- All of the following are valid indications for ICSI EXCEPT:

A. Severe oligoasthenoteratozoospermia (OAT)

B. Previous total fertilization failure with IVF

C. Surgically retrieved sperm (PESA, TESA, Micro-TESE)

D. Advanced maternal age with normal sperm parameters

E. Azoospermia with sperm retrieval

339- All of the following are TRUE about IMSI EXCEPT:

A. IMSI involves selecting sperm under very high magnification (≈6000x) to detect subtle morphological defects.

B. IMSI may be useful in cases of recurrent IVF/ICSI failure.

C. IMSI allows embryologists to avoid sperm with large vacuoles or head abnormalities.

D. IMSI requires advanced microscopy equipment compared to standard ICSI.

E. IMSI completely eliminates the risk of using sperm with DNA fragmentation.

340- Which of the following statements is TRUE regarding mature oocytes (Metaphase II, MII) compared to Metaphase I (MI)?

A. MII oocytes are arrested in metaphase of first meiotic division.

B. MI oocytes are the ones used for ICSI because they are fully mature.

C. Both MI and MII oocytes can be inseminated successfully with equal fertilization potential.

D. MII oocytes have extruded the first polar body.

E. MII oocytes contain diploid chromosome content.

341- A 32-year-old woman undergoes oocyte retrieval after ovarian stimulation. The embryologist reports that most of the retrieved oocytes are at Metaphase I (MI) stage, with no polar body visible. What is the BEST next step?

A. Use MI oocytes directly for ICSI, as they are fully competent

B. Culture MI oocytes in vitro to allow maturation to MII before ICSI

C. Discard all MI oocytes, only keep germinal vesicle oocytes

D. Perform IVF insemination with MI oocytes immediately

E. Freeze MI oocytes for future transfer without maturation

342- All of the following are TRUE characteristics of a Metaphase II (MII) oocyte EXCEPT:

A. Arrested at the second meiotic division (metaphase II stage)

B. Extrusion of the first polar body is a key marker of maturity

C. Contains haploid set of chromosomes ready for fertilization

D. Has higher fertilization potential compared to MI oocytes

E. Can be fertilized equally well whether or not the first polar body is visible

343- A 29-year-old woman undergoes oocyte retrieval after controlled ovarian stimulation. The embryologist reports that most retrieved oocytes are at the Germinal Vesicle (GV) stage, with an intact nucleus visible. What is the MOST appropriate interpretation/next step?

A. GV oocytes are fully mature and ready for ICSI

B. GV oocytes are the same as MII oocytes with first polar body extruded

C. GV oocytes are immature and cannot be fertilized directly

D. GV oocytes are more suitable for IVF than ICSI

E. GV oocytes can be used immediately for PGT

344- All of the following statements about oocyte maturation stages are TRUE EXCEPT:

A. Germinal Vesicle (GV) oocytes are immature, with an intact nucleus and no fertilization potential.

B. Metaphase I (MI) oocytes have initiated meiosis, no polar body yet, and are still immature.

C. Metaphase II (MII) oocytes have extruded the first polar body and are fertilization-competent.

D. Both MI and GV oocytes can be directly used for ICSI with the same success as MII.

E. Only MII oocytes are normally selected for insemination in IVF/ICSI.

345-Which of the following correctly describes the cleavage stage embryo?

A. Typically seen on Day 5–6

B. Composed of ~2–8 blastomeres

C. Has a blastocoel cavity

D. Consists of inner cell mass and trophectoderm

E. Results only after compaction

346- The morula stage of embryo development is characterized by:

A. Presence of blastocoel cavity

B. Around 16–32 cells with compaction

C. Differentiated inner cell mass and trophectoderm

D. Occurs on Day 2

E. Readiness for embryo transfer

347- All of the following are true regarding the blastocyst stage EXCEPT:

A. Occurs on Day 5–6 after fertilization

B. Has a blastocoel cavity

C. Differentiates into inner cell mass and trophectoderm

D. Cannot implant unless zona pellucida remains intact

E. Is the preferred stage for PGT biopsy

348- All of the following are features of the cleavage stage embryo EXCEPT:

A. Seen on Day 2–3 after fertilization

B. Typically has 2–8 cells (blastomeres)

C. Shows compaction of blastomeres

D. Cells remain totipotent at this stage

E. Grading is based on symmetry and fragmentation

349- All of the following describe differences between cleavage and blastocyst stage embryos EXCEPT:

A. Cleavage stage = Day 2–3, Blastocyst = Day 5–6

B. Cleavage embryos are graded by fragmentation, blastocysts by ICM & TE quality

C. Cleavage embryos have no blastocoel, blastocysts do

D. Cleavage embryos have higher implantation potential than blastocysts in most cases

E. Blastocyst transfer reduces risk of multiple pregnancy when SET is used

350- Which of the following statements about morula and blastocyst stages is NOT true?

A. Morula stage shows compaction, blastocyst shows cavity formation

B. Morula usually occurs at Day 4, blastocyst at Day 5–6

C. Morula stage already has a distinct inner cell mass and trophectoderm

D. Blastocyst stage is suitable for PGT biopsy

E. Morula represents the transition from cleavage to blastocyst

351- All of the following are correct about hatching EXCEPT:

A. Occurs around Day 6–7 post-fertilization

B. Is essential for implantation

C. Assisted hatching can be performed in IVF labs

D. Hatching means embryo remains inside zona pellucida for better attachment

E. Zona thinning or rupture is part of the process

352- A 38-year-old woman with repeated IVF failure has embryos reaching the blastocyst stage, but no implantation. Lab reports show thick zona pellucida. Which intervention is most appropriate?

A. Culture embryos to Day 3 only

B. Perform assisted hatching before transfer

C. Switch to IUI cycle

D. Use donor sperm

E. Cancel transfer cycle

353- All of the following are criteria of normal fertilization EXCEPT:

A. Presence of 2 pronuclei

B. 2 polar bodies

C. Equal-sized pronuclei

D. More than 3 pronuclei

E. Alignment of pronuclei before cleavage

354- Which of the following indicates abnormal fertilization?

A. 2 pronuclei and 2 polar bodies

B. 1 pronucleus only

C. 3 pronuclei

D. Both B and C

E. All of the above

355- All are causes of failed fertilization after ICSI EXCEPT:

A. Oocyte activation failure

B. Poor sperm quality

C. Abnormal zona pellucida hatching

D. Cytoplasmic immaturity of oocyte

E. Technical error during ICSI

356- Which of the following is TRUE regarding fertilization check in IVF lab?

A. Done after 2–4 hours of insemination

B. Normal fertilization is confirmed at ~16–18 hours post-insemination

C. Presence of 3PN is acceptable for transfer

D. Fertilization check requires embryo biopsy

E. No difference between IVF and ICSI fertilization checks

357- A 34-year-old woman with male factor infertility undergoes ICSI. At fertilization check, none of the injected oocytes show pronuclei. Which next step is most reasonable for the next cycle?

A. Assisted oocyte activation (e.g., calcium ionophore)

B. Repeat ICSI without changes

C. Transfer embryos despite no fertilization

D. Switch to natural intercourse

E. Perform ERA test

358- A 38-year-old woman undergoes IVF. Fertilization check reveals normal 2PN embryos but only 20% cleaved to 2-cell stage. What is the most likely explanation?

A. Failed fertilization

B. Embryo arrest after fertilization

C. Poor sperm injection technique

D. Morula compaction

E. Normal expected finding

359- All of the following are causes of failed fertilization in conventional IVF EXCEPT:

A. Poor sperm motility or count

B. Thickened zona pellucida

C. Failure of sperm-oocyte binding

D. Oocyte activation defect

E. Technical error in embryo transfer

360- All of the following may lead to failed fertilization after ICSI EXCEPT:

A. Oocyte cytoplasmic immaturity

B. Defective oocyte activation (Ca^{2+} oscillations)

C. Sperm head decondensation failure

D. Micromanipulation technique error

E. Blocked fallopian tube

361- All of the following are laboratory-related causes of failed fertilization EXCEPT:

A. Incorrect culture media pH

B. Incubator CO_2 imbalance

C. Inadequate temperature control

D. Endometrial receptivity defect

E. Prolonged exposure of gametes to room air

362- All of the following are patient-related causes of fertilization failure EXCEPT:

A. Severe oligoasthenoteratozoospermia

B. Sperm DNA fragmentation

C. Oocyte cytoplasmic immaturity

D. Deficiency of oocyte activation factors

E. Wrong gas mixture in incubator

363- All of the following may improve fertilization outcomes in recurrent ICSI failure EXCEPT:

A. Assisted oocyte activation (Ca^{2+} ionophore)

B. Use of testicular sperm in severe DNA damage cases

C. IMSI (high magnification sperm selection)

D. Artificial zona hardening

E. Optimizing ovarian stimulation for better oocyte quality

364- Which of the following is the main advantage of vitrification over slow freezing?

A. Cheaper procedure

B. Prevents ice crystal formation

C. Requires no special equipment

D. Lower post-thaw survival rates

E. Only suitable for sperm

365- All of the following can be cryopreserved EXCEPT:

A. Cleavage-stage embryos

B. Blastocysts

C. Oocytes

D. Endometrial tissue

E. Sperm

366- Which of the following is NOT an indication for embryo cryopreservation?

A. Surplus embryos after IVF

B. Risk of OHSS

C. Elective fertility preservation

D. Recurrent miscarriage due to uterine factors

E. Oncology patients before chemotherapy

367- A 35-year-old woman undergoes IVF. On Day 5, 3 blastocysts are formed. She prefers single embryo transfer (SET). What should be done with the remaining embryos?

A. Discard them immediately

B. Freeze them by vitrification

C. Transfer all embryos to reduce wastage

D. Culture to Day 7 before decision

E. Donate without consent

368- A man with non-obstructive azoospermia undergoes micro-TESE, and few sperm are retrieved. What is the best next step?

A. Use fresh sperm only, discard if not used

B. Freeze retrieved sperm for later ICSI

C. Repeat micro-TESE immediately

D. Switch to IUI

E. Cancel ICSI attempt

369- All of the following are valid indications for embryo cryopreservation EXCEPT:

A. Surplus embryos after IVF

B. Prevention of OHSS by freeze-all strategy

C. Fertility preservation before chemotherapy

D. Recurrent implantation failure due to poor endometrium

E. Desire for elective single embryo transfer

370- All of the following are indications for sperm cryopreservation EXCEPT:

A. Before chemotherapy or radiotherapy in men

B. Severe oligoasthenoteratozoospermia (backup sample)

C. Prior to surgical sperm retrieval (TESE, PESA)

D. Male factor infertility with azoospermia

E. Recurrent miscarriage due to uterine septum

371- All of the following are advantages of cryopreservation EXCEPT:

A. Prevents OHSS by avoiding fresh transfer

B. Provides backup gametes for future ART cycles

C. Allows elective fertility preservation

D. Guarantees 100% live birth in subsequent cycles

E. Enables donor programs (oocyte, sperm)

372- Lab report: 10 oocytes retrieved → 7 MII, 2 MI, 1 GV. After ICSI, 5 show 2PN, 1 shows 3PN, 1 unfertilized.

Interpretation?

A. Fertilization rate is 100%

B. 3PN embryo is abnormal, should not be transferred

C. Only 1PN embryos are normal

D. MI oocytes are mature and can be used directly

E. GV oocytes have highest implantation potential

373- Day 3 report: 6 embryos, all 8-cell, equal blastomeres, <10% fragmentation.

Best interpretation?

A. Poor quality cleavage embryos

B. High-quality cleavage embryos suitable for transfer or freezing

C. Arrested embryo development

D. Signs of polyspermy

E. Embryos should be discarded

374- Day 5 report: Blastocyst grading → 4AA, 3AB, 2CC.

Which embryo has best implantation potential?

A. 2CC

B. 3AB

C. 4AA

D. All equal

E. None are suitable

375- Lab report after fertilization check: All oocytes show 0 PN (no pronuclei). Most likely explanation?

A. Oocyte activation failure

B. Normal fertilization

C. Early cleavage embryos

D. Zona hatching failure

E. Blastocyst collapse

376- Patient report: 8 oocytes retrieved, 6 fertilized normally (2PN), 2 abnormal (3PN). On Day 5 → 3 blastocysts suitable for freezing. Counseling point for patient?

A. No embryos are suitable for transfer

B. Good prognosis since blastocyst development occurred

C. All abnormal embryos can be transferred safely

D. Only GV oocytes give best results

E. Need donor eggs immediately

377- All of the following are used in cleavage-stage embryo grading EXCEPT:

A. Number of blastomeres (cell count)

B. Symmetry of blastomeres

C. Degree of fragmentation

D. Quality of inner cell mass

E. Multinucleation of blastomeres

378- All of the following parameters are used in blastocyst grading EXCEPT:

A. Expansion of blastocoel cavity

B. Quality of inner cell mass (ICM)

C. Quality of trophectoderm (TE)

D. % fragmentation of blastomeres

E. Stage of zona hatching

379- All of the following are TRUE regarding embryo grading EXCEPT:

A. 8-cell embryo with <10% fragmentation on Day 3 is high quality

B. Blastocyst 4AA is considered top quality

C. Embryos with 3PN can be transferred if no other embryos are available

D. Symmetry of blastomeres is a good prognostic sign

E. Good-quality blastocysts can be frozen for later use

ANSWERS

310	B	345	B
311	B	346	B
312	C	347	D
313	D	348	C
314	D	349	D
315	D	350	C
316	E	351	D
317	D	352	B
318	D	353	D
319	E	354	E
320	B	355	C
321	B	356	B
322	C	357	A
323	B	358	B
324	D	359	E
325	E	360	E
326	C	361	D
327	C	362	E
328	B	363	D
329	D	364	B
330	D	365	D
331	C	366	D
332	E	367	B
333	D	368	B
334	A	369	D
335	E	370	E
336	E	371	D
337	C	372	B
338	D	373	B
339	E	374	C
340	D	375	A
341	B	376	B
342	E	377	D
343	C	378	D
344	D	379	C

OVARIAN HYPERSTIMULATION SYNDROME (OHSS)

380- All of the following are risk factors for OHSS EXCEPT:

A. PCOS

B. High AMH

C. High estradiol >3500 pg/ml

D. Low antral follicle count

E. hCG trigger

381- Which of the following is FALSE about OHSS?

A. Caused by increased vascular permeability via VEGF

B. More common with agonist trigger

C. May be worsened by pregnancy due to endogenous hCG

D. May be associated with enlarged ovaries and ascites

E. Can lead to thromboembolic events

382- All of the following are strategies to prevent OHSS EXCEPT:

A. Use of GnRH agonist trigger in antagonist cycles

B. Freeze-all embryos strategy

C. Coasting by withholding gonadotropins

D. Routine use of high-dose hCG for luteal support

E. Dopamine agonists (cabergoline)

383- A 26-year-old woman with PCOS undergoes ovarian stimulation. On trigger day, estradiol is 4800 pg/ml and >20 follicles are seen. What is the best strategy to reduce OHSS risk?

A. Proceed with hCG trigger and fresh ET

B. Cancel cycle

C. Use GnRH agonist trigger and freeze-all embryos

D. Give high-dose hCG and transfer multiple embryos

E. Proceed with IUI

384- A 30-year-old IVF patient develops abdominal distension, ascites on ultrasound, hematocrit 50%, oliguria, and dyspnea. What is the correct interpretation?

A. Mild OHSS

B. Moderate OHSS

C. Severe OHSS

D. Critical OHSS

E. No OHSS, normal stimulation

385- A patient developed moderate OHSS. Which of the following is NOT part of her management?

A. Careful fluid and electrolyte balance

B. Prophylactic anticoagulation

C. Outpatient monitoring if stable

D. Use of hCG for luteal phase support

E. Paracentesis if tense ascites

386- A 28-year-old woman after oocyte retrieval presents with abdominal distension, nausea, vomiting, and mild ascites on ultrasound. Hematocrit is 38%, urine output is normal. What is the likely diagnosis?

A. Mild OHSS

B. Moderate OHSS

C. Severe OHSS

D. Critical OHSS

E. No OHSS

387- A patient develops severe OHSS after hCG trigger. Which of the following is the MOST appropriate management?

A. High-dose oral fluids only

B. Hospitalization, fluid balance, thromboprophylaxis, paracentesis if needed

C. Immediate embryo transfer to relieve symptoms

D. Stop all medications and discharge

E. Start GnRH agonist daily

388- A 35-year-old IVF patient with OHSS is noted to have an ongoing pregnancy. Which statement is correct?

A. OHSS will resolve faster due to rising endogenous hCG

B. Pregnancy may prolong or worsen OHSS symptoms

C. Termination of pregnancy is mandatory

D. Switching to IUI is advisable

E. Pregnancy has no effect on OHSS course

389- All of the following are features of severe OHSS EXCEPT:

A. Tense ascites

B. Hematocrit >45%

C. Ovaries >12 cm

D. Oliguria

E. Normal abdominal scan with no ascites

390- All of the following are possible complications of OHSS EXCEPT:

A. Thromboembolism

B. Acute respiratory distress syndrome (ARDS)

C. Ovarian torsion

D. Chronic kidney disease years later

E. Pleural effusion

391- 31-year-old woman with severe OHSS presents with abdominal distension, tense ascites, dyspnea, and left leg swelling. Doppler confirms DVT. What is the MOST appropriate management?

A. Discharge on oral fluids only

B. Hospitalization + anticoagulation + fluid balance

C. Immediate fresh embryo transfer

D. Stop all treatment and observe

E. Coasting with gonadotropin withdrawal

392- A 29-year-old woman with OHSS develops oliguria (urine <200 ml/day), rising creatinine, and tense ascites. What is the next best step?

A. Give more hCG to improve corpus luteum support

B. Discharge home with oral hydration

C. Immediate embryo transfer

D. Ignore as this is mild OHSS

E. Careful IV fluids + consider paracentesis

393- A 33-year-old IVF patient with OHSS presents with dyspnea and chest pain. CXR shows pleural effusion and suspicion of pulmonary embolism. What is the most urgent step?

A. High-dose hCG support

B. Anticoagulation and supportive management in hospital

C. Discharge home as pleural effusion is expected

D. IVF cycle cancellation

E. Increase estradiol monitoring

394- A 26-year-old woman with critical OHSS presents with anuria, tense ascites, hemoconcentration (Hct 58%), and hypoxemia. What is the classification?

A. Mild OHSS

B. Moderate OHSS

C. Severe OHSS

D. Critical OHSS

E. No OHSS

395- Which of the following is the main mediator of increased vascular permeability in OHSS?

A. Estradiol

B. Progesterone

C. VEGF

D. LH

E. FSH

396- All of the following are TRUE about VEGF in OHSS EXCEPT:

A. Secreted from luteinized granulosa cells

B. Upregulated by hCG trigger

C. Causes increased vascular permeability

D. Prevents fluid extravasation into third spaces

E. Target for prevention with dopamine agonists

397-Which of the following drugs reduces VEGF-mediated OHSS?

A. Cabergoline

B. Estradiol valerate

C. Clomiphene citrate

D. Progesterone

E. Dexamethasone

398- All of the following statements are TRUE about antagonist protocol compared to long agonist protocol EXCEPT:

A. Associated with lower risk of OHSS

B. Allows ovulation trigger with GnRH agonist instead of hCG

C. Has shorter duration of stimulation

D. Provides consistently higher pregnancy rates in all patients

E. Is preferred in women with PCOS or high ovarian reserve

399- All of the following are features of mild OHSS EXCEPT:

A. Abdominal bloating

B. Ovarian enlargement up to 8 cm

C. Normal urine output

D. Hematocrit >50%

E. Managed with observation and fluids

400- A 28-year-old woman after IVF presents with mild abdominal discomfort and bloating. Ultrasound shows bilateral ovarian enlargement ~7 cm, no ascites. Hematocrit 36%. What is the diagnosis?

A. No OHSS

B. Mild OHSS

C. Moderate OHSS

D. Severe OHSS

E. Critical OHSS

401- A 29-year-old IVF patient with mild OHSS asks about treatment. Which is MOST appropriate?

A. Hospitalization and IV fluids

B. Paracentesis and anticoagulation

C. Outpatient follow-up, oral fluids, analgesia

D. Embryo transfer immediately to resolve symptoms

E. High-dose hCG for luteal support

402- A 30-year-old woman develops severe OHSS after IVF. She presents with massive abdominal distension, tense ascites, oliguria, and dyspnea. Hematocrit = 52%. Despite IV fluids, her symptoms persist. What is the MOST appropriate next step?

A. Continue oral fluids and discharge home

B. Give high-dose hCG for luteal support

C. Insert pigtail catheter for ascitic drainage

D. Repeat ovarian stimulation cycle

E. Perform IUI instead of IVF

403- Which of the following is the main indication for pigtail catheter in OHSS?

A. Mild abdominal bloating

B. Moderate OHSS with mild ascites

C. Severe OHSS with tense ascites and dyspnea

D. To stimulate implantation after embryo transfer

E. For routine management of all IVF patients

404- All of the following are advantages of using a pigtail catheter in OHSS EXCEPT:

A. Provides continuous drainage of ascites

B. Reduces intra-abdominal pressure

C. Improves renal perfusion and urine output

D. Prevents the need for hospitalization in severe OHSS

E. Avoids repeated paracentesis procedures

405- All of the following are TRUE about coasting EXCEPT:

A. Used when estradiol levels are very high (>3500 pg/ml)

B. Aimed at reducing risk of OHSS

C. Involves withholding gonadotropins while continuing GnRH analogue

D. Safe even if continued beyond 7 days

E. Helps small follicles undergo atresia

406- What is meant by "GnRH antagonist rescue" in IVF stimulation protocols?

A. Withholding gonadotropins when E2 is high

B. Switching from agonist to antagonist protocol mid-cycle to allow agonist trigger

C. Using cabergoline to block VEGF

D. Freezing all embryos after stimulation

E. Using high-dose hCG trigger to avoid OHSS

407- All of the following are advantages of GnRH antagonist rescue EXCEPT:

A. Allows use of GnRH agonist trigger instead of hCG

B. Reduces risk of OHSS in high responders

C. Involves stopping agonist and starting antagonist mid-cycle

D. Improves oocyte yield without affecting OHSS risk

E. Can be combined with freeze-all strategy

408- Which of the following statements about metformin in PCOS patients undergoing IVF is TRUE?

A. Increases risk of OHSS

B. May Reduces OHSS risk, especially in long agonist protocol cycles

C. Completely prevents OHSS better than antagonist protocol

D. Contraindicated in PCOS women during stimulation

E. Worsens insulin resistance

409- A 29-year-old woman with severe OHSS presents with tense ascites, oliguria, and hematocrit 50%. Despite crystalloids, urine output is poor.

What IV fluid may be added to improve intravascular volume?

A. Dextrose 5%

B. Hydroxyethyl starch (Hesteril)

C. Distilled water

D. Estradiol valerate

E. High-dose hCG infusion

410- Which of the following statements correctly differentiates between early and late OHSS?

A. Early OHSS is related to pregnancy hCG, while late OHSS is due to exogenous hCG trigger

B. Early OHSS occurs only in antagonist protocol, while late OHSS occurs only in agonist protocol

C. Early OHSS is milder, while late OHSS is always critical

D. Early OHSS is prevented by freeze-all, while late OHSS cannot be prevented

E. Early OHSS occurs 3–7 days after hCG trigger, while late OHSS occurs 10–17 days after due to endogenous hCG from pregnancy

411- What is the main reason why hCG should be avoided for luteal phase support in IVF?

A. hCG decreases progesterone secretion

B. hCG reduces follicular growth

C. hCG increases VEGF release and risk of OHSS

D. hCG has no luteotrophic effect

E. hCG impairs embryo implantation

412- A 27-year-old woman with PCOS has 22 follicles and E2 = 3900 pg/ml. The clinician decides to use a reduced dose (5,000 IU) hCG for ovulation trigger. What is the purpose of this approach?

A. To increase number of retrieved oocytes

B. To reduce severity of OHSS risk

C. To replace luteal phase support

D. To prevent premature LH surge

E. To improve blastocyst quality

413- All of the following are TRUE regarding OHSS in simple ovulation induction compared to IVF EXCEPT:

A. OHSS is less common in simple induction cycles than in IVF

B. hCG trigger plays a major role in causing OHSS in both IVF and simple induction

C. Severe OHSS can occur in simple induction if pregnancy happens (endogenous hCG)

D. Estradiol levels are always > 3500 pg/ml in simple induction OHSS

E. PCOS patients are at higher risk in both scenarios

414- Which of the following statements regarding estradiol (E2) levels in OHSS during simple ovulation induction is TRUE?

A. OHSS cannot occur unless E2 > 5000 pg/ml

B. OHSS may occur at E2 levels > 1700 pg/ml, especially with hCG and pregnancy

C. E2 levels are irrelevant in OHSS risk

D. OHSS in simple induction always requires E2 > 8000 pg/ml

E. OHSS is independent of hCG use in induction cycles

415- A 25-year-old woman with PCOS undergoes ovulation induction with gonadotropins. On ultrasound, 8 follicles >14 mm are seen, and E2 is 1800 pg/ml. What is the BEST next step to reduce OHSS risk?

A. Proceed with standard hCG trigger

B. Cancel the cycle

C. Add luteal hCG support

D. Switch to IVF immediately

E. Continue stimulation for more follicle growth

416- According to ASRM 2023 guidelines, which of the following statements regarding the use of volume expanders (albumin, hydroxyethyl starch, mannitol) in OHSS prevention is TRUE?

A. Strongly recommended for all high-risk patients to prevent OHSS

B. Recommended only in severe OHSS with ascites

C. Not recommended in patients at high risk of moderate or severe OHSS

D. Considered the first-line strategy in antagonist protocols

E. Required for luteal phase support in PCOS patients

417- According to ASRM 2023 guidelines, which of the following is correct regarding letrozole use in OHSS prevention?

A. Strongly recommended to reduce moderate-to-severe OHSS

B. Can be routinely used for luteal support to prevent OHSS

C. Recommended only in PCOS patients as first-line prevention

D. Considered the gold standard strategy in antagonist protocol cycles

E. Not recommended as an intervention to reduce moderate-to-severe OHSS

418- A 33-year-old retrieval day complicated by OHSS symptoms: tense ascites, Hct 50%, oliguria. Team planned fresh ET. Best plan now?

A. Fresh ET to “use up” hormones

B. Cancel ET; freeze-all and manage OHSS

C. Proceed with single ET only

D. Give luteal hCG and transfer

E. Discharge with oral fluids

419- All of the following are situations where cycle cancellation is advised to reduce OHSS risk EXCEPT:

A. >20 follicles with E2 > 3500 pg/ml and no access to agonist trigger or freeze-all

B. Multiple mature follicles in simple induction for IUI (risk of multiples + OHSS)

C. Symptomatic patient with abdominal distension, rising hematocrit, and E2 > 5000 pg/ml before hCG

D. PCOS patient with 2 mature follicles and E2 = 400 pg/ml on simple induction

E. Oocyte donor with >30 follicles and E2 > 5000 pg/ml where only fresh transfer is possible

LOW RESPONDER

420- A 38-year-old woman undergoes ovarian stimulation with 300 IU gonadotropins. On day 10, only 2 follicles >16 mm are seen, E2 = 450 pg/ml. What is the MOST appropriate interpretation?

A. Normal responder

B. Poor responder (low ovarian reserve / Bologna criteria)

C. Hyper-responder

D. Cycle cancellation mandatory

E. OHSS risk high

421- A 36-year-old Low responder with previous IVF cycle showing 3 oocytes retrieved. Which protocol may be considered to improve yield?

A. Long agonist protocol with hCG luteal support

B. Antagonist protocol with dual stimulation

C. Cancel without options

D. Use only clomiphene citrate

E. Freeze-all strategy for OHSS

422- All of the following are part of the Bologna criteria for low ovarian response EXCEPT:

A. Advanced maternal age (≥40 years) or other risk factors

B. Previous poor ovarian response (<3 oocytes retrieved)

C. Abnormal ovarian reserve test (low AMH/AFC)

D. Low fertilization rate despite adequate oocytes (quality issue)

E. Meeting at least 2 of the above 3 criteria

423- All of the following are correct differences between Bologna and Poseidon criteria EXCEPT:

A. Bologna defines poor responders broadly with 3 risk factors

B. Poseidon focuses on stratifying by age and oocyte quality/quantity

C. Bologna criteria include fertilization and embryo quality as diagnostic factors

D. Poseidon groups help predict prognosis and tailor stimulation

E. Bologna criteria require ≥2 of 3 conditions (age, past response, ovarian reserve)

424- All of the following are TRUE regarding poor ovarian responders EXCEPT:

A. Bologna criteria require at least 2 defining features

B. Poseidon subdivides patients by age and ovarian reserve

C. Both Bologna and Poseidon agree that all poor responders have the same prognosis

D. Poseidon aims to better individualize treatment and prognosis

E. Poor ovarian response may be due to both quantity and quality of oocytes

425- A 30-year-old woman, AMH 3.0 ng/ml, AFC 12, undergoes stimulation with 300 IU gonadotropins. Retrieval yields only 2 oocytes. Which Poseidon group does she belong to?

A. Group 1

B. Group 2

C. Group 3

D. Group 4

426- A 40-year-old woman with AMH 0.6 ng/ml and AFC 2 undergoes antagonist stimulation, retrieval yields 2 oocytes. Which Poseidon group?

A. Group 1

B. Group 2

C. Group 3

D. Group 4

427- A 34-year-old woman with AMH 3.2 ng/ml, AFC 14, previously had retrieval of 8 oocytes, but only 1 fertilized. Which classification applies?

A. Bologna criteria poor responder

B. Poseidon Group 1

C. Poseidon Group 2

D. Poor oocyte quality (Poseidon functional poor prognosis)

E. Hyper-responder

428- Which of the following is NOT typically recommended as a protocol for Low responders?

A. Microdose flare agonist protocol

B. Antagonist protocol with dual stimulation

C. PPOS protocol

D. Standard low-dose clomiphene alone

E. Estrogen priming with antagonist

429- A 39-year-old woman, AMH 0.6 ng/ml, AFC 4, previously failed long agonist protocol with 2 oocytes retrieved. Which stimulation strategy is MOST appropriate next cycle?

A. Antagonist protocol

B. Continue same long agonist protocol

C. Cancel cycle and no further attempts

D. Use only clomiphene citrate 50 mg

E. Double Stimulation Protocol (DuoStim)

430- Which statement about gonadotropin dosing for low responders is correct, according to ESHRE guidelines?

A. Doses above 300 IU/day yield significantly higher live birth rates

B. Daily FSH doses over 300 IU are not recommended

C. Optimal dose is 450–600 IU/day for poor responders

D. High doses always prevent cycle cancellation

E. Lower doses (<150 IU) are recommended in normal responders

431- A 40-year-old woman with AMH 0.5 ng/ml and AFC 3 undergoes antagonist stimulation. On retrieval day, only 2 follicles >18 mm are seen. What is the role of follicular flushing in her case?

A. Strongly contraindicated

B. May be considered to maximize oocyte yield

C. Always guarantees improved pregnancy rate

D. Unnecessary; cancel retrieval

E. First-line strategy in all IVF cycles

432- A 40-year-old woman, AMH 0.5 ng/ml, AFC 3, previously retrieved only 2 oocytes with high-dose antagonist stimulation. She is counseled about double stimulation (DuoStim). Which of the following is the MAIN advantage of this approach?

A. Reduces cost and medication use

B. Accumulates more oocytes in a shorter time

C. Prevents OHSS completely

D. Increases endometrial receptivity

E. Avoids the need for cryopreservation

433- Which statement about double stimulation (DuoStim) in low responders is TRUE?

A. Involves stimulation in luteal phase only

B. Always guarantees higher live birth rates

C. Contraindicated in poor responders

D. Used only in high responders to avoid OHSS

E. Recommended as protocol for low responder in ESHRE 2025 guidelines

434- Which statement best reflects the findings of the PRIMA trial for poor ovarian responders?

A. Mild stimulation resulted in significantly lower ongoing pregnancy rates

B. Mild stimulation was non-inferior to conventional stimulation with shorter duration and lower gonadotropin use

C. Mild stimulation had a much higher oocyte yield

D. Conventional stimulation had fewer cancellations

E. Mild stimulation resulted in no pregnancies

435- A 36-year-old woman with an AFC of 6 and AMH of 0.5 ng/ml is planned for IVF. You're deciding between "mild stimulation" (150 IU FSH + antagonist) and conventional (450 IU HMG + long agonist). Based on the PRIMA trial, what can you tell her about the likely outcomes?

A. Mild stimulation will result in significantly fewer pregnancies

B. She can expect similar ongoing pregnancy rates with fewer medications and shorter stimulation in mild stimulation.

C. Conventional stimulation will guarantee better results

D. Mild stimulation is not suitable for her age

E. Cancellation risk is much higher with mild stimulation

436- What follows immediately after the first oocyte retrieval in DuoStim?

A. Cycle cancellation

B. Natural luteal phase

C. Second ovarian stimulation (luteal phase stimulation)

D. Embryo transfer fresh

E. hCG administration only

437- Which of the following best describes the sequence of DuoStim?

A. Luteal stimulation → retrieval → follicular stimulation → retrieval

B. Continuous stimulation with no break → double retrieval same day

C. Natural cycle followed by one stimulation

D. Follicular stimulation → retrieval → luteal stimulation → retrieval

E. Two separate menstrual cycles needed

438- Which of the following is correct regarding agonist vs antagonist protocols in Low responders?

A. Agonist always produces higher live birth rate

B. Antagonist protocol always guarantees ≥10 oocytes

C. Agonist protocol prevents all cycle cancellations

D. Antagonist protocol is contraindicated in low responders

E. Antagonist & Agonist protocols are equally recommended

439- Which of the following statements about growth hormone in Low responders is FALSE?

A. It has been studied as an adjuvant to stimulation

B. Evidence for live birth improvement is still controversial

C. It is part of standard recommended protocol by guidelines

D. It may improve oocyte competence in some cases

E. It is administered with gonadotropins

440- Which of the following is correct regarding ESHRE/ASRM on LH supplementation?

A. Strongly recommended for all IVF patients

B. Recommended only for PCOS patients

C. Contraindicated in low responders

D. Replaces the need for FSH completely

E. May be considered in Low responders and older women

441- When is LH usually added during stimulation in low responders?

A. From the luteal phase before stimulation

B. At the start or mid-follicular phase

C. After oocyte retrieval only

D. During luteal support

E. After embryo transfer

442- Which guideline statement is MOST accurate regarding testosterone supplementation in Low responders?

A. It is routinely recommended for IVF patients

B. Considered investigational adjuvant with limited evidence

C. Only used for OHSS prevention

D. Contraindicated in women >35 years

E. Replaces gonadotropin stimulation

443- Which of the following is FALSE regarding DHEA use in low responders?

A. It is given orally before IVF cycles

B. Evidence of benefit is still controversial

C. It may improve oocyte yield and embryo quality

D. It is a standard mandatory therapy for all IVF patients

E. Some studies show improved pregnancy rates

444- For how long is DHEA usually given before IVF stimulation in Low responders?

A. 2–3 days

B. 2–3 weeks

C. 6–12 weeks

D. Only during luteal support

E. After embryo transfer

445- Which of the following is FALSE about Co Q10 in Low responders?

A. It may enhance mitochondrial function in oocytes

B. Some studies suggest improvement in oocyte yield and embryo quality

C. It is usually taken orally before IVF stimulation

D. It is considered an adjuvant therapy with limited evidence

E. It is a mandatory part of IVF protocols

446- For how long is Coenzyme Q10 often given before IVF stimulation in Low responders?

A. 2–3 days

B. 1–2 weeks

C. 2–3 months

D. Only during luteal support

E. After embryo transfer

IVF/ICSI WITH ENDOMETRIOSIS & ADENOMYOSIS

447- All of the following are true regarding endometriosis and ICSI outcomes EXCEPT:

A. Advanced endometriosis can reduce oocyte yield and quality

B. Endometriosis may impair implantation

C. Surgery is always mandatory before ICSI in all cases

D. Endometriosis can coexist with adenomyosis

E. Mild endometriosis may not need pretreatment before IVF

448- A 37-year-old woman with recurrent endometrioma surgery, AMH 0.6 ng/ml, and infertility >4 years. Best reproductive option?

A. Repeat surgery

B. IVF/ICSI directly

C. Ovulation induction with timed intercourse

D. IUI

E. Expectant management

449- All of the following are indications for IVF/ICSI in women with endometriosis EXCEPT:

A. Bilateral tubal occlusion due to endometriosis

B. Severe male factor infertility associated with endometriosis

C. Repeated failed IUI in minimal/mild endometriosis

D. Advanced endometriosis with markedly reduced ovarian reserve

E. As first-line treatment in all cases of stage I endometriosis with open tubes

450- All of the following statements about laparoscopy in the management of endometriosis-associated infertility according to ESHRE 2022 are true EXCEPT:

A. Laparoscopy is no longer the diagnostic gold standard.

B. Laparoscopy can be offered to improve natural conception in stage I/II endometriosis.

C. Decision for surgery should consider pain symptoms, ovarian reserve, and EFI score.

D. Laparoscopy is routinely recommended prior to IVF in all cases of endometriosis to improve outcomes.

E. Imaging is preferred for diagnosis unless imaging fails or empirical treatment fails.

451- Which of these is NOT aligned with ESHRE 2022 recommendations on IVF/ICSI protocols in endometriosis?

A. Both GnRH-agonist and antagonist protocols can be used interchangeably based on preference

B. Extended GnRH-agonist downregulation is explicitly not recommended

C. Prolonged COC or progestogen pre-treatment is not recommended to improve live birth rates

D. Laparoscopic confirmation of endometriosis is required before IVF

E. Ovarian suppression after surgery should not be solely for fertility enhancement

452- All of the following are consistent with ESHRE 2022 recommendations on managing endometriomas before IVF/ICSI EXCEPT:

A. Surgery is not routinely recommended for endometriomas.

B. Surgery may be considered to relieve pain or aid follicle access during oocyte retrieval.

C. Routine surgical removal of all endometriomas prior to IVF is strongly recommended.

D. Surgery for endometrioma may reduce ovarian reserve and should be individualized.

E. Surgery should be reserved for cases with suspected malignancy or technical retrieval issues.

453- All of the following are potential risks of performing endometrioma surgery prior to IVF EXCEPT:

A. Reduced ovarian reserve (lower AMH / AFC)

B. Increased cumulative live birth rate after IVF

C. Risk of surgical complications (adhesions, ovarian damage)

D. May require higher gonadotropin doses for subsequent stimulation

E. These risks necessitate case-by-case decision-making.

454- Which of the following is NOT an indication for surgical removal of endometrioma as per ESHRE 2022?

A. Severe pain or symptoms caused by the cyst

B. Rapid growth or suspicion of malignancy

C. Easy access to follicles for retrieval

D. To improve ovarian reserve before IVF

E. Large cyst interfering with retrieval technique

455- A 30-year-old woman has a 3 cm endometrioma, AMH 1.2 ng/ml, no pain, and patent tubes. She is preparing for IVF. What is the next step?

A. Surgery to improve ovarian reserve

B. Direct IVF/ICSI without surgery

C. Aspiration of endometrioma

D. Medical suppression with progestin only

E. Cancel IVF attempt

456- A 39-year-old woman with bilateral recurrent endometriomas, prior two surgeries, AMH 0.5 ng/ml, infertility 6 years. What is the best option now?

A. Repeat cystectomy

B. Direct IVF/ICSI without further surgery

C. Cancel IVF and continue suppression

D. Natural conception attempts

E. Tuboplasty

457- A 36-year-old with a 4 cm right ovarian endometrioma, no pain, but the cyst is blocking access to follicles during transvaginal scan. She is about to undergo IVF. What should be done?

A. IVF directly without intervention

B. Surgical removal to facilitate follicle access

C. Expectant management

D. GnRH agonist suppression for 6 months

E. Cancel IVF and advise donor egg

458- All of the following statements are true regarding the role of laparoscopy in minimal–mild endometriosis (rASRM I/II) according to ESHRE 2022 EXCEPT:

A. Laparoscopic treatment may be considered to improve chances of natural conception in selected cases

B. Decision for laparoscopy should consider symptoms, age, ovarian reserve, and EFI score

C. Non-invasive imaging (TVUS/MRI) may suffice in some cases without immediate laparoscopy

D. Diagnostic laparoscopy is not recommended solely to prove the diagnosis if imaging is conclusive or empirical treatment is effective

E. Laparoscopy is routinely recommended in all infertile women solely to enhance pregnancy rates

459- A 34-year-old woman with stage IV endometriosis, bilateral tubo-ovarian adhesions, infertility for 5 years. What is the role of IUI?

A. Strongly recommended

B. May be tried for 6 cycles

C. IVF/ICSI indicated

D. As effective as IVF in this case

E. Improves pregnancy rate compared to surgery alone

460- A 31-year-old with minimal endometriosis and open tubes has been infertile for 2 years. Semen analysis is normal. What is the most evidence-based treatment option before IVF?

A. Clomiphene citrate only

B. Stimulated IUI

C. Laparotomy for adhesiolysis

D. IVF/ICSI immediately

E. Expectant management for 2 more years

461- A 36-year-old woman with diffuse adenomyosis, infertility 4 years, two failed IUI attempts. Husband's semen is normal. Best next step?

A. Repeat IUI

B. IVF/ICSI

C. Expectant management

D. Adenomyomectomy first in all cases

E. Clomiphene citrate cycles

IVF/ICSI IN PATIENTS WITH MEDICAL DISEASES

462- Which of the following is a recognized indication for choosing ICSI over conventional IVF in HBV/HCV patients?

A. To reduce the risk of viral transmission via seminal fluid

B. To completely eliminate the need for viral screening

C. To avoid the need for embryo cryopreservation

D. To increase risk of OHSS

E. To bypass ovarian stimulation

463- A 37-year-old man with Hepatitis C carrier status, low sperm count, planned for ICSI. What lab precaution is essential?

A. Use the same incubator and dishware as all other patients

B. Segregated cryopreservation tank for his samples

C. No need for viral testing of his partner

D. Proceed with natural cycle only

E. Embryo discard after fertilization

464- Which of the following investigations should be routinely performed before IVF/ICSI regarding Hepatitis?

A. HBsAg, Anti-HCV, HIV screening

B. Liver biopsy for all patients

C. Only ALT/AST without serology

D. Hepatitis serology only if symptomatic

E. No viral testing required

465- Which thyroid investigation is routinely required before IVF/ICSI?

A. Only T3

B. Only T4

C. TSH (± free T4 if abnormal)

D. Thyroid ultrasound for all patients

E. Thyroid antibody panel in every case

466- What is the recommended TSH target in hypothyroid women undergoing IVF/ICSI?

A. <5.0 mIU/L

B. <4.5 mIU/L

C. <2.5–3.0 mIU/L

D. <6.0 mIU/L

E. No specific target

467- Which of the following is TRUE about hypothyroidism in IVF/ICSI?

A. It has no impact on implantation

B. It can increase miscarriage risk if untreated

C. Levothyroxine should only be started after pregnancy

D. TSH monitoring is unnecessary during stimulation

E. Mild hypothyroidism always requires stopping IVF

468- A 29-year-old woman with subclinical hypothyroidism (TSH 4.8 mIU/L, normal T4), positive anti-TPO antibodies, failed 2 IVF cycles. What is the most appropriate management?

A. Levothyroxine supplementation before next IVF attempt

B. Continue IVF without thyroid therapy

C. Hysteroscopy only

D. Donor egg program

E. Stop ART

469- All of the following are potential risks of uncontrolled hyperthyroidism in IVF/ICSI EXCEPT:

A. Increased miscarriage rate

B. Risk of thyrotoxic crisis during pregnancy

C. Adverse impact on implantation

D. Reduced risk of OHSS

E. Obstetric complications

470- A 34-year-old woman with Graves' disease is controlled on PTU, TSH 2.0 mIU/L, free T4 normal. She is scheduled for ICSI. What should be done?

A. Cancel IVF cycle

B. Proceed with ICSI as planned

C. Stop PTU immediately

D. Delay until pregnancy occurs naturally

E. Switch to levothyroxine

471- Which of the following is NOT a routine part of pre-IVF evaluation in SLE patients?

A. Disease activity assessment (clinical/lab)

B. Antiphospholipid antibody testing

C. Renal function assessment

D. Liver biopsy in all cases

E. Complete blood count and clotting profile

472- All of the following are risks in IVF/ICSI for SLE patients EXCEPT:

A. Flare of disease with hormonal stimulation

B. Increased risk of thrombosis

C. Miscarriage associated with antiphospholipid antibodies

D. Increased OHSS risk requiring preventive strategies

E. Guaranteed contraindication to pregnancy in all SLE patients

473- Which of the following drugs is considered relatively safe to continue in SLE patients undergoing IVF?

A. Hydroxychloroquine

B. Methotrexate

C. Cyclophosphamide

D. Mycophenolate mofetil

E. Leflunomide

474- A 34-year-old woman with active lupus nephritis is asking about IVF. What is the best advice?

A. Proceed immediately with stimulation

B. Delay IVF until disease remission is achieved

C. IVF is contraindicated forever

D. Natural conception only

E. Start gonadotropins directly

475- A 36-year-old woman with SLE, recurrent miscarriage, positive lupus anticoagulant, planning ICSI. What is the most important additional management?

A. Anticoagulation with heparin + aspirin during ART and pregnancy

B. No additional therapy needed

C. High-dose steroids only

D. Embryo transfer cancellation

E. Tuboplasty

476- Which is the preferred method of luteal phase support in SLE patients after IVF/ICSI?

A. High-dose hCG injections

B. Natural Progesterone (vaginal /injectable)

C. No luteal phase support is needed

D. Estrogen only

E. Oral Synthetic progesterone

477- A 35-year-old woman with SLE, positive antiphospholipid antibodies, infertility × 4 years, scheduled for ICSI. Which stimulation approach is safest?

A. High-dose gonadotropins with long agonist protocol

B. Antagonist protocol with prophylactic anticoagulation

C. Expectant management

D. IVF contraindicated

E. Dual stimulation protocol always required

478- A 36-year-old with SLE and history of thrombosis, now stable on aspirin + heparin. Planned for IVF. What trigger should be chosen to minimize thrombotic risk?

A. hCG only

B. GnRH agonist trigger

C. Dual trigger with high-dose hCG

D. No trigger needed

E. Oocyte pick-up without stimulation

479- Regarding anticoagulation in SLE patients undergoing oocyte retrieval, which of the following is TRUE?

A. Heparin should be continued without interruption during oocyte retrieval

B. Heparin should be stopped 1 hour before retrieval and resumed immediately after

C. Heparin is contraindicated in all IVF cycles

D. Heparin should only be stopped if the patient develops OHSS

E. Heparin must be stopped 24 hours before retrieval and resumed 12 hours after the procedure

480- A 32-year-old woman with stable SLE, positive antiphospholipid antibodies, scheduled for embryo transfer. What is the recommended strategy?

A. Transfer two embryos to improve chance of pregnancy

B. Cancel transfer

C. Transfer three embryos if blastocysts

D. Single embryo transfer due to high-risk maternal status

E. No role for ART in SLE

481- In a poorly controlled diabetic patient undergoing IVF/ICSI stimulation, which is the most critical risk?

A. Poor ovarian response

B. OHSS

C. Miscarriage risk

D. Implantation failure

E. No significant risk

482- The optimal HbA1c before starting IVF/ICSI is:

A. < 7%

B. < 8%

C. < 6%

D. < 6.5%

E. > 8% acceptable

483- In a Type 1 diabetic patient on insulin pump, when is the best time to optimize glycemic control before IVF?

A. On the day of stimulation start

B. Before embryo transfer

C. At least 3 months before protocol initiation

D. On oocyte retrieval day

E. During pregnancy only

484- Which IVF drug requires caution in diabetic patients with diabetic retinopathy?

A. hCG trigger

B. GnRH agonist

C. Dexamethasone

D. Progesterone luteal support

E. Metformin

485- A 32-year-old woman with Type 2 diabetes, HbA1c = 9%, requesting IVF. Best decision is:

A. Proceed with stimulation

B. Delay IVF until glycemic control

C. Switch to insulin only on retrieval day

D. Use frozen embryo transfer immediately

E. Ignore HbA1c if age < 35

486- A Type 2 diabetic patient on Metformin + Insulin undergoing IVF shows thin endometrium. The most accurate explanation is:

A. Metformin reduces endometrial thickness

B. GnRH analogues are the main cause

C. Diabetes has no relation

D. Poor glycemic control affects endometrium

E. Progesterone luteal support toxicity

487- In a patient with severe heart disease undergoing IVF/ICSI, the main risk during ovarian stimulation is:

A. Thromboembolism

B. OHSS

C. Poor ovarian response

D. Anemia

E. Endometritis

488- Which cardiac condition is considered a strong contraindication for IVF/ICSI until optimized?

A. Controlled hypertension

B. NYHA class III–IV heart failure

C. Mild mitral regurgitation

D. Stable angina

E. PVCs (premature ventricular contractions)

489- The preferred trigger for final oocyte maturation in a woman with high cardiac risk is:

A. hCG trigger

B. Dual trigger (hCG + GnRH agonist)

C. GnRH agonist trigger

D. Natural LH surge only

E. No trigger needed

490- Which medication during IVF should be used with caution in patients on anticoagulation for cardiac disease?

A. Progesterone

B. Estradiol valerate

C. Aspirin

D. LMWH

E. Dexamethasone

491- During IVF/ICSI in women with prosthetic heart valves, the major concern is:

A. Poor ovarian reserve

B. Endometritis

C. Anticoagulation management

D. Risk of OHSS

E. Egg quality reduction

492- A 34-year-old woman with peripartum cardiomyopathy (EF 30%) seeks IVF. Best management is:

A. Start stimulation with close echo monitoring

B. Surrogacy or oocyte donation advised

C. Use natural cycle IVF

D. Proceed with minimal stimulation protocol

E. No contraindication if young age

493- A woman with congenital cyanotic heart disease presents for IVF. Which is most likely during stimulation?

A. Ovarian hyperstimulation

B. High implantation rate

C. Increased oocyte yield

D. No special risk

E. Severe hypoxia and hemodynamic instability

494- A 30-year-old with mechanical mitral valve on warfarin requests IVF. The safest anticoagulation strategy is:

A. Continue warfarin throughout stimulation

B. Stop anticoagulation until transfer

C. Use aspirin only

D. Switch to LMWH during stimulation

E. No anticoagulation needed

495- A 28-year-old with controlled arrhythmia on beta-blockers is undergoing IVF. Which statement is correct?

A. IVF contraindicated

B. Ovarian response will be poor

C. Beta-blockers may be continued with monitoring

D. Switch to digoxin before stimulation

E. Stop all cardiac drugs

496- In a cardiac high-risk patient, the trigger of choice for oocyte maturation is:

A. hCG trigger

B. Dual trigger (hCG + GnRH agonist)

C. No trigger (natural LH only)

D. GnRH agonist trigger

E. Random trigger

497- Which luteal support is safest in patients with cardiac disease?

A. High-dose oral estrogen

B. Vaginal progesterone

C. Injectable hCG

D. GnRH agonist support

E. Corticosteroids only

498- In a patient with prosthetic valve on anticoagulation, the key step in IVF protocol modification is:

A. Stop anticoagulation completely during stimulation

B. Convert warfarin to LMWH during stimulation

C. Use aspirin only

D. Delay IVF until off anticoagulation

E. Proceed without change

499- A 35-year-old woman with dilated cardiomyopathy (EF 35%) desires IVF. Which stimulation protocol is safest?

A. Long agonist protocol with high-dose gonadotropins

B. Antagonist protocol with low-dose gonadotropins

C. Natural cycle without monitoring

D. Dual stimulation protocol

E. No need to modify protocol

500- Patient with arrhythmia on beta-blockers, IVF planned. Which protocol modification is correct?

A. Antagonist protocol with GnRH agonist trigger

B. Long agonist protocol with hCG trigger

C. Short protocol with high gonadotropin doses

D. Natural cycle only

E. IVF contraindicated

501- During stimulation, a patient with heart disease develops shortness of breath. The protocol step to minimize recurrence in future cycles is:

A. Antagonist protocol + freeze-all strategy

B. Long agonist protocol + fresh transfer

C. Increase gonadotropin doses

D. Continue with same stimulation

E. Avoid progesterone support

502- Which strategy is best for a woman with mechanical valve on anticoagulation and significant cardiac risk?

A. Transfer two embryos to increase chance in one cycle

B. Freeze-all strategy and elective SET later

C. Always fresh double embryo transfer

D. Avoid embryo freezing

E. No transfer at all

503- A 32-year-old with congenital heart disease, EF 40%, requesting IVF. What is the safest embryo transfer strategy?

A. Double embryo transfer in fresh cycle

B. Triple embryo transfer if age < 35

C. Elective single embryo transfer (eSET)

D. Random transfer depending on embryo quality

E. Transfer only blastocysts in pairs

504- Why is single embryo transfer (SET) strongly recommended in IVF/ICSI for women with heart disease?

A. To increase chance of twins

B. To reduce risk of multiple pregnancy and cardiac overload

C. To improve ovarian response

D. To shorten stimulation period

E. To avoid luteal support

FERTILITY PRESERVATION

505- Which of the following is considered the standard fertility preservation technique in postpubertal women according to ESHRE?

A. Embryo cryopreservation

B. Ovarian tissue cryopreservation

C. GnRH agonist co-treatment only

D. IVF with immediate transfer

E. Oocyte cryopreservation

506- In prepubertal girls, the only established fertility preservation option:

A. Oocyte cryopreservation

B. Embryo cryopreservation

C. Ovarian tissue cryopreservation

D. In vitro maturation of follicles

E. Ovarian suppression with GnRH agonist

507- In young boys (prepubertal), ESHRE recommends which option for fertility preservation?

A. Sperm cryopreservation

B. Embryo cryopreservation

C. Testicular tissue cryopreservation

D. GnRH agonist suppression

E. Oocyte freezing

508- A 28-year-old woman with breast cancer (ER+) requiring chemotherapy in 2 weeks, which is the most suitable FP option?

A. Ovarian tissue cryopreservation only

B. Random-start ovarian stimulation for oocyte cryopreservation

C. Delay chemotherapy until luteal phase stimulation

D. Use GnRH agonist only

E. No fertility preservation possible

509- Which of the following is NOT considered an established fertility preservation method by ESHRE?

A. Oocyte cryopreservation

B. Embryo cryopreservation

C. Ovarian tissue cryopreservation

D. In vitro maturation (IVM) of oocytes as stand-alone

E. Sperm cryopreservation

510- A 31-year-old woman with severe endometriosis, not yet ready for pregnancy, but concerned about ovarian reserve. Best option?

A. Ovarian suppression with GnRH agonists

B. Oocyte cryopreservation (social FP)

C. IVF with fresh embryo transfer

D. Ovarian tissue cryopreservation only

E. No preservation recommended

511- Which is the main limitation of ovarian tissue cryopreservation in hematologic malignancies?

A. High cost

B. Risk of malignant cell reintroduction

C. Poor ovarian reserve

D. Low pregnancy rates

E. High OHSS risk

512- A 30-year-old with estrogen-receptor positive breast cancer needs urgent oocyte cryopreservation. Which stimulation protocol is recommended?

A. Standard FSH only

B. Random-start with aromatase inhibitor (letrozole) co-stimulation

C. No stimulation allowed

D. hMG + hCG trigger only

E. GnRH agonist suppression alone

513- A 34-year-old woman wishes elective (social) fertility preservation. According to ESHRE, the recommended method is:

A. Oocyte cryopreservation

B. Ovarian tissue cryopreservation

C. Embryo freezing without partner

D. GnRH agonist only

E. No option indicated for social reasons

514- What is the main rationale for using double stimulation (DuoStim) in fertility preservation?

A. To increase number of embryos per transfer

B. To obtain more oocytes in a short time frame

C. To reduce medication doses

D. To prevent OHSS

E. To avoid luteal support

515- Which two phases are used in double stimulation protocol?

A. Follicular phase only

B. Luteal phase only

C. Follicular and luteal phases in the same menstrual cycle

D. Mid-cycle and post-ovulation

E. Any two random cycles

516- In which patients is DuoStim most often indicated for fertility preservation?

A. Women with good ovarian reserve

B. Prepubertal girls

C. Cancer patients with urgent chemotherapy start

D. Women with PCOS

E. Surrogates only

517- A 29-year-old with breast cancer, chemotherapy planned within 6 weeks. Which stimulation approach maximizes oocyte yield?

A. Single follicular stimulation

B. Natural cycle IVF

C. Double stimulation (DuoStim)

D. GnRH agonist suppression

E. Embryo cryopreservation only

518- What is a key advantage of luteal phase stimulation in DuoStim protocols?

A. Produces better-quality embryos than follicular phase

B. Shortens time to chemotherapy without losing oocytes

C. Requires no gonadotropins

D. Avoids anesthesia

E. Eliminates need for cryopreservation

519- Which of the following is a limitation of DuoStim protocols?

A. Cannot be used in cancer patients

B. Higher cost and need for lab flexibility

C. Only applicable in prepubertal girls

D. Contraindicated in low responders

E. Not compatible with embryo freezing

520- A 35-year-old woman with diminished ovarian reserve and urgent fertility preservation. Which protocol provides the best oocyte yield before gonadotoxic therapy?

A. Long GnRH agonist protocol

B. Short flare protocol

C. Antagonist protocol single stimulation

D. DuoStim (double stimulation in one cycle)

E. Natural cycle IVF

521- Which factor most strongly determines the optimal number of oocytes needed for fertility preservation success?

A. AMH alone

B. Age at cryopreservation

C. Stimulation protocol type

D. Trigger used

E. Luteal support type

522- A 29-year-old freezing oocytes for social reasons, wishes one future child. Target number of mature oocytes to be relatively safe is:

A. 3–5

B. 6–10

C. 12–15

D. 20–25

E. >30

523- Which of the following is true regarding oocyte yield and live birth probability?

A. Number of oocytes required decreases with age

B. Number of oocytes required increases with age

C. Oocyte number has no relation to success

D. Only embryo cryopreservation determines outcome

E. 5 oocytes are always sufficient regardless of age

524- According to ESHRE, fertility preservation in women with overt POI is:

A. Strongly recommended

B. Optional in all cases

C. Not recommended

D. Only with GnRH agonists

E. Only with DuoStim protocols

525- A 22-year-old virgin with Hodgkin's lymphoma requires urgent fertility preservation. Which approach is safest for oocyte retrieval?

A. Transvaginal puncture with hymen disruption

B. Transabdominal ultrasound-guided retrieval

C. Ovarian wedge resection

D. Oocyte pick-up via hysteroscopy

E. No fertility preservation possible

526- A virgin patient with low ovarian reserve, needs maximum oocyte yield quickly. Which strategy is appropriate?

A. Transvaginal oocyte pick-up with hymen rupture

B. Transabdominal aspiration + DuoStim protocol

C. Only embryo cryopreservation

D. No preservation possible unless married

E. Wait until menopause

527- Main concern with trans-rectal oocyte retrieval is:

A. Oocyte damage

B. Risk of rectal infection or fistula formation

C. Poor embryo quality

D. Difficulty with ovarian stimulation

E. Contraindication in all cancer patients

528- A 24-year-old virgin, ovaries located deep in pelvis, transabdominal aspiration not feasible. Which retrieval approach can be considered?

A. Standard vaginal puncture despite hymen

B. Laparoscopic ovarian wedge resection

C. Trans-rectal ultrasound–guided oocyte retrieval

D. No fertility preservation possible

E. Only ovarian tissue cryopreservation

529- Which of the following is true about ovarian tissue cryopreservation?

A. Only experimental with no live births reported

B. Established method with >200 live births worldwide

C. Contraindicated in prepubertal girls

D. Requires ovarian stimulation first

E. Not allowed for cancer patients

530- A 30-year-old woman froze 15 mature oocytes. Estimated chance of at least one live birth is around:

A. <20%

B. ~40–50%

C. ~60%

D. ~90%

E. Guaranteed 100%

531- According to ESHRE/ASRM data, optimal number of mature oocytes to bank before age 35 to achieve ~70% chance of live birth is:

A. 5–8

B. 10–15

C. 15–20

D. 25–30

E. >40

532- A 40-year-old woman freezes 10 mature oocytes. Approximate chance of live birth is:

A. <10%

B. 20–30%

C. 40–50%

D. 60–70%

E. >80%

533- Which of the following statements is correct about pregnancy after oocyte freezing?

A. Success is independent of age at freezing

B. Oocyte number and age at freezing determine outcome

C. Every oocyte guarantees one embryo

D. Frozen oocytes have higher implantation than fresh

E. Pregnancy is guaranteed if >10 oocytes are frozen

RECURRENT IMPLANTATION FAILURE (RIF) & ADD-ONS

534- A woman with 3 failed IVF cycles had embryos that reached cleavage stage but never implanted. PGT-A showed euploid embryos. What is the most likely explanation?

A. Embryo factor remains the main cause

B. Uterine/endometrial factor is the main cause

C. Maternal age >35 is the main cause

D. Genetic abnormality not detected by PGT-A

535- A 34-year-old with 3 failed transfers of euploid embryos. Next best investigation is:

A. Semen analysis

B. Repeat ovarian stimulation

C. Empirical aspirin therapy

D. Stop IVF attempts

E. Uterine cavity evaluation (hysteroscopy)

536- Which of the following is *not* a proven cause of RIF?

A. Thin endometrium

B. Embryo aneuploidy

C. Chronic endometritis

D. Paternal karyotype abnormality

E. Luteal support with progesterone

537- A 29-year-old with RIF, endometrial thickness 6 mm at transfer. Which intervention may improve outcomes?

A. Endometrial scratching only

B. High-dose gonadotropins

C. Hysteroscopic metroplasty

D. Strategies to optimize endometrial growth

E. GnRH agonist suppression

538- Which of the following tests is most useful in evaluating embryonic factors in RIF?

A. AMH testing

B. Preimplantation genetic testing for aneuploidy (PGT-A)

C. Vitamin D level

D. Doppler uterine artery flow

E. LH surge monitoring

539- A woman with RIF, normal uterus, recurrent biochemical pregnancies, antiphospholipid antibodies positive. Cause is most likely:

A. Embryo fragmentation

B. Thin endometrium

C. IVF lab error

D. Poor sperm DNA quality

E. Maternal thrombophilia

540- Which intervention is NOT routinely recommended by ESHRE 2023 for RIF?

A. PGT-A in advanced maternal age

B. Correction of intrauterine pathology

C. Empirical immunotherapy (e.g. IVIG, steroids)

D. Endometrial cavity assessment

E. Consideration of blastocyst transfer

541- Patient with RIF, normal hysteroscopy, good endometrium, euploid embryos. According to ESHRE, which remains controversial?

A. Endometrial receptivity array (ERA)

B. Correction of polyps

C. PGT-A in advanced age

D. Screening for uterine adhesions

E. Thin endometrium optimization

542- Which of the following endocrine tests is advised in RIF evaluation as per ESHRE?

A. TSH, thyroid antibodies

B. NK cell function

C. ERA receptivity panel

D. Coagulation genetic screening for all

E. Vitamin D level only

543- A 35-year-old woman with recurrent implantation failure has normal investigations. Which intervention is evidence-based and most likely to improve implantation?

A. Low molecular weight heparin

B. Endometrial scratching

C. Blastocyst transfer with PGT-A

D. Intralipid infusion

E. ERA test

544- Woman with RIF and antiphospholipid antibody syndrome. According to ESHRE:

A. Anticoagulation indicated only if APS confirmed

B. Anticoagulation for all RIF patients

C. Immunotherapy superior to heparin

D. No role for anticoagulation

E. IVF contraindicated

545- Which of the following is *recommended* in the investigation of recurrent implantation failure (RIF) according to ESHRE 2023?

A. Vitamin D testing

B. Lifestyle factors reassessment

C. Microbiome profiling

D. Uterine NK cell testing

E. HLA-C compatibility

546- A 29-year-old with RIF, hysteroscopy normal, embryos euploid, endometrium good. Which of the following is NOT recommended by ESHRE?

A. Vitamin D testing

B. Chronic endometritis testing

C. Progesterone levels in luteal phase

D. Lifestyle reassessment

E. Endometrial thickness reassessment

547- Which immunological tests are NOT recommended in RIF work-up according to ESHRE 2023?

A. NK cell testing (peripheral and uterine)

B. Blood cytokine profiling

C. HLA-C compatibility

D. Uterine T lymphocyte testing

E. All of the above

548- Woman with RIF, clinician suggests sperm DNA fragmentation testing. According to ESHRE, this is:

A. Recommended for all cases

B. Only if male factor infertility present

C. Not recommended

D. Alternative to PGT-A

E. First-line after 2 failed cycles

549- A 35-year-old woman with 3 failed euploid blastocyst transfers is referred for recurrent implantation failure (RIF) work-up. According to ESHRE 2023, which of the following steps are RECOMMENDED in her evaluation and management?

A. Lifestyle reassessment and optimization

B. Endometrial thickness reassessment and possible estradiol adjustment

C. Genetic counselling ± PGT if chromosomal abnormality detected

D. Uterine evaluation with hysteroscopy/3D US

E. All of the above

550- A 32-year-old with unexplained RIF is seeking "extra" interventions. According to ESHRE 2023, which of the following are NOT RECOMMENDED as routine interventions?

A. Vitamin D testing and supplementation in all cases

B. Immunological therapies (IVIG, intralipid, PBMC infusion)

C. Intrauterine biologics (PRP, hCG, G-CSF)

D. Endometrial scratching or assisted hatching

E. All of the above

551- According to ESHRE, which of the following add-ons is classified as "not recommended"?

A. DNA fregmentation test

B. Time-lapse incubation

C. Immunological treatments (intralipid, IVIG)

D. Endometrial scratching

E. All of the above

552- A 36-year-old with recurrent implantation failure requests endometrial scratching before next transfer. According to ESHRE:

A. Strongly recommended

B. Can be considered in all women

C. Not recommended due to lack of benefit

D. Equivalent to blastocyst transfer

E. Increases miscarriage rate

553- Which laboratory add-on is considered safe and may improve logistics, but not proven to improve live birth rate?

A. Time-lapse imaging/incubation

B. ERA testing

C. PRP intrauterine infusion

D. PGT-A in all patients

E. Intralipid infusion

554- A couple asks about "immune therapy" (IVIG/intralipid) as an add-on to IVF. ESHRE recommendation is:

A. Strong evidence of benefit

B. Optional in all patients

C. Not recommended

D. Recommended only with PCOS

E. Improves oocyte quality

555- According to ESHRE/ASRM, elective freeze-all in all IVF cycles is:

A. Strongly recommended for all patients

B. Not routinely recommended, only in specific indications

C. Contraindicated in young women

D. Replaces fresh embryo transfer as gold standard

E. Mandatory after PGT-A

556- Embryo glue refers to transfer medium enriched with:

A. Progesterone

B. Hyaluronic acid

C. Growth hormone

D. Albumin

E. Estrogen

557- A 33-year-old with unexplained infertility asks about embryo glue to improve implantation. Current guideline stance is:

A. Clear evidence supports use in all patients

B. Evidence limited, may be considered but not routine

C. Proven to be superior to blastocyst transfer

D. Replaces luteal support

E. Only useful in oocyte donors

558- A 32-year-old with 3 failed embryo transfers asks about intrauterine hCG infusion before transfer. What is the correct counselling?

A. It guarantees improved live birth rate

B. It replaces progesterone luteal support

C. It is superior to blastocyst transfer

D. It is experimental with inconsistent evidence

E. It is mandatory in RIF patients

559- A 35-year-old with RIF asks about intralipid infusion before embryo transfer. Appropriate counselling is:

A. Strong evidence it improves live birth

B. Evidence insufficient, not recommended outside research

C. It replaces luteal progesterone support

D. Works only with fresh embryo transfers

E. It guarantees implantation

560- Platelet-rich plasma (PRP) intrauterine infusion is:

A. Established therapy

B. Mandatory in thin endometrium

C. Equivalent to embryo glue

D. Replaces estradiol treatment

E. Experimental add-on with insufficient evidence

561- ERA (Endometrial Receptivity Array) testing is:

A. Controversial, not routine, may be considered in RIF

B. Recommended for all IVF patients

C. Mandatory in PCOS

D. Equivalent to PGT-A

E. Replaces hysteroscopy

562- A 34-year-old with RIF and persistent thin endometrium (<7 mm) asks about PRP infusion before transfer. Correct counselling is:

A. PRP is established therapy with proven live birth benefit

B. PRP guarantees improvement in endometrial thickness

C. PRP eliminates the need for estradiol support

D. PRP reduces miscarriage directly

E. PRP is experimental, with limited and inconsistent evidence

563- Which of the following is the main rationale for sperm DNA fragmentation (SDF) testing in IVF/ICSI?

A. To assess sperm motility only

B. To evaluate chromatin integrity linked to embryo development and miscarriage

C. To measure testosterone levels

D. To predict OHSS risk

E. To assess endometrial receptivity

564- According to ESHRE 2023, routine use of sperm DNA fragmentation testing in IVF/ICSI is:

A. Strongly recommended for all infertile couples

B. Optional in all patients with unexplained infertility

C. Not recommended

D. Mandatory in donor sperm cycles

E. Replaces semen analysis

565- Which of the following statements regarding sildenafil use in ART is most accurate?

A. It is routinely recommended in all IVF/ICSI patients

B. It is only useful in women with recurrent miscarriage

C. Its use is experimental with limited evidence on improving live birth rates

D. It replaces the need for estrogen therapy in endometrial preparation

E. It is effective as adjuvant in treatment of thin endometrium

566- A 32-year-old woman with poor ovarian reserve is about to start IVF stimulation. She asks if taking low-dose aspirin before stimulation will improve her response. According to guidelines, the correct recommendation is:

A. Aspirin improves ovarian response and is recommended

B. Aspirin should be used only in poor responders

C. Aspirin use is not recommended in low responders

D. Aspirin must be started in all IVF cycles to improve implantation

567- A 36-year-old woman with Low ovarian response (POSEIDON group 4) is considering intra-ovarian PRP before her next IVF cycle. According to current evidence, what is the most accurate statement?

A. PRP consistently improves live birth rates in poor responders

B. PRP is experimental with limited evidence on reproductive outcomes

C. PRP is strongly recommended by ESHRE in poor responders

D. PRP has proven superiority over DHEA and growth hormone

E. PRP Equivalent to oocyte donation in terms of efficacy

COMMON CHALLENGES OF IVF/ICSI

568- In which situation is myomectomy before IVF most strongly recommended?

A. Intramural fibroid 2.5 cm not distorting the cavity

B. Subserosal fibroid 5 cm

C. Submucosal fibroid distorting the cavity

D. Intramural fibroid 3.5 cm without cavity distortion

E. Cervical fibroid

569- A 34-year-old woman has multiple intramural fibroids, the largest measuring 3.8 cm, none distorting the cavity. She is preparing for IVF. What is the most evidence-based management?

A. Mandatory laparoscopic myomectomy

B. Proceed with IVF without surgery

C. Pre-treatment with GnRH agonist for 3 months

D. Hysteroscopic resection

E. Uterine artery embolization

570- Which of the following is least appropriate as a management strategy for women with fibroids undergoing IVF?

A. Expectant management for subserosal fibroid 2 cm

B. Hysteroscopic removal of submucosal fibroid distorting cavity

C. Myomectomy for symptomatic fibroid with cavity distortion

D. Uterine artery embolization before IVF

E. Proceeding with IVF in patient with stable intramural fibroid 3 cm not affecting cavity

571- A 32-year-old woman underwent myomectomy for a large intramural fibroid. The operative note states: "Endometrial cavity was entered during surgery." She asks when she can proceed with IVF/ICSI. What is the most appropriate recommendation?

A. IVF can be started immediately in the next cycle regardless of cavity entry

B. Wait at least 1 month before IVF in all cases of myomectomy

C. Wait 3 months if cavity was not entered, 6 months if cavity was entered

D. Wait 6 months after surgery irrespective of cavity status

E. IVF should only be attempted after 12 months post-myomectomy

572- A patient forgets to administer the trigger injection (hCG) at the instructed time before oocyte retrieval. What is the main risk?

A. Empty follicle syndrome

B. Embryo aneuploidy

C. Poor endometrial receptivity

D. Multiple pregnancy

E. Thin endometrium

573- A patient undergoing IVF forgets to administer the hCG trigger injection at the instructed time before oocyte retrieval. What is the most appropriate management?

A. Proceed with oocyte retrieval at the planned time without trigger

B. Administer the hCG as soon as remembered and reschedule oocyte retrieval accordingly

C. Double the hCG dose the next morning and keep retrieval on schedule

D. Cancel the cycle immediately and restart stimulation next month

E. Replace hCG with progesterone and continue as planned

574- A woman undergoing IVF stimulation with daily FSH injections forgets her dose on day 5 of stimulation. What is the most appropriate advice?

A. Double the next day's dose to compensate

B. Skip the missed dose and continue as normal

C. Contact the clinic for further instructions

D. Take the missed dose at the same time the next day

E. Take the missed dose as soon as she remembers, then continue as scheduled

575- Which of the following IVF medications is most critical in terms of timing, where a missed or delayed dose may completely compromise the cycle?

A. Estradiol supplementation in FET cycles

B. Progesterone luteal phase support

C. Gonadotropin injections (FSH)

D. GnRH antagonist during stimulation

E. Prenatal vitamins

576- A patient in an antagonist IVF protocol forgets to take her GnRH antagonist dose on stimulation day 7. What is the main risk?

A. Poor follicular growth

B. Premature LH surge and ovulation

C. Reduced oocyte quality

D. Increased ovarian hyperstimulation

E. Thin endometrium

577- During ovarian stimulation for IVF, which of the following findings most strongly suggest a premature LH surge and possible ovulation?

A. Rising estradiol levels with multiple growing follicles

B. Sudden fall in estradiol levels with collapsed follicles on ultrasound

C. Persistently low progesterone during stimulation

D. Endometrium remaining thin despite adequate estrogen support

E. Stable LH levels and unruptured follicles on scan

578- A woman undergoing ovarian stimulation for IVF is found to have a sudden fall in estradiol with evidence of collapsed follicles on ultrasound, suggesting premature LH surge and ovulation. What is the most appropriate management?

A. Continue stimulation and schedule trigger as planned

B. Cancel the cycle and plan a new stimulation protocol with GnRH antagonist/agonist cover

C. Give higher dose of gonadotropins and continue stimulation

D. Proceed directly with embryo transfer without oocyte retrieval

E. Start luteal phase progesterone support immediately and attempt oocyte retrieval

579- A woman undergoing IVF stimulation was instructed to take her hCG trigger at 10:00 pm for oocyte retrieval 36 hours later. She mistakenly took it at 1:00 am (≈3 hours delay). What is the most appropriate management?

A. Cancel the cycle because timing of hCG was missed

B. Proceed with oocyte retrieval at the originally scheduled time (36 hours after planned trigger)

C. Adjust oocyte retrieval timing to 35–36 hours after the actual Hcg administration

D. Give an extra dose of hCG in the morning and keep retrieval on schedule

E. Convert the cycle to intrauterine insemination (IUI) instead of retrieval

580- A woman undergoing IVF forgets to take her vaginal progesterone dose on day 3 after embryo transfer. She remembers the next morning. What is the most appropriate management?

A. Skip the missed dose and continue as scheduled

B. Double the next dose to compensate for the missed one

C. Take the missed dose as soon as she remembers and continue regular dosing

D. Stop progesterone completely since it will not affect the outcome

E. Restart the entire luteal support protocol from day 1

581- A woman undergoing IVF has luteal support with progesterone. She presents with vaginal bleeding on day 10 after embryo transfer. What is the most appropriate action?

A. Stop luteal support immediately

B. Continue progesterone and perform pregnancy test on scheduled day

C. Switch to oral progesterone only

D. Add estrogen therapy immediately

E. Cancel the cycle and plan a new stimulation

582- A woman becomes pregnant after IVF and is on estradiol tablets plus vaginal progesterone for luteal support. She develops severe hyperemesis gravidarum and cannot tolerate oral medications. What is the most appropriate management?

A. Stop all hormonal support immediately since pregnancy is established

B. Continue only vaginal progesterone and discontinue estradiol tablets

C. Switch estradiol to transdermal or vaginal route and continue progesterone

D. Replace oral estradiol with high-dose oral progesterone

E. Stop estradiol but double the progesterone dose vaginally

583- Which congenital uterine anomaly is most consistently associated with implantation failure and miscarriage in IVF/ICSI?

A. Arcuate uterus

B. Septate uterus

C. Bicornuate uterus

D. Didelphys uterus

E. Unicornuate uterus

584- A 30-year-old woman with a diagnosed arcuate uterus is planning IVF. What is the most appropriate management?

A. Hysteroscopic metroplasty before IVF

B. Proceed with IVF without surgical intervention

C. Laparotomy with uterine reconstruction

D. Uterine artery embolization

E. Cancel IVF and advise natural conception

585- Which of the following statements about bicornuate uterus and IVF is most accurate?

A. Always requires surgical correction before IVF

B. Does not typically impair implantation but increases obstetric complications

C. Has the same prognosis as septate uterus

D. Should be reclassified as arcuate in IVF context

E. Improves pregnancy rates after hysteroscopic metroplasty

586- In a patient with unicornuate uterus undergoing IVF, which outcome is most likely?

A. Normal implantation and live birth rates identical to controls

B. Always requires metroplasty before IVF

C. Higher chance of multiple gestation

D. Reduced ovarian reserve due to uterine anomaly

E. Increased risk of miscarriage and preterm delivery

587- Which uterine anomaly has the strongest evidence that surgical correction improves IVF outcomes?

A. Bicornuate uterus

B. Arcuate uterus

C. Septate uterus

D. Didelphys uterus

E. Unicornuate uterus

588- Which of the following best describes the effect of endometrial polyps on IVF outcomes?

A. B. May reduce implantation and pregnancy rates depending on size and number

B. Always prevents implantation

C. Improves endometrial receptivity

D. No association with pregnancy outcomes

E. Increases oocyte retrieval rates

589- A 32-year-old woman scheduled for IVF is found to have a 1.8 cm endometrial polyp on ultrasound. What is the most appropriate management?

A. Proceed directly with IVF without intervention

B. Hysteroscopic polypectomy before IVF

C. High-dose estrogen therapy

D. Uterine artery embolization

E. Myomectomy

590- Which of the following endometrial polyp characteristics is most likely to impair IVF implantation?

A. Small sessile polyp <5 mm

B. Large polyp >1.5 cm protruding into uterine cavity

C. Multiple polyps confined to endocervical canal

D. Asymptomatic polyp detected incidentally during stimulation

E. Calcified endometrial polyp >1 mm

591- A patient underwent oocyte retrieval and a fresh transfer was planned, but a newly diagnosed endometrial polyp is detected during endometrial assessment. What is the best management?

A. Proceed with fresh transfer as planned

B. Cancel embryo transfer and perform polypectomy, then freeze embryos

C. Ignore the finding because polyps do not affect implantation

D. Increase luteal support to overcome implantation defect

E. Start GnRH agonist therapy instead of transfer

592- Which of the following is the most appropriate method for definitive diagnosis and treatment of endometrial polyps before IVF?

A. Saline infusion sonohysterography

B. Blind dilation and curettage

C. Hysteroscopy with resection

D. MRI pelvis

E. Endometrial biopsy

593- Which of the following best describes the impact of a cesarean scar defect (niche) on IVF outcomes?

A. No effect on implantation or pregnancy

B. Always causes uterine rupture during stimulation

C. May be associated with lower implantation and pregnancy rates

D. Improves endometrial receptivity by increasing vascularity

E. Has the same prognosis as arcuate uterus

594- A 34-year-old woman with a history of two cesarean sections is preparing for IVF. Transvaginal ultrasound shows a cesarean scar defect with fluid collection in the niche & Postmenstrual spotting . What is the most appropriate management before embryo transfer?

A. Proceed with embryo transfer without intervention

B. Perform correction of the scar defect

C. Start high-dose estrogen therapy only

D. Ignore the finding and increase luteal support

E. Repeat cesarean section before IVF

595- Which is the gold standard diagnostic method for cesarean scar defect before IVF?

A. Hysterosalpingography (HSG)

B. MRI pelvis only

C. Transabdominal ultrasound only

D. Endometrial biopsy

E. hysteroscopy

596- In a patient with a previous cesarean section undergoing IVF assessment, which is the correct method for measuring the size of a cesarean scar defect (niche) on transvaginal ultrasound or saline infusion sonohysterography?

A. Measure only the length of the hypoechoic area parallel to the endometrial cavity

B. Assess niche size using uterine volume measurements alone

C. Evaluate endometrial thickness above the cesarean scar only

D. Measure niche depth, width, and length, and calculate residual myometrial thickness (RMT)

E. Use Doppler flow indices as the primary tool for size determination

597- In women with a cesarean scar defect (niche) undergoing IVF, which statement regarding residual myometrial thickness (RMT) is most accurate?

A. RMT has no clinical relevance in IVF outcomes

B. An RMT <2.5–3 mm is associated with higher risk of fluid accumulation and poor implantation

C. RMT >1 mm is always safe for embryo transfer

D. RMT measurement is only important during pregnancy, not before IVF

E. RMT should be assessed by MRI rather than ultrasound for IVF planning

598- Which of the following is NOT recommended as a treatment option for cesarean scar niche before IVF?

A. Hysteroscopic resection

B. Laparoscopic niche repair

C. Vaginal niche repair

D. Expectant management if asymptomatic and no fluid

E. Myomectomy of the scar site

599- In which situation is laparoscopic or vaginal niche repair preferred over hysteroscopic resection before IVF?

A. Niche with residual myometrial thickness (RMT) >5 mm

B. Small asymptomatic niche without fluid accumulation

C. Niche with RMT <2.5–3 mm and large defect

D. Niche detected only during pregnancy

E. All niches regardless of thickness

600- In women with a cesarean scar defect (niche) preparing for IVF, in which situation is hysteroscopic correction most appropriate?

A. Symptomatic niche with fluid collection and residual myometrial thickness >3 mm

B. Asymptomatic small niche with residual myometrial thickness <2 mm

C. Large niche with residual myometrial thickness <2.5 mm

D. Any cesarean scar niche regardless of symptoms or thickness

E. Niche detected only during pregnancy in second trimester

601- A woman with previous cesarean deliveries is undergoing IVF. During endometrial assessment, persistent fluid is noted in the cavity arising from the scar niche. What is the best next step?

A. Proceed with fresh transfer

B. Freeze all embryos and correct the scar defect before transfer

C. Add aspirin and heparin to improve implantation

D. Administer antibiotics and continue with transfer

E. Cancel IVF treatment permanently

602- After hysteroscopic niche resection, when is it generally considered safe to proceed with embryo transfer in IVF?

A. Immediately in the next cycle

B. After 2–3 cycles to allow healing

C. After 6 months minimum

D. Only after hysterectomy

E. No waiting period is needed

ANSWERS

380	D	415	B
381	B	416	C
382	D	417	E
383	C	418	B
384	C	419	D
385	D	420	B
386	B	421	B
387	B	422	D
388	B	423	C
389	E	424	C
390	D	425	A
391	B	426	D
392	E	427	D
393	B	428	D
394	D	429	E
395	C	430	B
396	D	431	B
397	A	432	B
398	D	433	E
399	D	434	B
400	B	435	B
401	C	436	C
402	C	437	D
403	C	438	E
404	D	439	C
405	D	440	E
406	B	441	B
407	D	442	B
408	B	443	D
409	B	444	C
410	E	445	E
411	C	446	C
412	B	447	C
413	D	448	B
414	B	449	E

450	D	485	B
451	D	486	D
452	C	487	A
453	B	488	B
454	D	489	C
455	B	490	B
456	B	491	C
457	B	492	B
458	E	493	E
459	C	494	D
460	B	495	C
461	B	496	D
462	A	497	B
463	B	498	B
464	A	499	B
465	C	500	A
466	C	501	A
467	B	502	B
468	A	503	C
469	D	504	B
470	B	505	E
471	D	506	C
472	E	507	C
473	A	508	B
474	B	509	D
475	A	510	B
476	B	511	B
477	B	512	B
478	B	513	A
479	E	514	B
480	D	515	C
481	C	516	C
482	C	517	C
483	C	518	B
484	A	519	B

520	D	555	B
521	B	556	B
522	C	557	B
523	B	558	D
524	C	559	B
525	B	560	E
526	B	561	A
527	B	562	E
528	C	563	B
529	B	564	C
530	C	565	C
531	C	566	C
532	B	567	B
533	B	568	C
534	B	569	B
535	E	570	D
536	E	571	C
537	D	572	A
538	B	573	B
539	E	574	C
540	C	575	D
541	A	576	B
542	A	577	B
543	C	578	B
544	A	579	C
545	B	580	C
546	A	581	B
547	E	582	C
548	C	583	B
549	E	584	B
550	E	585	B
551	E	586	E
552	C	587	C
553	A	588	A
554	C	589	B

590	591	592	593	594	595	596	597	598	599	600	601	602
B	B	C	C	B	E	D	B	E	C	A	B	B

PART 2

TRUE/FALSE QUESTIONS IN IVF/ICSI

1. Regarding ovarian stimulation in IVF/ICSI:

A. GnRH agonists can be used for pituitary downregulation ( )

B. Antagonist protocols completely eliminate the risk of OHSS ( )

C. Clomiphene citrate is commonly used for controlled ovarian stimulation ( )

D. Gonadotropins are the mainstay drugs for stimulation ( )

E. Monitoring is usually done by ultrasound and estradiol measurement ( )

2. With respect to Oocyte retrieval:

A. It is usually performed 30 hours after hCG trigger ( )

B. Transvaginal ultrasound-guided aspiration is the standard method ( )

C. General anesthesia is always required ( )

D. Empty follicle syndrome may occasionally occur ( )

E. Oocyte retrieval carries a risk of pelvic infection ( )

3. Concerning fertilization and ICSI:

A. ICSI bypasses the zona pellucida penetration step ( )

B. ICSI guarantees 100% fertilization ( )

C. Conventional IVF may fail in cases of poor sperm motility ( )

D. Oocyte quality influences fertilization success ( )

E. ICSI is indicated in mild male factor infertility ( )

4. Regarding embryo culture:

A. Embryos are typically cultured to day 3 (cleavage stage) or day 5 (blastocyst) ( )

B. Sequential culture media support prolonged embryo development ( )

C. Extended culture always guarantees higher live birth rates ( )

D. Blastocyst transfer may allow better selection ( )

E. Culture conditions must mimic the in-vivo environment ( )

5. With respect to embryo transfer:

A. Ultrasound guidance improves success rates ( )

B. Single embryo transfer reduces risk of multiple pregnancy ( )

C. Embryo transfer is always done under general anesthesia ( )

D. Endometrial thickness is one factor influencing success ( )

E. Transfer of poor-quality embryos never results in pregnancy ( )

6. Concerning luteal phase support in IVF/ICSI:

A. Progesterone supplementation is standard practice ( )

B. hCG may be used with safety for luteal support ( )

C. Luteal support is unnecessary in antagonist cycles ( )

D. Vaginal progesterone is commonly used ( )

E. Duration of support may extend until confirmation of pregnancy ( )

7. In relation to OHSS (ovarian hyperstimulation syndrome):

A. It is characterized by decrease vascular permeability ( )

B. Mild OHSS may cause ascites and hemoconcentration ( )

C. GnRH antagonist protocols eliminate the risk completely ( )

D. “Coasting” can be used to reduce risk ( )

E. Use of a GnRH agonist trigger in antagonist cycles can reduce OHSS risk ()

8. Regarding cryopreservation:

A. Vitrification is not the preferred method for oocyte and embryo freezing ( )

B. Slow freezing is superior to vitrification ( )

C. Cryopreservation may be used for fertility preservation in cancer patients ( )

D. Frozen embryo transfer (FET) can achieve live birth rates comparable to fresh transfer ( )

E. Sperm cannot be cryopreserved indefinitely ( )

9. With respect to preimplantation genetic testing (PGT):

A. PGT-A is used for aneuploidy screening ( )

B. PGT-M is for monogenic disease ( )

C. Biopsy may be performed at cleavage stage only ( )

D. PGT guarantees a healthy live birth ( )

E. Mosaicism can complicate interpretation ( )

10. Concerning fertilization failure:

A. Not occur in normal semen analysis ( )

B. Total fertilization failure is more common in conventional IVF than ICSI ( )

C. Artificial oocyte activation may be used in selected cases ( )

D. ICSI completely prevents fertilization failure ( )

E. Oocyte-related abnormalities are never implicated in failed fertilization

11. Regarding poor ovarian response:

A. Defined as retrieval of fewer than 3 oocytes in a stimulation cycle ( )

B. Advanced maternal age is not a risk factor ( )

C. Increasing gonadotropin dose always overcomes poor response ( )

D. AMH and AFC are predictors of ovarian response ( )

E. Low responders have lower pregnancy rates ( )

12. With respect to embryo grading:

A. Embryo morphology is not a predictor of implantation ( )

B. Blastocyst grading includes assessment of inner cell mass and trophectoderm ( )

C. All poor morphology embryos are non-viable ( )

D. Time-lapse imaging increase pregnancy & live birth rate ( )

E. Fragmentation is one of the grading criteria ( )

13. Concerning complications of IVF/ICSI:

A. OHSS is the most specific iatrogenic complication ( )

B. Multiple pregnancy is the most common complication ( )

C. Ectopic pregnancy risk is reduced after IVF ( )

D. Ovarian torsion may occur after stimulation ( )

E. Miscarriage rates are not influenced by maternal age ( )

14. Regarding success rates in IVF/ICSI:

A. Female age is the strongest predictor of success ( )

B. Implantation rates decline with advanced maternal age ( )

C. Live birth rates are identical at all ages ( )

D. Male age has no impact on outcomes ( )

E. Embryo quality strongly influences success ( )

15. With respect to embryo implantation:

A. The "window of implantation" occurs in the follicular phase ( )

B. Endometrial receptivity is influenced by progesterone ( )

C. Chronic endometritis has no effect on implantation ( )

D. Thin endometrium may reduce implantation rates ( )

E. Immunological factors has major role in implantation ( )

16. Concerning natural cycle IVF:

A. Uses minimal or no stimulation ( )

B. Yields higher oocyte numbers than stimulated cycles ( )

C. May be useful in women with very low ovarian reserve ( )

D. Carries no risk of OHSS ( )

E. Is widely used as standard IVF practice ( )

17. Regarding indications for ICSI:

A. Severe oligoasthenoteratozoospermia ( )

B. History of fertilization failure in previous IVF ( )

C. Male partner with obstructive azoospermia ( )

D. Unexplained infertility where sperm is normal ( )

E. Mild male factor with normal fertilization in past cycles ( )

18. With respect to multiple pregnancy in ART:

A. The risk increases with multiple embryo transfer ( )

B. Single embryo transfer reduces the risk ( )

C. Multiple pregnancy carries increased maternal and neonatal risks ( )

D. Multiple pregnancy is the desired outcome of ART ( )

E. National guidelines often recommend elective single embryo transfer in young women ( )

19. Concerning ovarian reserve and ART outcomes:

A. AMH reflects the number of the antral follicle pool ( )

B. Low AFC predicts high ovarian response ( )

C. High AMH is associated with lower risk of OHSS ( )

D. Ovarian reserve tests perfectly predict pregnancy outcomes ( )

E. Basal FSH is used as an indirect marker of ovarian reserve ( )

20. Regarding sperm retrieval techniques:

A. TESE involves testicular sperm extraction ( )

B. PESA refers to percutaneous epididymal sperm aspiration ( )

C. MESA is microsurgical epididymal sperm aspiration ( )

D. Sperm retrieval is only possible in obstructive azoospermia ( )

E. Retrieved sperm can be used with IVF ( )

21. With respect to endometrial preparation for frozen embryo transfer (FET):

A. Can be natural or hormone replacement based ( )

B. Estrogen is used to build up endometrium ( )

C. hCG safe to support luteal phase ( )

D. Endometrial thickness of >14 mm is generally favorable ( )

E. No monitoring is required at all ( )

22. Concerning add-on therapies in IVF:

A. Endometrial scratching is universally proven to improve outcomes ( )

B. Use of growth hormone recommended in Low responders ( )

C. Assisted hatching may benefit selected cases ( )

D. Immunotherapy is established standard practice ( )

E. Most add-ons lack strong evidence ( )

23. Regarding complications of oocyte retrieval:

A. Pelvic infection is a common complication ( )

B. Ovarian bleeding may occur ( )

C. Ureteric injury is a common complication ( )

D. Injury to pelvic vessels is impossible ( )

E. The procedure is generally considered safe ( )

24. Regarding lab conditions in IVF/ICSI:

A. Stable temperature and pH are essential ( )

B. High oxygen tension enhances embryo development ( )

C. CO_2 incubators are commonly used ( )

D. Volatile organic compounds can harm embryos ( )

E. Culture media must be quality controlled ( )

25. With respect to ICSI risks:

A. May decrease risk of imprinting disorders ( )

B. Bypasses natural sperm selection ( )

C. Completely eliminates risk of genetic transmission ( )

D. Requires careful counseling of couples ( )

E. Increases fertilization rate in male factor infertility ( )

26. Concerning blastocyst transfer:

A. Improves selection of viable embryos ( )

B. Reduces multiple pregnancy when combined with SET ( )

C. Guarantees implantation ( )

D. Not requires good embryo culture systems ( )

E. May lead to fewer embryos available for freezing ( )

27. Regarding ovarian hyperstimulation syndrome (OHSS):

A. Caused by increase Gonadotropins dose > 225 ( )

B. VEGF plays a role in pathophysiology ( )

C. Triggering with GnRH agonist increase risk in antagonist cycles ( )

D. Always occurs in natural cycles ( )

E. Severe cases may require hospitalization ( )

28. With respect to donor oocytes:

A. Useful in women with premature ovarian insufficiency ( )

B. Success mainly depends on donor age ( )

C. Recipients require endometrial preparation ( )

D. Donor age has no impact on outcomes ( )

E. Indicated in repeated poor ovarian response ( )

29. Concerning embryo selection technologies:

A. Morphology is not the basic selection method ( )

B. Time-lapse imaging can monitor cleavage patterns ( )

C. Artificial intelligence may assist embryo ranking ( )

D. All methods guarantee successful implantation ( )

E. Non-invasive testing of spent media is evidence based ( )

30. Regarding sperm DNA fragmentation:

A. High levels may impair fertilization ( )

B. May increased miscarriage rates ( )

C. Cannot be assessed by laboratory tests ( )

D. May be improved by lifestyle changes ( )

E. Is higher in smokers ( )

31. According to Eshre Guidelines, ART in endometriosis:

A. Long protocol is the best in endometriosis ( )

B. Endometriomas always need surgical removal before IVF ( )

C. Ovarian reserve not affected by endometriosis ( )

D. Fertility outcomes may be the same to unexplained infertility ( )

E. Medical suppression with GnRH agonists prior to IVF may help ( )

32. Concerning multiple failed IVF cycles:

A. Maternal age is an important prognostic factor ( )

B. Recurrent implantation failure may be related to uterine factors ( )

C. Changing stimulation protocol always ensures success ( )

D. PGT not recommended at all ( )

E. Lifestyle factors should be reassessed ( )

33. Regarding complications in pregnancy after ART:

A. Risk of multiple pregnancy is higher ( )

B. Ectopic pregnancy is more common than in spontaneous conceptions ( )

C. Miscarriage risk is unaffected by maternal age ( )

D. Preterm birth is less frequent ( )

E. Hypertensive disorders are less common ( )

34. Concerning luteal phase in ART:

A. Corpus luteum function is impaired after controlled ovarian stimulation ( )

B. Progesterone deficiency may compromise implantation ( )

C. Estrogen alone is sufficient for luteal support ( )

D. Vaginal progesterone is commonly prescribed ( )

E. Luteal support improves pregnancy outcomes ( )

35. With respect to cryopreserved embryo transfer (FET):

A. FET avoids risk of OHSS ( )

B. Endometrial preparation can be only medicated ( )

C. Live birth rates can be comparable to fresh transfer ( )

D. Frozen embryos have higher risk of congenital anomalies ( )

E. Embryos can be stored indefinitely ( )

36. Concerning the PPOS (Progestin-Primed Ovarian Stimulation) protocol:

A. Uses oral progestins to prevent premature LH surge ( )

B. Can be combined with gonadotropins for stimulation ( )

C. Requires GnRH antagonist for pituitary suppression ( )

D. Embryos are cryopreserved due to endometrial effects ( )

E. Considered an alternative for high responders ( )

37. Regarding sperm preparation techniques:

A. Swim-up method selects motile sperm ( )

B. Density gradient centrifugation separates normal sperm ( )

C. Preparation reduces infection risk ( )

D. All techniques completely eliminate abnormal sperm ( )

E. Preparation is required before IUI and IVF ( )

38. Concerning IVM (In Vitro Maturation):

A. Involves retrieval of immature oocytes from unstimulated or minimally stimulated ovaries ( )

B. Oocytes are matured in culture before fertilization ( )

C. Increase the risk of OHSS ( )

D. Is widely used as the standard ART protocol ( )

E. May be useful in women with PCOS ( )

39. Concerning embryo transfer technique:

A. Transfer should be atraumatic ( )

B. Ultrasound guidance not improves pregnancy rates ( )

C. Tenaculum is always required ( )

D. Catheter choice may influence outcomes ( )

E. Difficult transfers not reduce success ( )

40. Regarding sperm cryopreservation:

A. Used in cancer patients before chemotherapy ( )

B. Can be done for men undergoing vasectomy ( )

C. Freezing damages all sperm irreversibly ( )

D. Post-thaw sperm can be used for ICSI ( )

E. Cryoprotectants are used to prevent ice damage ( )

41. With respect to ART laboratory safety:

A. Air quality in the lab is not necessary ( )

B. Exposure to volatile organic compounds can harm gametes ( )

C. Embryologists should use strict aseptic technique ( )

D. Temperature fluctuations have no effect on embryos ( )

E. Lab accreditation and quality control are important ( )

42. Concerning cumulative live birth rates:

A. Cumulative rates steady with multiple embryo transfers ( )

B. Freeze-all strategies may contribute to lower cumulative rates ( )

C. Maternal age has no effect on cumulative outcomes ( )

D. Use of donor oocytes not improves cumulative success ( )

E. Cumulative live birth rate is a better measure than per-cycle success ( )

43. Regarding elective single embryo transfer (eSET):

A. Reduces risk of multiple pregnancy ( )

B. Is especially recommended in old women with good prognosis ( )

C. Guarantees higher live birth rate than double embryo transfer ( )

D. Success depends on embryo quality ( )

E. Supported by national and international guidelines ( )

44. With respect to ovarian stimulation monitoring:

A. Serial ultrasound not necessary to assess follicle growth ( )

B. Estradiol levels have no value in monitoring the response ( )

C. Monitoring prevents OHSS in all cases ( )

D. Premature LH surge is possible without suppression ( )

E. Follicle size is used to time the trigger ( )

45. Concerning "empty follicle syndrome":

A. Refers to absence of oocytes despite normal follicular development ( )

B. May be related to failure of hCG trigger ( )

C. Is a common occurrence in IVF cycles ( )

D. Can be genuine or false depending on cause ( )

E. Repeat trigger and retrieval may help in false cases ( )

46. Regarding sperm selection in ICSI:

A. Morphologically normal sperm are preferred ( )

B. Motility is not considered during selection ( )

C. Genetic testing is performed on each sperm ( )

D. IMSI allows higher magnification selection ( )

E. Sperm DNA fragmentation is directly visible under microscope ( )

47. With respect to ART and ethics:

A. Consent is not mandatory before treatment ( )

B. Embryo storage has legal limitations in many countries ( )

C. All countries allow embryo donation ( )

D. Counseling is not recommended for all couples ( )

E. Ethical issues may include embryo selection and disposal ( )

48. Concerning advanced maternal age and ART:

A. Oocyte quality declines with age ( )

B. Aneuploidy risk increases with age ( )

C. Donor oocytes can overcome age-related infertility ( )

D. Success rates remain constant irrespective of age ( )

E. Miscarriage risk increases with advanced age ( )

49.Regarding the use of platelet-rich plasma (PRP) in IVF/ICSI according to ESHRE guidelines:

A. PRP is currently considered an experimental therapy ( )

B. Evidence strongly supports PRP for improving endometrial receptivity ( )

C. ESHRE guidelines state there is insufficient evidence for use ( )

D. PRP should only be offered within research or clinical trials ( )

E. PRP is established as standard treatment for recurrent implantation failure ()

50. Regarding future directions in ART:

A. Artificial intelligence may assist embryo selection ( )

B. Uterine transplantation is being explored ( )

C. Gene editing is standard clinical practice ( )

D. Stem cell–derived gametes are under research ( )

E. Advances aim to improve safety and efficacy ( )

ANSWERS

Q	A	B	C	D	E
1	T	F	F	T	T
2	F	T	F	T	T
3	T	F	T	T	F
4	T	T	F	T	T
5	T	T	F	T	F
6	T	F	F	T	T
7	F	F	F	T	T
8	F	F	T	T	F
9	T	T	F	F	T
10	F	T	T	F	F
11	T	F	F	T	T
12	F	T	F	F	T
13	T	T	F	T	F
14	T	T	F	F	T
15	F	T	F	T	F
16	T	F	T	T	F
17	T	T	T	T	F
18	T	T	T	F	T
19	T	F	F	F	T
20	T	T	T	F	T
21	T	T	F	F	F
22	F	F	T	F	T
23	F	T	F	F	T
24	T	F	T	T	T
25	F	T	F	T	T
26	T	T	F	F	T
27	F	T	F	F	T
28	T	T	T	F	T
29	F	T	T	F	F
30	T	T	F	T	T
31	F	F	F	F	F
32	T	T	F	F	T
33	T	T	F	F	F
34	T	T	F	T	T
35	T	F	T	F	T

Q	A	B	C	D	E
36	T	T	F	T	T
37	T	T	T	F	T
38	T	T	F	F	T
39	T	F	F	T	F
40	T	T	F	T	T
41	F	T	T	F	T
42	T	F	F	F	T
43	T	F	F	T	T
44	F	F	F	T	T
45	T	T	F	T	T
46	T	F	F	T	F
47	F	T	F	F	T
48	T	T	T	F	T
49	T	F	T	T	F
50	T	T	F	T	T

PART 3

Extended Matching Questions (EMQs) IN IVF/ICSI

EMQ 1

Options:

A. Semen analysis of the partner
B. Screening for infectious diseases (HIV, Hepatitis B & C, syphilis)
C. Baseline hormonal profile (FSH, LH, AMH, TSH, Prolactin, AFC)
D. Cervical smear (Pap test)
E. Hysteroscopy / saline sonography for uterine cavity assessment
F. Lifestyle optimization (weight, smoking cessation, folic acid supplementation)
G. Blood grouping and hemoglobin
H. Thrombophilia and karyotyping (selected cases)

Scenarios:

1. A 32-year-old woman scheduled for IVF; requires assessment of ovarian reserve before starting stimulation.
2. A 35-year-old man; first-line mandatory test before proceeding with ICSI.
3. A 29-year-old woman; needs evaluation of uterine cavity to rule out intrauterine adhesions or submucous fibroids.
4. A 30-year-old couple; both require blood tests to exclude HIV and Hepatitis B & C prior to IVF.

EMQ 2

Options:

A. Age of the woman
B. Antral follicle count (AFC) by transvaginal ultrasound
C. Anti-Müllerian Hormone (AMH) level
D. Low ovarian response
E. Previous ovarian response to stimulation
F. BMI and lifestyle factors
G. Ovarian volume on ultrasound
H. Estradiol level on day 3
I. Family history of premature ovarian insufficiency
J. Ovarian surgery history

Scenarios:

1. A 32-year-old woman with infertility; most reliable biochemical marker to assess ovarian reserve and predict response.
2. A 30-year-old woman; transvaginal ultrasound shows 16 small follicles in both ovaries together, suggesting good prognosis.
3. A 39-year-old woman; her main negative prognostic factor for ovarian stimulation outcome is this.
4. A 35-year-old woman with high day 3 FSH and low estradiol; interpretation?
5. A 28-year-old woman; her sister was diagnosed with premature ovarian insufficiency at age 32 — risk factor in her evaluation.
6. A 34-year-old woman with history of bilateral ovarian cystectomy; most relevant surgical factor affecting predicted response.

EMQ 3

Options:

A. Pituitary desensitization
B. Suppression of LH surge
C. Short agonist Protocol
D. PPOS Protocol
E. Improves follicular synchronization
F. Antagonist Protocol
G. Longer duration, more injections
H. Mid-luteal long agonist protocol
I. Not preferred in poor responders
J. IVF/ICSI

Scenarios:

1. A 30-year-old woman undergoing IVF; started on GnRH agonist in mid-luteal phase of the previous cycle.
2. In the long agonist protocol, the purpose of starting GnRH agonist early is to achieve this pituitary effect.
3. Disadvantage of this protocol is Asynchronization of growing follicles.
4. A 31-year-old with severe endometriosis
5. One limitation of this protocol is the need for freeze all embryos.

EMQ 4

Options:

A. Immediate suppression of LH surge
B. Start GnRH antagonist on day 5–6 of stimulation
C. No initial flare effect
D. Shorter duration, fewer injections
E. Reduced risk of OHSS
F. DouStim Protocol
G. GnRH agonist trigger
H. Risk of premature LH surge if antagonist missed
I. Indicated in PCOS patients undergoing IVF
J. Antagonist Protocol

Scenarios:

1. A 29-year-old woman undergoing IVF; GnRH antagonist is introduced in the mid-follicular phase to prevent this event.
2. A 31-year-old patient on antagonist protocol; one advantage is.
3. A 27-year-old woman with PCOS at high risk of OHSS; antagonist protocol is chosen for safety.
4. A 33-year-old low responder; appropriate protocol.
5. A 32-year-old undergoing IVF; high responder, appropriate trigger.
6. A 35-year-old woman; counseling includes that this protocol achieves pregnancy outcomes similar to the Long agonist protocol.

EMQ 5

Options

A. GnRH agonist trigger
B. hCG trigger
C. Dual trigger (GnRH agonist + hCG)
D. Freeze-all strategy
E. Mild stimulation protocol
F. Antagonist protocol
G. Double Stimulation Protocol
H. Natural cycle IVF
I. Progesterone
J. Cycle cancellation

Scenarios

1. A 39-year-old poor responder undergoing IVF is advised to have two stimulations within the same cycle to maximize oocyte yield.
2. A patient in the luteal phase after embryo transfer; what is the standard hormonal support?
3. A patient undergoing an oocyte donation program; the aim is to collect many oocytes while minimizing OHSS risk.
4. A woman undergoing IVF cycle but shows no ovarian response to stimulation; what is the suitable step?
5. A patient who wants a simple, low-cost cycle without stimulation drugs, just natural ovulation monitoring.
6. A patient undergoing stimulation who needs effective LH surge prevention with a short, simple protocol.

EMQ 6

Options

A. Follicular phase stimulation
B. Luteal phase stimulation
C. Random Start
D. Antagonist Protocol
E. Requires "freeze-all" strategy
F. Two stimulation cycles within one menstrual cycle
G. Higher oocyte yield compared to conventional single stimulation
H. Increased risk of OHSS compared to antagonist protocol

Scenarios

1. A 28-year-old woman newly diagnosed with breast cancer requires urgent fertility preservation before chemotherapy; this protocol is chosen to retrieve more oocytes quickly.
2. In DuoStim, the first stimulation is started during this phase of the menstrual cycle.

3. In DuoStim, the second stimulation is started during this phase after oocyte retrieval.
4. A 35-year-old woman is counseled that fresh transfer is not possible in DuoStim.
5. Start of IVF Protocol in many oncology patients

EMQ 7

Options:

A. FSH (urinary or recombinant)
B. LH supplementation
C. HMG (human menopausal gonadotropin)
D. Low-dose step-up protocol
E. Step-down protocol
F. High-dose gonadotropins
G. Ovarian hyperstimulation syndrome (OHSS)
H. Maximum Gonadotropins dose 300 IU
I. Minimum Gonadotropins dose 75 IU
J. Monitoring by serum estradiol & follicular scan

Scenarios:

1. A 34-year-old woman with hypogonadotropic hypogonadism; requires additional supplementation during stimulation.
2. A 32-year-old woman undergoing IVF; received gonadotropins which provides both FSH and LH activity.
3. A 27-year-old woman with PCOS; stimulation started with a very low FSH dose to reduce risk of OHSS.
4. A 36-year-old woman with diminished ovarian reserve; What is the maximum dose of gonadotropins?
5. A 30-year-old undergoing IVF; most important method to titrate gonadotropin dose and avoid complications.

EMQ 8

Options:

A. hCG trigger
B. GnRH agonist trigger
C. Risk of OHSS
D. Premature LH surge
E. Follicles <3 after stimulation
F. Follicles >20 with very high estradiol
G. Cycle cancellation due to poor response
H. Cycle cancellation due to excessive response
I. Dual trigger (hCG + GnRH agonist)
J. Empty follicle syndrome

Scenarios:

1. A 27-year-old PCOS patient at high risk of OHSS; safest option for triggering ovulation.
2. A 30-year-old woman; with mid-luteal long agonist protocol >20 follicles and very high estradiol level, safest option is
3. A 35-year-old woman undergoing IVF; no oocytes retrieved despite adequate follicular growth and triggering.
4. A 31-year-old poor responder; doctor considers using both hCG and GnRH agonist to improve oocyte maturity.
5. A 29-year-old woman undergoing IVF; standard medication used to mimic LH surge and trigger final oocyte maturation.

EMQ 9

Options:

A. Transvaginal ultrasound-guided aspiration
B. 34–36 hours after ovulation trigger
C. Local anesthesia with sedation
D. General anesthesia
E. Empty follicle syndrome
F. Risk of pelvic infection
G. Ovarian hyperstimulation syndrome (OHSS)
H. Bleeding from ovary/vaginal wall
I. Luteal phase support

Scenarios:

1. A 29-year-old woman received hCG trigger; retrieval is scheduled optimally at this interval after injection.
2. A 31-year-old woman complains of abdominal pain and distension after retrieval; diagnosis is.
3. A 28-year-old woman after oocyte retrieval develops fever and lower abdominal pain; complication suspected.
4. A 30-year-old woman undergoing IVF; oocyte retrieval is usually performed by this technique.
5. A 27-year-old woman after retrieval; advised to start progesterone supplementation for this reason.
6. A 33-year-old woman with severe pelvic adhesions undergoes oocyte retrieval, which anesthesia instead of sedation.
7. A 35-year-old woman develops significant hemoperitoneum and vaginal wall bleeding after retrieval; complication suspected.

EMQ 10

Options:

A. Oral dydrogesterone
B. Intramuscular progesterone
C. hCG for luteal support
D. Combination of progesterone + estrogen
E. Start on the evening of the day of oocyte retrieval
F. 10–12 weeks gestation if pregnant
G. OHSS
H. Vaginal progesterone
I. Improves implantation rates
J. No LPS needed in natural cycles

Scenarios:

1. A 29-year-old woman after IVF oocyte retrieval; most commonly used agent for luteal support.

2. A 31-year-old woman receives hCG for luteal support; major disadvantage is increased risk of this complication.
3. A 32-year-old woman; luteal support is initiated after this time relative to the procedure.
4. A 30-year-old woman who became pregnant after IVF; luteal support should be continued until this gestational age.
5. A 28-year-old undergoing IVF; rationale for LPS is to improve implantation and maintain early pregnancy.
6. A 26-year-old woman in a natural cycle IUI; Role of luteal support in this setting.

EMQ 11

Options:
A. Cleavage stage transfer
B. Blastocyst transfer
C. Transabdominal ultrasound guidance
D. Soft catheter for transfer
E. Single embryo transfer (SET)
F. Multiple embryo transfer
G. Luteal phase progesterone support
H. Complication: multiple pregnancy
I. Difficult transfer
J. Frozen embryo transfer (FET)

Scenarios:

1. A 29-year-old woman undergoing IVF; embryo transfer is done under this imaging guidance to ensure correct placement.
2. A 30-year-old patient with high risk of twins; recommended strategy to minimize multiple pregnancy.
3. A 31-year-old woman; embryo transfer performed on day 5 after fertilization.
4. A 28-year-old woman; embryo transfer performed earlier at Day 3

5. A 33-year-old woman; embryo transfer complicated due to cervical stenosis, requiring special techniques.
6. A 32-year-old woman after embryo transfer; advised to continue this medication to support implantation.

EMQ 12

Options:
A. Modified natural cycle (hCG trigger)
B. Artificial cycle with estradiol + progesterone
C. GnRH agonist pretreatment
D. Luteal phase progesterone support
E. Endometrial thickness ≥7 mm
F. Endometrial scratching (experimental)
G. Natural cycle FET
H. Cancellation if no dominant follicle in natural cycle
I. Flexible scheduling with artificial protocol
J. Monitoring with ultrasound + serum estradiol/progesterone

Scenarios:

1. A 29-year-old woman with regular ovulatory cycles; simplest approach is to use her spontaneous cycle for FET.
2. A 32-year-old woman with irregular cycles; endometrial preparation with estradiol followed by progesterone is chosen.
3. A 30-year-old woman; ovulation monitored with ultrasound, then hCG used to trigger and schedule transfer.
4. A 31-year-old woman; no follicle developed in natural cycle monitoring.
5. A 33-year-old woman; counseling includes that in artificial cycles, transfer can be timed flexibly for convenience.

EMQ 13

Options:
A. Preimplantation Genetic Testing (PGT)
B. Sperm sorting (flow cytometry / MicroSort)
C. Ethical indication – prevention of X-linked genetic disease

D. Non-medical / social sex selection
E. Embryo transfer of selected sex only
F. Contraindicated by law in many countries
G. Chorionic villus sampling (CVS) – after natural conception
H. Amniocentesis – after natural conception
I. Risk of embryo damage during biopsy

Scenarios:

1. A 32-year-old couple, both carriers of Duchenne muscular dystrophy, request sex selection to avoid an affected male child.
2. A 30-year-old couple undergoing IVF; embryos are biopsied at blastocyst stage and tested before transfer.
3. A 28-year-old couple request sex selection for “family balancing,” although both are healthy and fertile.
4. A 34-year-old woman; counseling includes for sex selection.
5. A 31-year-old couple; sex selection attempted by separating X-bearing from Y-bearing sperm before insemination.
6. A 29-year-old woman after embryo biopsy for PGT; main procedural risk explained during consent.

EMQ 14

Options:

A. Indication – monogenic disorder
B. Indication – chromosomal translocation
C. Indication – X-linked disease
D. Trophectoderm biopsy at blastocyst stage (day 5)
E. Cleavage-stage biopsy at day 3 (less common now)
F. Embryo freezing until results available
G. Transfer of unaffected embryo only
H. Risk of embryo damage
I. Alternative – prenatal diagnosis by CVS or amniocentesis
J. Ethical consideration and counseling required

Scenarios:

1. A 30-year-old couple, both carriers of cystic fibrosis, request genetic testing of embryos before transfer.

2. A 33-year-old man has a balanced chromosomal translocation; couple seeks IVF with embryo testing.
3. A 28-year-old woman, family history of Duchenne muscular dystrophy; wants to avoid having an affected male child.
4. A 32-year-old couple undergoing IVF; embryos biopsied at day 5 from trophectoderm cells.
5. A 29-year-old couple; embryos are frozen until genetic testing results are back.
6. A 34-year-old woman; counseling includes small but real risk to the embryo during biopsy procedure.

EMQ 15

Options:
A. Oligospermia (low count)
B. Asthenospermia (low motility)
C. Teratospermia (abnormal morphology)
D. Oligoasthenoteratospermia (OAT syndrome)
E. Azoospermia (no sperm in ejaculate)
F. Obstructive azoospermia (e.g., post-vasectomy)
G. Non-obstructive azoospermia (testicular failure)
H. Varicocele
I. Y-chromosome microdeletion
J. Testicular sperm extraction (TESE)

Scenarios:

1. A 32-year-old man with semen analysis showing complete absence of sperm; testicular biopsy confirms spermatogenic failure.
2. A 30-year-old man, semen analysis reveals low concentration, poor motility, and abnormal morphology.
3. A 28-year-old man, infertility for 2 years, scrotal exam shows dilated pampiniform plexus veins.
4. A 35-year-old man, azoospermia, FSH normal, testes normal size, history of vasectomy 5 years ago.

5. A 29-year-old man, semen analysis reveals sperm count <10 million/ml, normal motility and morphology.
6. A 31-year-old man, infertility, karyotype and genetic testing show AZFc deletion on Y chromosome.

EMQ 16

Options:

A. Germinal vesicle (GV) oocyte
B. Metaphase I (MI) oocyte
C. Metaphase II (MII) oocyte
D. Normal fertilization
E. Abnormal fertilization
F. Day 3 cleavage stage embryo
G. Day 5 blastocyst stage
H. Embryo grading based on cell number & fragmentation
I. Vitrification (rapid freezing)
J. Slow freezing (conventional method)

Scenarios:

1. A 29-year-old woman undergoing oocyte retrieval; the mature oocyte stage suitable for ICSI is identified.
2. A 31-year-old IVF patient; fertilization check 16–18 hours later shows 2 pronuclei (2PN) — this indicates.
3. A 32-year-old woman; embryologist reports 3 pronuclei (3PN) after insemination — represents.
4. A 28-year-old patient; embryo transfer is planned at day 3, when embryo has 6–8 cells.
5. A 30-year-old patient; embryo culture extended to day 5 blastocyst transfer for better selection.
6. A 33-year-old woman; embryos assessed by grading system that evaluates fragmentation and cell number.
7. A 27-year-old couple; surplus good-quality embryos are frozen by vitrification, the modern cryopreservation method.

8. A 35-year-old IVF case; older method of cryopreservation used, associated with higher ice crystal damage.

EMQ 17

Options:

A. Day 3 cleavage stage grading (cell number, symmetry, fragmentation)
B. Day 5 blastocyst grading (expansion, ICM & TE quality)
C. Embryo morphology under light microscope
D. Time-lapse monitoring (morphokinetics)
E. Preimplantation Genetic Testing (PGT-A)
F. Assisted hatching (selected cases)
G. Transfer of single best-quality embryo (SET)
H. Embryo compaction at morula stage
I. Cytoplasmic appearance and multinucleation assessment
J. Clinical factor: patient age and previous IVF history

Scenarios:

1. A 29-year-old woman; clinic uses type of incubator to assess exact timing of cell divisions for embryo selection.
2. A 34-year-old woman; PGT-A performed to exclude embryos with aneuploidy before transfer.
3. A 31-year-old woman; embryologist reports multinucleation in blastomeres, which lowers embryo quality.
4. A 30-year-old woman; embryo selection also considers female age and previous IVF attempts.
5. A 28-year-old woman; during embryo culture, compaction at the morula stage is assessed before blastocyst formation.
6. A 32-year-old patient; embryologist evaluates embryos under a light microscope for morphology before further grading.

EMQ 18

Options:

A. hCG trigger as the main precipitating factor
B. High estradiol & multiple follicles (>20)
C. Increased vascular permeability & third spacing
D. Enlarged multicystic ovaries
E. Ascites & hemoconcentration
F. Thromboembolic risk

G. Withholding hCG / cycle cancellation (prevention)
H. GnRH agonist trigger (in antagonist cycles)
I. Cabergoline
J. Supportive management with fluids, albumin, thromboprophylaxis

Scenarios:

1. A 27-year-old woman with PCOS develops severe abdominal pain and distension after ovulation trigger; main drug responsible.
2. A 30-year-old woman with OHSS develops ascites, hemoconcentration, and dyspnea — main underlying pathophysiology.
3. A 28-year-old woman with OHSS; ultrasound shows bilateral enlarged ovaries with multiple cysts.
4. A 32-year-old develops moderate OHSS; physician explains risk of this vascular complication.
5. A 26-year-old high-risk patient on antagonist protocol; safest ovulation trigger to reduce OHSS risk.
6. A 31-year-old PCOS patient; prophylaxis with this dopamine agonist reduces incidence of OHSS.
7. A 30-year-old woman admitted with severe OHSS; best approach includes IV fluids, albumin, and thromboprophylaxis.

EMQ 19

Options:
A. Conventional IVF insemination
B. Intracytoplasmic sperm injection (ICSI)
C. Physiological ICSI (PICSI; hyaluronan-binding)
D. Intracytoplasmic morphologically selected sperm injection (IMSI)
E. Testicular sperm extraction (TESE)
F. Percutaneous epididymal sperm aspiration (PESA)
G. Rescue ICSI after fertilization failure
H. Artificial oocyte activation (calcium ionophore)
I. Assisted hatching (selected cases)
J. In-vitro maturation (IVM) of oocytes

Scenarios:

1. A 35-year-old man with severe oligoasthenoteratozoospermia; fertilization requires direct sperm injection.
2. A 33-year-old man with obstructive azoospermia after vasectomy; motile sperm to be retrieved from epididymis.
3. A 31-year-old man with non-obstructive azoospermia; testicular retrieval planned for use in the lab.
4. A 30-year-old couple with normozoospermia; 12 mature oocytes retrieved—standard insemination planned.
5. Previous cycle had 0/10 oocytes showing 2PN after conventional IVF; lab proceeds with late microinjection same day.
6. Recurrent ICSI fertilization failure; suspected oocyte activation deficiency—adjunct planned to improve activation.
7. High sperm DNA fragmentation; lab uses hyaluronan-binding selection before microinjection.
8. Recurrent ICSI failure with severe teratozoospermia; center uses high-magnification sperm selection (≥6000×).

EMQ 20

Options:

A. Reduced oocyte quality in endometriosis
B. Distorted tubo-ovarian anatomy
C. Inflammatory peritoneal environment impairing fertilization
D. Adenomyosis → impaired implantation
E. Lower IVF/ICSI success rates compared to controls
F. Long agonist protocol
G. Pretreatment with GnRH agonists for adenomyosis
H. Surgical removal of large endometrioma (>4 cm) before ICSI
I. Risk of reduced ovarian reserve after cystectomy
J. Counseling about lower pregnancy and higher miscarriage rates

Scenarios:

1. A 32-year-old woman with severe endometriosis undergoing ICSI; her oocytes retrieved are fewer and of lower quality.
2. A 30-year-old woman with adenomyosis; main mechanism of infertility is defective endometrial receptivity and implantation.
3. A 34-year-old woman with stage III endometriosis; IVF outcomes discussed.
4. A 29-year-old woman with adenomyosis planned for ICSI
5. A 31-year-old woman with a 6 cm endometrioma; surgery considered before ICSI.
6. A 33-year-old woman with endometriosis-related infertility: Which GnRH agonist protocol can be used?

EMQ 21

Options:

A. Preconception cardiology assessment (echo, ECG)
B. Multidisciplinary team management (cardiology + reproductive medicine + anesthesia)
C. High-risk lesions (severe pulmonary hypertension, Eisenmenger's, severe aortic stenosis) – pregnancy contraindicated
D. Anticoagulation adjustment (e.g., heparin instead of warfarin)
E. Cycle cancellation if cardiac decompensation occurs
F. Avoid OHSS – antagonist protocol + GnRH agonist trigger
G. Frozen embryo transfer in natural/modified cycles to avoid high estrogen exposure
H. Day surgery / anesthesia risk assessment before oocyte retrieval
I. Strict fluid balance and thromboprophylaxis in stimulation cycles
J. Counseling about maternal and fetal risks

Scenarios:

1. A 32-year-old woman with congenital heart disease presents for IVF; first essential step is.
2. A 34-year-old patient with mechanical mitral valve on warfarin; requires anticoagulation adjustment before ovarian stimulation.

3. A 29-year-old with severe pulmonary hypertension seeks fertility treatment; she is counseled that pregnancy is absolutely contraindicated.
4. A 31-year-old woman with dilated cardiomyopathy scheduled for oocyte retrieval; anesthesia team involvement is mandatory.
5. A 28-year-old woman with cardiac disease undergoing IVF; stimulation protocol chosen to minimize OHSS risk.
6. A 33-year-old with heart disease; safest embryo transfer approach is to use frozen embryos.
7. A 30-year-old woman with cardiac disease undergoing IVF; counseling includes potential maternal morbidity and adverse fetal outcomes.

EMQ 22

Options:

A. Antiphospholipid antibody screening (aPL, lupus anticoagulant, anticardiolipin)
B. Risk of thrombosis during ovarian stimulation
C. Disease should be quiescent ≥ 6 months before IVF/ICSI
D. Use of antagonist protocol with GnRH agonist trigger to reduce OHSS
E. Hydroxychloroquine continuation is safe and recommended
F. Avoid estrogen exposure in active disease → use minimal stimulation / natural FET
G. Anticoagulation (heparin + low-dose aspirin) if aPL positive
H. Multidisciplinary care (rheumatology + reproductive medicine + hematology)
I. High-risk for pregnancy loss and preeclampsia
J. Counseling about maternal and fetal risks

Scenarios:

1. A 29-year-old woman with SLE planning IVF; advised to delay treatment until disease activity is controlled.
2. A 31-year-old woman undergoing IVF; screening for this autoimmune antibody panel is mandatory due to risk of miscarriage and thrombosis.

3. A 32-year-old SLE patient with positive aPL antibodies; requires prophylaxis with anticoagulation in addition to aspirin during ART and pregnancy.
4. A 30-year-old woman with SLE undergoing ovarian stimulation; Which protocol chosen to reduce risk of OHSS and thrombosis.
5. A 28-year-old with SLE on hydroxychloroquine; advised to continue medication during IVF and pregnancy.
6. A 34-year-old woman with SLE; counseling includes.
7. A 33-year-old SLE patient; IVF management requires joint input from rheumatology, reproductive medicine, and hematology.

EMQ 23

Options:

A. Optimize HbA1c < 6.5% before conception
B. Preconception counseling about maternal & fetal risks
C. Screening and management of diabetic complications (renal, retinal, cardiac)
D. Switch oral hypoglycemics to insulin before IVF
E. Lifestyle modification and weight reduction in obese T2DM
F. Folic acid high dose (5 mg/day) preconception
G. Higher risk of miscarriage and congenital malformations with poor control
H. Increased obstetric risks: preeclampsia, macrosomia, stillbirth
I. Multidisciplinary care (endocrinology + reproductive medicine + obstetrics)
J. Frozen embryo transfer (FET) after achieving optimal metabolic control

Scenarios:

1. A 32-year-old woman with type1 DM scheduled for IVF; her HbA1c is 8.2%. Treatment must be postponed until this target is achieved.
2. A 34-year-old woman with poorly controlled diabetes; counseling includes.
3. A 30-year-old woman with type 2 DM on metformin and sulfonylurea; requires transition to this therapy before IVF and pregnancy.

4. A 29-year-old obese woman with type 2 DM; advised to lose weight and improve glycemic control before IVF.
5. A 31-year-old woman with diabetes planning IVF; requires preconception folate supplementation at this dosage.
6. A 35-year-old woman with diabetes; advised to undergo eye, kidney, and cardiac assessment before starting ART.
7. A 33-year-old woman with uncontrolled diabetes; safest option is to freeze embryos and delay transfer until optimal metabolic control.
8. A 28-year-old woman with diabetes undergoing IVF; her care requires combined input from endocrinology, reproductive medicine, and obstetrics.

EMQ 24

Options:
A. Embryo cryopreservation
B. Oocyte cryopreservation (freezing)
C. Ovarian tissue cryopreservation
D. Sperm cryopreservation
E. GnRH agonists during chemotherapy (ovarian suppression)
F. Testicular tissue freezing (experimental)
G. Indication: malignancy requiring gonadotoxic chemo/radiotherapy
H. Indication: elective fertility preservation (social freezing, advanced age)
I. Prepubertal boy with cancer – only option currently experimental
J. Counseling about future success rates and risks

Scenarios:
1. A 28-year-old unmarried woman with breast cancer scheduled for chemotherapy; best established method of fertility preservation if time allows.
2. A 30-year-old woman with a partner, facing chemotherapy; embryos are created via IVF and frozen for future use.
3. A 26-year-old woman with lymphoma, no time for ovarian stimulation; option is cryopreservation of ovarian cortical tissue.

4. A 15-year-old boy with leukemia, prepubertal; fertility preservation offered but only available as experimental.
5. A 29-year-old man with testicular cancer, planned for orchiectomy and chemotherapy; standard preservation method.
6. A 34-year-old healthy woman, delaying childbearing for career reasons; requests elective fertility preservation.
7. A 31-year-old woman with cancer; GnRH agonist given during chemotherapy to reduce ovarian damage.
8. A 27-year-old woman referred for fertility preservation; counseling includes realistic expectations about pregnancy chances and risks.

EMQ 25

Options:
A. Embryo aneuploidy (chromosomal abnormalities)
B. Uterine factor (fibroid, polyp, adhesions, septum)
C. Chronic endometritis
D. Advanced maternal age & poor oocyte quality
E. Thrombophilia / antiphospholipid syndrome
F. Immune dysfunction (abnormal NK cells, controversial)
G. Preimplantation Genetic Testing (PGT-A)
H. Hysteroscopy to evaluate uterine cavity
I. Endometrial receptivity testing (ERA – experimental)
J. Counseling about limited evidence and realistic expectations

Scenarios:

1. A 37-year-old woman with repeated failed IVF cycles; main age-related factor reducing implantation success.
2. A 32-year-old woman with RIF; uterine cavity evaluation shows intrauterine adhesions.
3. A 34-year-old couple; recurrent IVF failure due to chromosomally abnormal embryos — option to improve selection.
4. A 30-year-old woman with RIF; hysteroscopy reveals endometrial polyp, which may impair implantation.

5. A 31-year-old woman with positive antiphospholipid antibodies; associated with thrombosis and implantation failure.
6. A 29-year-old woman with RIF; biopsy suggests endometritis.
7. A 35-year-old woman with RIF; clinic offers endometrial receptivity assay, but counseling includes limited evidence for routine use.
8. A 33-year-old woman with multiple failed cycles; counseling emphasizes uncertain benefit of many adjuvant therapies.

EMQ 26

Options:

A. PRP = autologous platelet concentrate rich in growth factors
B. Intra-ovarian PRP
C. Intrauterine PRP
D. Experimental / not yet standard of care
E. May improve endometrial receptivity
F. Proposed to enhance ovarian stem cell activation
G. Indication: recurrent implantation failure (RIF) with thin endometrium
H. Endometrial cavity
I. Limited evidence & need for more RCTs
J. Established options (e.g., hysteroscopy, estrogen therapy for thin endometrium)

Scenarios:

1. A 32-year-old woman with recurrent thin endometrium despite high-dose estrogen; offered this intrauterine intervention which is not evidence-based.
2. A 35-year-old low responder with very low AMH; experimental therapy proposed involves intra-ovarian injection.
3. A 30-year-old woman with persistent thin endometrium, clinician advises prioritizing established options.
4. A 28-year-old patient asks how PRP works — doctor explains it is.
5. A 33-year-old couple counseled about PRP; informed that its role in IVF/ICSI.

6. A 34-year-old woman with thin endometrium undergoing IVF; PRP infusion is administered into this site.

EMQ 27

Options:

A. This type of fibroid has no impact on fertility
B. Intramural fibroid ≥ 5 cm may impair IVF outcome
C. Submucous fibroid → reduces implantation and pregnancy rates
D. Hysteroscopic myomectomy for submucous fibroid
E. Laparoscopic or open myomectomy for large intramural fibroid
F. Risk of uterine rupture in future pregnancy after myomectomy
G. Delay in IVF for surgical recovery after myomectomy
H. Fibroids may increase miscarriage risk
I. Pre-IVF assessment with transvaginal ultrasound ± hysteroscopy
J. Counseling: management individualized based on size, type, and symptoms

Scenarios:

1. A 32-year-old woman with infertility; hysteroscopy shows submucous fibroid distorting the uterine cavity.
2. A 35-year-old woman; ultrasound shows intramural fibroid 5 cm, compressing the endometrium, before IVF.
3. A 30-year-old woman with 3 cm subserosal fibroid; doctor reassures her it won't affect implantation.
4. A 33-year-old woman undergoing IVF; submucous fibroid removed by this surgical approach.
5. A 36-year-old woman with large intramural fibroid; laparoscopic myomectomy planned but IVF delayed for healing.
6. A 34-year-old woman with fibroids; counseled that they increase risk of
7. A 31-year-old woman with infertility; pre-IVF workup includes

EMQ 28

Options:

A. Assisted hatching
B. Time-lapse embryo monitoring (morphokinetics)
C. Embryo glue (hyaluronic acid–enriched transfer medium)
D. Endometrial scratching
E. Immunotherapy (IVIG, intralipid – experimental)
F. Aneuploidy (PGT-A)
G. Physiological ICSI (PICSI – sperm selection with hyaluronic acid)
H. IMSI (intracytoplasmic morphologically selected sperm injection)
I. Mitochondrial transfer / PRP (experimental)
J. Lack strong evidence, use with caution

Scenarios:

1. A 29-year-old couple; clinic offers genetic testing to exclude aneuploid embryos before transfer.
2. A 36-year-old man with severe teratozoospermia; lab proposes high-magnification sperm selection.
3. A 35-year-old woman; counseled that most IVF "add-ons" are
4. A 32-year-old woman with recurrent implantation failure; offered zona pellucida thinning to aid hatching.
5. A 30-year-old couple; continuous culture with a system that records exact timing of embryo cleavages.
6. A 31-year-old woman; transfer performed using a hyaluronic acid–enriched medium.
7. A 34-year-old woman with repeated IVF failure; clinic suggests endometrial procedure despite limited evidence.
8. A 33-year-old man with high sperm DNA fragmentation; sperm selection via hyaluronan binding before ICSI.

EMQ 29

Options:

A. Take as soon as remembered, don't double GNs dose next day
B. Risk of premature LH surge
C. May lead to pituitary flare / loss of suppression
D. Missed hCG trigger → cycle cancellation if not corrected in time
E. Luteal phase deficiency
F. Double dosing accidentally → risk of OHSS if gonadotropins overdosed
G. Contact clinic immediately for advice
H. Some medications have strict timing (hCG, GnRH antagonist), others more flexible
I. Documented missed trigger → may reschedule retrieval or cancel cycle
J. Counseling patients about strict compliance before starting treatment

Scenarios:

1. A 35-year-old woman advised that some IVF meds (e.g., hCG and antagonist) require strict timing, while others like FSH allow limited flexibility.
2. A 33-year-old overstimulated patient accidentally doubled her gonadotropin dose; risks need to be discussed.
3. A 30-year-old patient forgot to take hCG at the scheduled time; how to manage.
4. A 32-year-old patient on antagonist protocol misses her cetrorelix injection.
5. A 34-year-old woman on a long GnRH agonist protocol missed her downregulation dose.
6. A 28-year-old woman delays starting progesterone by five days after oocyte retrieval.
7. A 29-year-old woman forgets her daily FSH injection and remembers later the same day.
8. A 31-year-old woman starting IVF receives counseling emphasizing strict adherence and what to do if a dose is missed.

EMQ 30

Options:

A. Screen TSH before IVF/ICSI
B. Subclinical hypothyroidism (TSH >2.5–4.0 mIU/L) → treat with levothyroxine
C. Overt hypothyroidism → must be corrected before IVF
D. Hyperthyroidism (Graves') → stabilize before attempting pregnancy
E. Thyroid autoimmunity (anti-TPO antibodies) → risk of miscarriage and implantation failure
F. Close monitoring of thyroid function during stimulation and early pregnancy
G. Poor IVF outcomes if uncontrolled thyroid disease
H. Levothyroxine safe and continued throughout pregnancy
I. Antithyroid drugs (PTU first trimester, carbimazole/ methimazole after)
J. Multidisciplinary care (endocrinology + reproductive medicine)

Scenarios:

1. A 30-year-old woman planned for IVF; initial workup includes this test to exclude thyroid dysfunction.
2. A 32-year-old woman with TSH 6.5 mIU/L; IVF postponed until she starts levothyroxine and achieves normal thyroid function.
3. A 29-year-old woman with subclinical hypothyroidism (TSH 3.8 mIU/L); advised to start this treatment.
4. A 34-year-old woman with Graves' disease; IVF delayed until euthyroid state achieved.
5. A 31-year-old woman with positive anti-TPO antibodies; counseled about increased risk of miscarriage and lower implantation rates.
6. A 28-year-old woman with hypothyroidism on levothyroxine; told to continue it during IVF and pregnancy.
7. A 35-year-old woman with hyperthyroidism in first trimester after IVF; safest drug to use is.
8. A 33-year-old woman with thyroid disease undergoing IVF; requires joint management between endocrinology and reproductive medicine teams.

EMQ 31

Options:

A. Septate uterus – poor implantation & ↑ miscarriage risk
B. Bicornuate uterus – usually associated with preterm labor
C. Associated with infertility & adverse pregnancy outcome
D. Double uterine cavities, may carry pregnancy but↑ obstetric risks
E. Usually a normal variant, minimal impact
F. Hysteroscopic metroplasty
G. 3D ultrasound or MRI – best diagnostic imaging
H. HSG – initial but limited in differentiating anomalies
I. Counseling: anomaly-specific reproductive prognosis
J. Consider surrogacy if repeated IVF failures and uncorrectable anomaly

Scenarios:

1. A 30-year-old woman with recurrent IVF implantation failure; hysteroscopy shows a fibrous partition dividing the cavity.
2. A 32-year-old woman with infertility; HSG shows abnormal uterine contour, further assessment with.
3. A 28-year-old woman with recurrent miscarriage; diagnosis is septate uterus, treated with this surgical approach.
4. A 34-year-old woman with congenital anomaly; pregnancy possible but higher risk of preterm labor due to reduced uterine volume.
5. A 27-year-old woman undergoing IVF; arcuate uterus identified incidentally, doctor reassures.
6. A 31-year-old woman with unicornuate uterus; counseled about fertility and adverse pregnancy outcomes.
7. A 35-year-old with uterus didelphys; advised of possible pregnancy, but risk of obstetric complications is high.

EMQ 32

Options:

A. Niche / isthmocele = pouch-like defect at previous C.S scar
B. Postmenstrual spotting (brown discharge)
C. Dysmenorrhea & chronic pelvic pain
D. Secondary infertility due to altered uterine environment
E. Diagnosis by saline infusion sonohysterography (SIS) or hysteroscopy
F. Transvaginal ultrasound as initial screening
G. Hysteroscopic resection of fibrotic tissue (metroplasty)
H. Laparoscopic / combined repair in large/deep defects
I. Risk of impaired implantation and miscarriage in IVF/ICSI
J. Counseling about obstetric complications (scar ectopic, uterine rupture)

Scenarios:

1. A 34-year-old G2P2 after two lower-segment C.S reports rust-colored staining for 5–7 days after menses with otherwise normal exam and labs; intermenstrual bleeding is minimal.
2. A 32-year-old with secondary infertility post–C.S has an equivocal TVUS; early-follicular saline infusion imaging is requested to delineate an anechoic triangular pouch in the anterior isthmus.
3. A 30-year-old preparing for FET has persistent intracavitary fluid pooling from an anterior lower-segment defect; the possible cause is.
4. A 36-year-old with a large/deep cesarean-scar defect (defect depth 7 mm, residual myometrium 1.8 mm) is planned for repair; the surgeon favors an abdominal/combined approach.
5. A 33-year-old symptomatic patient with a shallow niche (residual myometrium ≥3.5 mm) and abnormal bleeding is scheduled for endoscopic correction via the cavity.
6. A 35-year-old with prior C.S seeks preconception counseling; discussion includes future risks unique to scar defects during pregnancy.

EMQ 33

Options:

A. Endometrial thickness <7 mm
B. Poor implantation and pregnancy rates
C. Causes: Asherman's syndrome (intrauterine adhesions)
D. Causes: prolonged clomiphene use
E. High-dose estrogen therapy
F. Vaginal sildenafil (off-label)
G. Intrauterine G-CSF infusion
H. PRP (platelet-rich plasma) infusion
I. Hysteroscopic adhesiolysis for intrauterine synechiae
J. Consider embryo cryopreservation (FET) until endometrium optimized

Scenarios:

1. A 31-year-old IVF patient with slow endometrial growth on artificial prep; the physician escalates to an intensified estrogen replacement regimen.
2. A 35-year-old with high-quality blastocysts but persistently thin lining; advised to bank embryos now and defer transfer until the lining improves.
3. A 28-year-old with refractory thin endometrium after excluding adhesions/infection; offered biologic intrauterine therapy that remains investigational (not standard of care).
4. A 29-year-old with suboptimal lining is prescribed an off-label vaginal vasodilator to augment uterine perfusion.
5. A 32-year-old on trigger day shows endometrial thickness 6.2 mm despite adequate estradiol and trilaminar pattern.
6. A 34-year-old post-D&C with hypomenorrhea; hysteroscopy confirms intrauterine synechiae requiring definitive treatment.
7. A 30-year-old asks why thin lining lowers success; you counsel about its association with reduced implantation and live-birth chances.

EMQ 34

Options:

A. Tubal factor – hydrosalpinx reflux
B. Chronic endometritis
C. Subclinical infection (e.g., chlamydia)
D. Endometrial atrophy / thin lining
E. Impaired implantation & reduced pregnancy rates
F. Transvaginal ultrasound – diagnosis
G. Antibiotic therapy if infection suspected
H. Salpingectomy or tubal disconnection for hydrosalpinx
I. Freeze-all strategy until cavity is clear
J. Cycle cancellation if persistent fluid on transfer day

Scenarios:

1. A 32-year-old in an IVF stimulation cycle: on trigger day, TVUS shows a small anechoic pocket within the endometrial cavity with an otherwise trilaminar lining and adequate thickness. The team debates the best initial diagnostic approach and documentation before altering the plan.
2. A 34-year-old with bilateral hydrosalpinx (classic "beads-on-a-string" appearance) is counseled before the next cycle about the physiologic mechanism by which fluid reaches the cavity and how this changes management.
3. A 30-year-old with recurrent intracavitary fluid across multiple cycles despite high-quality embryos is counseled that the key issue is reduced implantation and pregnancy rates rather than embryo competence per se.
4. A 28-year-old with cavity fluid and scant postmenstrual spotting undergoes hysteroscopy and biopsy: CD138-positive plasma cells and culture consistent with a low-grade endometrial inflammation. What is the most likely diagnosis?

5. A 31-year-old preparing for a fresh transfer still has persistent cavity fluid on the morning of ET; stable aspiration cannot be maintained. What is the most appropriate decision for this cycle?
6. A 35-year-old with unilateral hydrosalpinx and repeated IVF failures is weighing options prior to another transfer; discussion centers on definitive tubal intervention to improve outcomes.
7. A 29-year-old with intermittent cavity fluid has a new sexual partner within 3 months and mucopurulent cervical discharge on exam. What initial step should precede re-preparation for transfer?

EMQ 35

Options:
A. DHEA supplementation (25 mg TDS for ≥ 6–8 weeks)
B. May Improves ovarian reserve markers & Recruitment
C. Coenzyme Q10
D. May improve oocyte quality and embryo development
E. Used in poor ovarian responders (low AMH, low AFC)
F. Mechanism: enhances mitochondrial energy production in oocytes
G. Still considered adjuvant / experimental, not standard of care
H. Safe, well-tolerated supplements
I. Evidence: some RCTs show improved pregnancy/live birth, others inconclusive
J. Counseling: benefit uncertain, use with realistic expectations

Scenarios:
1. A 38-year-old low responder with low AMH; prescribed this androgen precursor for 2 months before IVF.
2. A 34-year-old with diminished ovarian reserve; given this supplement with antioxidant effect targeting mitochondrial function.
3. A 36-year-old IVF patient; advised both DHEA and CoQ10
4. A 37-year-old low responder; counseled that supplements are safe and well tolerated but not guaranteed to work.

5. A 39-year-old with repeated IVF failures; doctor explains some trials show better pregnancy outcomes; others are inconclusive.

EMQ 36

Options:

A. Success rates per cycle and cumulative live birth rate
B. Risk of multiple pregnancy (especially with double embryo transfer)
C. Risk of Ovarian Hyperstimulation Syndrome (OHSS)
D. Risk of miscarriage and ectopic pregnancy even after IVF
E. Counseling about cycle cancellation (poor or excessive response)
F. Possibility of needing donor gametes or embryos in poor responders
G. Discussion of legal/ethical aspects (embryo freezing, surplus embryos, sex selection limitations)
H. Counseling about pregnancy and obstetric risks (preterm birth, low birth weight, hypertensive disorders)
I. Psychological stress and need for support
J. Financial cost, repeated cycles may be required

Scenarios:

1. A 35-year-old primigravida-to-be asks whether IVF itself changes perinatal outcomes for a planned singleton; discussion covers higher rates of preeclampsia and medically indicated late-preterm birth compared with spontaneous conception.
2. A 29-year-old with elevated HADS-Anxiety scores worries about injections, failure, and stigma; you outline structured coping resources and when to refer for formal support.
3. A 31-year-old couple requests a forecast for "how many attempts" they should budget for; you frame expected spend given typical need for more than one stimulation/transfer.
4. A 36-year-old with AMH 0.3 ng/mL and ≤3 oocytes retrieved in two prior cycles asks about the next step if another cycle yields no blastocysts.

5. A 33-year-old signs consent; they must decide on storage limits and disposition of surplus embryos and are reminded of jurisdictional limits on sex selection.
6. A 34-year-old asks if transfer "guarantees" a pregnancy; counseling emphasizes residual risks that persist even with high-quality embryos.
7. A 28-year-old with PCOS (AFC 40, estradiol rapidly rising) is warned about an iatrogenic complication of stimulation and how protocol choices aim to mitigate it.
8. A 30-year-old requests two-embryo transfer "to improve odds"; counseling centers on balancing marginal gain vs. neonatal and maternal harms.

EMQ 37

Options:
A. Younger maternal age (<35 years)
B. Good ovarian reserve (AMH, AFC)
C. Normal BMI and healthy lifestyle (no smoking, no alcohol)
D. Adequate endometrial thickness (≥7–8 mm) at transfer
E. Good-quality blastocyst stage transfer (day 5)
F. Single embryo transfer (SET) to reduce multiple pregnancy risk
G. Use of donor oocytes in older women
H. Previous successful IVF cycle (cumulative success increases)
I. Experienced IVF laboratory and embryologist
J. Counseling & psychological support reducing stress

Scenarios:

1. A 31-year-old undergoes day-5 transfer of a 4AA embryo after extended culture for physiologic self-selection.
2. A 34-year-old conceived on her second IVF cycle previously; her current counseling references cumulative probability across attempts.
3. A 33-year-old couple compares clinics; they are advised to consider KPIs (blastulation rates, vitrification-warming survival, lab accreditation) when selecting a center.

4. A 40-year-old with AMH 0.2 ng/mL and prior poor ovarian response explores the option most likely to normalize age-related aneuploidy risk.
5. A 29-year-old nulligravida beginning IVF asks why her prognosis exceeds that of her 39-year-old sister, assuming all other variables equal.
6. A 32-year-old has AMH 3.2 ng/mL and AFC 15 on day-3 scan; the team anticipates robust follicular recruitment.
7. A 30-year-old with BMI 22, nonsmoker, no alcohol, adheres to exercise and Mediterranean-style diet; clinician highlights a modifiable prognostic edge.
8. A 28-year-old scheduled for FET once the lining reaches a trilaminar 8.2 mm; transfer is timed accordingly.

EMQ 38

Options:

A. AI-based embryo selection using morphokinetics (time-lapse imaging)
B. Deep learning analysis of embryo images for implantation prediction
C. AI to optimize stimulation protocols and drug dosing
D. AI prediction models for individualized success rates (age, AMH, BMI, history)
E. Automated sperm selection using AI-assisted imaging
F. AI for detecting abnormal embryo development patterns early
G. Reducing subjectivity and inter-observer variability in embryo grading
H. Integration with electronic medical records for personalized treatment planning
I. Still experimental, not standard of care
J. Ethical considerations – transparency, bias, patient consent

Scenarios:

1. A 32-year-old couple undergoing IVF; AI software used with time-lapse incubator to select the best embryo.

2. A 34-year-old patient; AI model analyzes large datasets to provide her personalized probability of live birth.
3. A 30-year-old man with severe teratozoospermia; clinic tests AI-assisted sperm selection for ICSI.
4. A 29-year-old woman; embryologist explains that AI helps to reduce subjectivity in embryo grading compared to human-only assessment.
5. A 33-year-old couple; AI flagged an abnormal embryo division pattern at early cleavage stage.
6. A fertility clinic pilot project uses AI to recommend ovarian stimulation doses individualized to patient characteristics.
7. A 35-year-old woman asks if AI is routine; doctor clarifies that it is.
8. A 31-year-old couple; counseling includes ethical considerations of using AI in reproductive medicine.

ANSWERS

EMQ	1	2	3	4	5	6	7	8
1	C	A	E	B	-	-	-	-
2	C	B	A	D	I	J	-	-
3	H	B	F	J	D	-	-	-
4	H	D	I	F	G	J	-	-
5	G	I	A	J	H	F	-	-
6	F	A	B	E	C	-	-	-
7	B	C	I	H	J	-	-	-
8	B	H	J	I	A	-	-	-
9	B	G	F	A	I	D	H	-
10	H	G	E	F	I	J	-	-
11	C	E	B	A	I	G	-	-
12	G	B	A	H	I	-	-	-
13	C	A	D	F	B	I	-	-
14	A	B	C	D	F	H	-	-
15	G	D	H	F	A	I	-	-
16	C	D	E	F	G	H	I	J
17	D	E	I	J	H	C	-	-
18	A	C	D	F	H	I	J	-
19	B	F	E	A	G	H	C	D
20	A	D	E	J	I	F	-	-
21	A	D	C	H	F	G	J	-
22	C	A	G	D	E	J	H	-
23	A	G	D	E	F	C	J	I
24	B	A	C	F	D	H	E	J
25	D	B	G	H	E	C	I	J
26	C	B	J	A	I	H	-	-
27	C	B	A	D	E	H	I	-
28	F	H	J	A	B	C	D	G
29	H	F	I	B	C	E	A	J
30	A	C	B	D	E	H	I	J
31	A	G	F	B	E	C	D	-
32	B	E	A	H	G	J	-	-
33	E	J	G/H	F	A	I	B	-
34	F	A	E	B	J	H	G	-
35	A	C	G	J	I	-	-	-
36	H	I	J	F	G	D	C	B
37	E	H	I	G	A	B	C	D
38	A	D	E	G	F	C	I	J

PART 4

CASE-BASED & SHORT ESSAY QUESTIONS IN IVF/ICSI

CASE NO. (1) COUNSELING FOR IVF/ICSI

A 34-year-old woman with 5 years of primary infertility, bilateral tubal block on HSG is planned for IVF/ICSI. She and her husband attend your clinic for counseling before starting the cycle.

1. What are the key points to include in counseling a couple before IVF/ICSI?
2. How do you explain the chances of success (live birth rate per cycle vs cumulative rate)?
3. What is the impact of female age on IVF/ICSI success?
4. How do you counsel regarding the risk of multiple pregnancy?
5. What are the risks of ovarian hyperstimulation syndrome (OHSS) and how can it be prevented?
6. How do you explain the possibility of cycle cancellation (low or high response)?
7. What are the risks of oocyte retrieval procedure?
8. How do you counsel about the risk of miscarriage and ectopic pregnancy after IVF?
9. How should couples be counseled about embryo freezing and surplus embryos?
10. What legal and ethical issues should be discussed before IVF/ICSI (e.g., gamete donation, sex selection restrictions)?
11. How do you counsel couples about the risk of congenital anomalies in IVF children?
12. What obstetric risks are increased after IVF/ICSI pregnancies (e.g., preterm birth, low birth weight, hypertensive disorders)?

13. How do you counsel about the possibility of using donor sperm/oocytes/embryos if needed?
14. What psychological and emotional support should be offered to couples undergoing IVF?
15. What financial considerations and expectations should be addressed before IVF/ICSI?
16. How do you counsel couples about experimental or "add-on" therapies in IVF/ICSI?
17. What advice should be given about lifestyle modifications before, during and after IVF?

CASE NO. (2) PATIENT PREPARATION BEFORE IVF/ICSI

A 32-year-old woman, married for 5 years, presents with primary infertility. She reports irregular menstrual cycles every 35–40 days. She has no chronic medical illnesses. How should this patient be prepared before starting an IVF/ICSI cycle?

1. What baseline investigations are required for the female partner before starting IVF/ICSI?
2. What baseline investigations are required for the male partner before IVF/ICSI?
3. Why is ovarian reserve testing (AMH, AFC, FSH) important before IVF/ICSI?
4. What infectious disease screening is mandatory before IVF/ICSI?
5. What is the role of cervical smear (Pap smear) and breast exam before IVF?

6. What systemic comorbidities should be optimized before IVF (thyroid disease, diabetes, hypertension, etc.)?
7. How does BMI affect IVF outcome and what is the recommended range before treatment?
8. What lifestyle modifications are recommended for both partners before IVF?
9. What vaccinations are recommended for women before starting IVF/ICSI?
10. What uterine evaluations should be performed before IVF (TVS, hysteroscopy, saline sonography)?
11. What is the role of treating hydrosalpinx before IVF?
12. Why is counseling about multiple pregnancy risk important before IVF?
13. What psychological preparation/support should be offered before IVF/ICSI?
14. What are the legal/ethical consents required before IVF (embryo freezing, number of embryos transferred, donor gametes if needed)?
15. What financial counseling should be provided before IVF/ICSI?

CASE NO. (3) ASSESSMENT OF THE PREDICTED RESPONSE TO CONTROLLED OVARIAN STIMULATION

A 30-year-old woman with a 4-year history of primary infertility is scheduled for IVF. She has regular cycles and no significant past medical history. On transvaginal ultrasound performed on day 3 of the cycle, both ovaries are visualized and the antral follicle count (AFC) is 22. How can her predicted response to ovarian stimulation be assessed?

1. Why is it important to predict ovarian response before starting stimulation in IVF/ICSI?
2. What are the characteristics of a low ovarian responder?
3. What are the characteristics of a high ovarian responder?
4. What are the clinical predictors of ovarian response (age, BMI, previous response)?
5. What is the role of baseline day 2–3 FSH and estradiol in predicting ovarian response?
6. What is the role of (AMH) in ovarian response prediction?
7. What is the role of (AFC) by transvaginal ultrasound?
8. How do AMH and AFC compare in predicting ovarian response?
9. What is the Bologna criteria for defining low ovarian response?
10. What is the POSEIDON classification and how does it differ from Bologna criteria?
11. How do ovarian reserve tests guide stimulation protocol choice?
12. How does ovarian reserve testing help in counseling patients before IVF/ICSI?
13. What are the limitations of ovarian reserve tests in predicting live birth rates?
14. How does prediction of high response help in preventing OHSS?
15. What other novel markers or tests are being studied for predicting ovarian response?

CASE NO. (4) LH SUPPRESSION

A 34-year-old woman is undergoing IVF treatment. On day 6 of controlled ovarian stimulation, serum LH level is found to be elevated. The treating team decides to start a GnRH antagonist to control the premature LH rise.

1. What is the physiological role of LH in the menstrual cycle?
2. Why is LH suppression important during controlled ovarian stimulation in IVF/ICSI?
3. What are the risks of a premature LH surge during ovarian stimulation?
4. How can premature LH surge affect IVF/ICSI outcomes?
5. What drugs are used to suppress LH in IVF protocols?
6. What is the difference between GnRH agonist and GnRH antagonist in LH suppression?
7. How does the long GnRH agonist protocol suppress LH?
8. How does the GnRH antagonist protocol suppress LH?
9. What is the effect of LH suppression on follicular development and oocyte quality?
10. What is the "flare effect" in GnRH agonist use?
11. In what situations is LH supplementation needed during stimulation?
12. How is LH suppression monitored during stimulation cycles?

CASE NO. (5) AGONIST PROTOCOLS

A 29-year-old woman with primary infertility is scheduled for IVF. She is started on a GnRH agonist in the mid-luteal phase of the previous cycle, followed by controlled ovarian stimulation with gonadotropins.

1. What is the mechanism of action of GnRH agonists?
2. What is the "flare effect" and how is it used in IVF protocols?
3. What is the difference between long and short agonist protocols?
4. How does the long agonist protocol achieve pituitary downregulation?
5. What is the typical timing of starting GnRH agonist in the long protocol?
6. What are the main advantages of the long agonist protocol?
7. What are the main disadvantages of the long agonist protocol?
8. In which patients is the short (flare) protocol commonly used?
9. What is the role of agonist protocols in low responders?
10. How do agonist protocols help in prevention of premature LH surge?
11. What are the risks of using GnRH agonists (e.g., hypoestrogenic side effects)?
12. How is ovarian stimulation with gonadotropins combined with agonist protocols?
13. What are the expected outcomes (oocyte yield, pregnancy rate) with long agonist vs antagonist protocol?
14. What is the role of GnRH agonist trigger instead of hCG in certain protocols?
15. How do you monitor patients during a long agonist protocol?
16. What are the clinical situations where agonist protocols are preferred over antagonist protocols?

CASE NO. (6) ANTAGONIST PROTOCOL

A 31-year-old woman with secondary infertility is planned for IVF. She is started on controlled ovarian stimulation with gonadotropins from day 2 of her cycle. On day 6 of stimulation, a GnRH antagonist is introduced. US monitoring shows multiple growing follicles with adequate estradiol levels.

1. What is the mechanism of action of GnRH antagonists?
2. How do antagonist protocols prevent premature LH surge?
3. What are the differences between agonist and antagonist protocols?
4. When is GnRH antagonist usually started during controlled ovarian stimulation?
5. What are the advantages of the antagonist protocol compared to the long agonist protocol?
6. What are the disadvantages or limitations of antagonist protocol?
7. Why is antagonist protocol preferred in patients at high risk of OHSS?
8. How is the timing of antagonist administration determined (fixed vs flexible protocol)?
9. What is the role of GnRH agonist trigger in antagonist cycles?
10. How does the antagonist protocol affect cycle duration and gonadotropin requirement?
11. What are the pregnancy and live birth rates in antagonist vs agonist cycles?
12. What is the role of antagonist protocol in low responders?
13. What are the side effects of GnRH antagonists?
14. What monitoring is needed during antagonist stimulation cycles?
15. In what clinical scenarios is antagonist protocol the first choice?

CASE NO. (7) PPOS PROTOCOL

A 33-year-old woman with polycystic ovary syndrome and primary infertility is scheduled for IVF. She is started on controlled ovarian stimulation with gonadotropins from day 2 of her cycle. From the same day, she receives daily oral progesterone (medroxyprogesterone acetate) to prevent a premature LH surge. Follicular growth is monitored by ultrasound and estradiol measurements, and a GnRH agonist trigger is planned once adequate follicular development is achieved.

1. What is the PPOS protocol in IVF/ICSI?
2. What is the mechanism of action of progestins in preventing premature LH surge?
3. How does PPOS differ from GnRH antagonist and agonist protocols?
4. What types of progestins are commonly used in PPOS?
5. What is the main indication for using PPOS protocol?
6. Why is fresh embryo transfer not recommended in PPOS cycles?
7. What is the role of "freeze-all strategy" in PPOS cycles?
8. How does PPOS affect oocyte yield and embryo quality compared to other protocols?
9. What are the advantages of PPOS protocol (simplicity, cost, oral medication)?
10. What are the disadvantages or limitations of PPOS protocol?
11. What groups of patients benefit most from PPOS (e.g., donors, PCOS, high responders)?
12. How is luteal phase support managed after PPOS if a fresh transfer is considered?
13. What is the role of PPOS in fertility preservation cycles?

14. How do outcomes (pregnancy rates, live birth rates) of PPOS compare with antagonist protocols?
15. What are the safety considerations of using progestins in IVF/ICSI cycles?

CASE NO. (8) DOUBLE STIMULATION PROTOCOL

A 36-year-old woman with diminished ovarian reserve and a history of poor response in previous IVF cycles is scheduled for double stimulation (DuoStim). She begins ovarian stimulation in the follicular phase of her menstrual cycle with gonadotropins, and several oocytes are retrieved. After oocyte pickup, stimulation is reinitiated in the luteal phase of the same cycle, leading to a second retrieval of mature oocytes. All embryos are planned for cryopreservation.

1. What is meant by double stimulation (DuoStim) protocol in IVF/ICSI?
2. What is the physiological basis of DuoStim (follicular and luteal waves of folliculogenesis)?
3. In which phases of the menstrual cycle can ovarian stimulation be initiated?
4. What are the main indications for DuoStim protocol?
5. Why is DuoStim particularly useful in low ovarian responders?
6. What is the role of DuoStim in fertility preservation (e.g., oncology patients)?
7. How is the first stimulation phase (follicular) performed in DuoStim?
8. How is the second stimulation phase (luteal) initiated?
9. What trigger is usually used in DuoStim cycles?
10. Why is “freeze-all strategy” mandatory in DuoStim?

11. How do oocyte yield and quality compare between follicular and luteal stimulations?
12. What are the advantages of DuoStim compared to conventional single stimulation?
13. What are the disadvantages and limitations of DuoStim?
14. What are the pregnancy and live birth outcomes after DuoStim?
15. What are the safety considerations of DuoStim (OHSS risk, patient burden)?
16. How do international guidelines view the role of DuoStim in ART practice?

CASE NO. (9) GONADOTROPINS IN IVF/ICSI

A 32-year-old woman with primary infertility is scheduled for IVF/ICSI. Controlled ovarian stimulation is initiated on day 2 of her menstrual cycle using recombinant FSH. During stimulation, human menopausal gonadotropin (hMG) is added to provide both FSH and LH activity, aiming to support follicular growth and estradiol production. Follicular development is monitored by serial transvaginal ultrasound and serum estradiol levels until the criteria for triggering final oocyte maturation are met.

1. What are gonadotropins and which hormones do they include?
2. What are the main types of gonadotropins used in ovarian stimulation?
3. What is the difference between urinary-derived and recombinant gonadotropins?
4. What is hMG (human menopausal gonadotropin) composed of?
5. What are the main clinical uses of FSH in IVF/ICSI cycles?

6. What is the role of LH in ovarian stimulation protocols?
7. In which situations is LH supplementation indicated during stimulation?
8. What are the advantages of recombinant FSH compared to urinary FSH?
9. What are the disadvantages of recombinant gonadotropins?
10. How is the starting dose of gonadotropins determined?
11. How do patient age and ovarian reserve affect gonadotropin dosing?
12. What are the risks associated with gonadotropin stimulation?
13. How is ovarian response monitored during gonadotropin stimulation?
14. What is the role of gonadotropins in antagonist protocols?
15. What is the role of gonadotropins in agonist protocols?
16. What are biosimilar gonadotropins and how do they compare with originals?
17. What are the predictors of gonadotropin dose adjustment during stimulation?
18. How do gonadotropins contribute to the risk of OHSS?
19. What are the differences in pregnancy outcomes between urinary and recombinant gonadotropins?
20. How do guidelines (e.g., ESHRE/ASRM) recommend using gonadotropins in ART cycles?

CASE NO. (10) TRIGGERING OF OVULATION

A 30-year-old woman undergoing IVF with controlled ovarian stimulation shows adequate follicular growth on day 10, with three leading follicles measuring 18–20 mm and serum estradiol levels within the expected range. To induce final oocyte maturation, ovulation is triggered using recombinant hCG.

1. What is meant by "triggering ovulation" in IVF/ICSI cycles?
2. What are the commonly used drugs for triggering ovulation?
3. How does hCG act as an ovulation trigger?
4. What is the difference between urinary hCG and recombinant hCG?
5. What is the role of GnRH agonist as a trigger in antagonist cycles?
6. What are the advantages of GnRH agonist trigger over hCG?
7. What is the main risk associated with hCG trigger?
8. Why is GnRH agonist trigger useful in patients at risk of OHSS?
9. What are the disadvantages of GnRH agonist trigger?
10. How is the timing of oocyte retrieval calculated after trigger?
11. What is the role of dual trigger (hCG + GnRH agonist)?
12. How do you decide the appropriate trigger in low responders vs high responders?
13. What is empty follicle syndrome and how is it related to ovulation trigger?
14. What monitoring is done before giving the trigger injection?
15. What happens if the trigger injection is missed or mistimed?
16. How does trigger choice influence luteal phase support requirements?
17. How do international guidelines (ESHRE/ASRM) recommend choosing an ovulation trigger?

CASE NO. (11) CYCLE CANCELLATION

A 35-year-old woman undergoing IVF is started on controlled ovarian stimulation with gonadotropins. Despite 10 days of stimulation, ultrasound monitoring shows minimal follicular growth with only one follicle measuring 10 mm, and serum estradiol remains very low. In another instance, a patient shows an excessive ovarian response with more than 25 developing follicles and very high estradiol levels, placing her at significant risk of ovarian hyperstimulation syndrome (OHSS). In both situations, the IVF cycle is cancelled to avoid poor outcome or serious complications.

1. What is meant by cycle cancellation in IVF/ICSI?
2. What are the common indications for IVF/ICSI cycle cancellation?
3. How does poor ovarian response lead to cycle cancellation?
4. What is the role of premature LH surge in cycle cancellation?
5. How does excessive ovarian response (risk of OHSS) lead to cancellation?
6. What are the criteria for cancellation due to inadequate follicular growth?
7. When is cancellation considered due to endometrial factors?
8. How does failed or mistimed trigger injection cause cycle cancellation?
9. What is the role of patient non-compliance in cycle cancellation?
10. What are the emotional and psychological impacts of cycle cancellation on couples?
11. What are the financial implications of cycle cancellation?
12. How do clinicians counsel patients about the possibility of cancellation before starting treatment?

13. What is the role of “freeze-all strategy” instead of cancellation in high responders?
14. How can cycle cancellation be prevented in low responders?
15. How can cycle cancellation be prevented in high responders at risk of OHSS?
16. What adjustments are made in subsequent cycles after cancellation?

CASE NO. (12) OOCYTE RETRIEVAL

A 29-year-old woman undergoing IVF has completed controlled ovarian stimulation with adequate follicular development. Thirty-six hours after ovulation trigger with recombinant hCG, she is scheduled for oocyte retrieval. The procedure is performed under transvaginal ultrasound guidance with conscious sedation. Follicular fluid is aspirated from both ovaries, and oocytes are identified in the embryology laboratory for subsequent fertilization.

1. What is oocyte retrieval and why is it performed in IVF/ICSI?
2. What is the optimal timing of oocyte retrieval after ovulation trigger?
3. What is the standard technique used for oocyte retrieval?
4. What type of anesthesia is commonly used for oocyte retrieval?
5. What are the possible complications of oocyte retrieval?
6. What is empty follicle syndrome?
7. How is infection risk minimized during oocyte retrieval?
8. How is bleeding during or after retrieval managed?
9. What is the average number of oocytes retrieved in a normal responder?
10. How is luteal phase supported after oocyte retrieval?

11. What is the difference between oocyte retrieval in agonist vs antagonist protocols?
12. How is oocyte retrieval performed in women with difficult pelvic anatomy or adhesions?
13. What are the risks of general anesthesia vs sedation in oocyte retrieval?
14. How long does the procedure usually take?
15. What is the impact of oocyte retrieval complications on future fertility or IVF cycles?

CASE NO. (13) LUTEAL PHASE SUPPORT

A 30-year-old woman undergoes IVF with controlled ovarian stimulation and oocyte retrieval. Following oocyte retrieval, she is started on luteal phase support to enhance endometrial receptivity and implantation. Vaginal micronized progesterone is administered daily, with the option of adding intramuscular progesterone or oral dydrogesterone.

1. Why is luteal phase support required in IVF/ICSI cycles?
2. What are the main causes of luteal phase defect in stimulated cycles?
3. What are the different forms of progesterone supplementation used for LPS?
4. What are the routes of progesterone administration (oral, vaginal, intramuscular, S.C)?
5. What are the advantages and disadvantages of vaginal vs intramuscular progesterone?
6. What is the role of hCG in luteal phase support? Why is it not recommended nowadays?
7. What is the role of estradiol supplementation in luteal support?

8. What is the evidence for using GnRH agonist as an adjunct in luteal support?
9. When should luteal support be started after oocyte retrieval/embryo transfer?
10. How long should luteal phase support be continued in IVF cycles?
11. What is the difference in luteal support needs between fresh and frozen embryo transfer cycles?
12. How is luteal phase support managed in GnRH agonist trigger cycles?
13. What complications can arise if luteal phase support is inadequate?
14. What do ESHRE/ASRM guidelines recommend as first-line luteal support in IVF/ICSI?
15. What is intensive luteal phase support and when is it used?
16. How do you counsel patients about the importance of adherence to luteal phase support?

CASE NO. (14) EMBRYO TRANSFER

A 32-year-old woman undergoing IVF has two good-quality blastocysts available for transfer. On day 5 after oocyte retrieval, a single blastocyst is selected for transfer to reduce the risk of multiple pregnancy. The procedure is performed under ultrasound guidance using a soft catheter, with care taken to minimize trauma to the endometrium. The remaining embryos are cryopreserved for future use.

1. What is embryo transfer and why is it a critical step in IVF/ICSI?
2. What are the different timings of embryo transfer (day 2–3 cleavage vs day 5 blastocyst)?

3. What are the advantages of blastocyst transfer compared to cleavage-stage transfer?
4. What factors influence the decision of single vs double embryo transfer?
5. What are the risks associated with multiple embryo transfer?
6. What are the characteristics of an optimal endometrium for embryo transfer?
7. What is the ideal endometrial thickness for transfer?
8. What are the steps of the embryo transfer procedure?
9. What is the role of ultrasound guidance during embryo transfer?
10. How does the type of catheter affect success rates in embryo transfer?
11. What is the difference between "easy" and "difficult" embryo transfer?
12. What are the possible complications during embryo transfer?
13. How does embryo transfer technique impact implantation and pregnancy outcomes?
14. What is the role of luteal phase support after embryo transfer?
15. What are the key counseling points for the patient after embryo transfer?

CASE NO. (15) ENDOMETRIAL PREPARATION FOR FROZEN EMBRYO TRANSFER

A 34-year-old woman with secondary infertility has three frozen blastocysts from a previous IVF cycle. She is scheduled for frozen embryo transfer. Endometrial preparation is started using oral estradiol from day 2 of her cycle to promote endometrial proliferation. After adequate thickness (> 8 mm) is achieved on ultrasound, vaginal progesterone is introduced to synchronize endometrial receptivity with embryo

development. Embryo transfer is planned on day 5 of progesterone supplementation, matching the blastocyst stage.

1. Why is endometrial preparation important before frozen embryo transfer?
2. What is the optimal endometrial thickness required for embryo implantation?
3. What are the methods of endometrial preparation for FET?
4. How does the natural (true ovulatory) cycle protocol work for FET?
5. What is the role of US and hormonal monitoring in natural cycle FET?
6. What is the hormone replacement therapy (HRT/artificial cycle) protocol for endometrial preparation?
7. What is the role of estradiol and progesterone in HRT-FET cycles?
8. How is the timing of progesterone initiation critical in HRT-FET cycles?
9. What is the modified natural cycle and when is it used?
10. What are the advantages and disadvantages of natural vs HRT cycles?
11. How is luteal phase support managed in FET cycles?
12. What are the factors associated with thin endometrium in FET cycles?
13. What are the possible adjuvant treatments for thin endometrium (e.g., sildenafil, PRP, G-CSF)?
14. What complications can arise from inadequate endometrial preparation?
15. How do ESHRE/ASRM guidelines recommend preparing the endometrium before FET?
16. What is the difference in pregnancy and live birth rates between fresh embryo transfer and frozen embryo transfer?
17. What is the freeze-all strategy in IVF, and what are its advantages and disadvantages

CASE NO. (16) SEX SELECTION

A 35-year-old couple with two daughters seeks IVF with preimplantation genetic testing (PGT) for the purpose of family balancing. The couple requests selection of a male embryo for transfer, despite having no medical or genetic indication. Embryos are created through IVF, biopsied at the blastocyst stage, and tested for chromosomal sex. A male embryo is chosen for transfer solely based on the couple's social preference, while the other embryos are cryopreserved.

1. What is sex selection and how can it be performed in IVF/ICSI?
2. What are the medical indications for sex selection?
3. What are the non-medical (social/family balancing) reasons for sex selection?
4. What is the role of preimplantation genetic testing (PGT) in sex selection?
5. What laboratory techniques are used to determine embryo sex before transfer?
6. What is sperm sorting and how is it related to sex selection?
7. What are the success rates and limitations of sperm sorting methods (e.g., MicroSort)?
8. What ethical issues are associated with sex selection for non-medical reasons?
9. What is the legal status of sex selection in different countries?
10. How do ESHRE and ASRM guidelines view sex selection?
11. What are the risks of discarding embryos based on sex?
12. How do you counsel a couple requesting sex selection for family balancing?

13. What are the psychosocial implications of sex selection practices?
14. What alternatives to sex selection may be offered for couples with genetic disease concerns?
15. What role does cultural and religious context play in decision-making about sex selection?

CASE NO. (17) PREIMPLANTATION GENETIC TESTING (PGT)

A 29-year-old woman and her 32-year-old husband are both carriers of the β-thalassemia gene mutation. They undergo IVF with intracytoplasmic sperm injection (ICSI) to create embryos. On day 5, trophectoderm biopsy is performed, and the cells are analyzed for the specific β-globin gene mutation using molecular genetic techniques. Only embryos free from the mutation are selected for transfer, while affected embryos are excluded to prevent transmission of the disease.

1. What is preimplantation genetic testing (PGT)?
2. How does PGD differ from preimplantation genetic testing for aneuploidy (PGT-A) and PGT-M?
3. What are the main indications for PGT?
4. What types of genetic disorders can be detected by PGD?
5. What are the methods of embryo biopsy used for PGT?
6. At what stage of embryo development is biopsy usually performed?
7. What laboratory techniques are used in PGT (e.g., FISH, PCR, NGS)?
8. What is the risk of embryo damage during biopsy?
9. How accurate is PGD in detecting genetic abnormalities?
10. What are the limitations of PGT?
11. What is mosaicism and how does it affect PGD results?
12. How does PGT affect implantation and pregnancy rates?

13. What are the ethical issues related to PGT ?
14. How is PGD used in sex-linked genetic disorders?
15. What is the difference between PGD and prenatal diagnosis (CVS, amniocentesis)?
16. How do you counsel couples regarding the benefits and limitations of PGT ?
17. What is the legal status of PGT in different countries?

CASE NO. (18) MALE FACTOR IN IVF/ICSI

A 35-year-old man with non-obstructive azoospermia undergoes testicular sperm extraction (TESE). Motile spermatozoa are successfully retrieved and cryopreserved for later use. His 30-year-old wife is then scheduled for IVF. Controlled ovarian stimulation is performed, followed by oocyte retrieval. The previously frozen-thawed testicular sperm are used for intracytoplasmic sperm injection (ICSI), and resulting embryos are cultured for transfer or cryopreservation.

1. What are the indications for using ICSI instead of conventional IVF in male factor infertility?
2. How does severe oligoasthenoteratozoospermia (OAT) affect the choice of IVF vs ICSI?
3. What is the role of surgical sperm retrieval (PESA, TESA, micro-TESE) in azoospermic men undergoing ICSI?
4. How does obstructive azoospermia differ from non-obstructive azoospermia in terms of sperm retrieval and outcome?
5. What is the impact of sperm DNA fragmentation on IVF/ICSI outcomes?

6. What are the laboratory methods available to select the best sperm for ICSI (e.g., IMSI, PICSI, MACS)?
7. What is the role of cryopreserved sperm in IVF/ICSI cycles?
8. How does the use of testicular sperm compare to ejaculated sperm in cases of high DNA fragmentation?
9. What are the expected fertilization and pregnancy rates with ICSI in severe male factor infertility?
10. How do genetic abnormalities (e.g., Y-chromosome microdeletions, Klinefelter syndrome, CFTR mutations) affect counseling before ICSI?
11. When should genetic counseling be offered to couples undergoing ICSI for male factor infertility?
12. What is the risk of transmitting genetic or chromosomal abnormalities to offspring with ICSI?
13. What is the role of sperm freezing before chemotherapy or gonadotoxic treatment in male infertility and IVF/ICSI?
14. How does advanced paternal age affect ART outcomes and embryo quality in IVF/ICSI?
15. What are the ethical considerations of using donor sperm in IVF/ICSI when no viable sperm is retrieved?

CASE NO. (19) IVF LAB

A 31-year-old woman undergoes controlled ovarian stimulation and oocyte retrieval. The collected oocytes are immediately transferred to the IVF laboratory, where they are assessed for maturity. In the lab, oocytes are either inseminated with prepared motile sperm for conventional IVF or injected directly with a single sperm in intracytoplasmic sperm injection (ICSI). Fertilization is confirmed by the presence of two

pronuclei, and embryos are cultured in a controlled environment with regulated temperature, humidity, and gas concentrations. Embryo development is monitored daily until transfer or cryopreservation.

1. What are the main functions of the IVF laboratory?
2. What are the ideal environmental conditions in an IVF lab (temperature, pH, CO_2, O_2)?
3. What culture media are used for gametes and embryos in IVF?
4. How are oocytes classified after retrieval (mature MII, MI, GV, degenerated)?
5. How is sperm prepared for IVF/ICSI in the lab?
6. What is the difference between conventional IVF and ICSI in terms of lab procedure?
7. How is fertilization assessed in the IVF lab?
8. What are the signs of normal fertilization (2PN stage)?
9. How are embryos graded at the cleavage stage (day 2–3)?
10. How are embryos graded at the blastocyst stage (day 5–6)?
11. What is embryo compaction and when does it occur?
12. What are the criteria for selecting the best embryo for transfer?
13. What are the different methods of embryo cryopreservation?
14. What is vitrification and why is it preferred over slow freezing?
15. What are the survival rates of embryos after thawing?
16. How is sperm cryopreservation performed in the IVF lab?
17. What are the risks of contamination or infection in the IVF laboratory?
18. What is the role of time-lapse incubators in embryo culture and selection?
19. What is the role of AI in embryo grading and selection in the IVF lab?
20. What quality control measures are essential in an IVF laboratory?

CASE NO. (20) HOW TO SELECT THE BEST EMBRYO

A 32-year-old woman undergoes IVF with ICSI. After oocyte retrieval and fertilization, 8 embryos are available for culture. On day 3, embryo grading shows:

- **3 embryos, Grade A (8-cell, equal blastomeres, minimal fragmentation)**
- **2 embryos, Grade B (6–7 cells, moderate fragmentation)**
- **3 embryos, Grade C (poor cell symmetry, heavy fragmentation)**

Culture is continued to day 5. Three blastocysts develop:

- **1 blastocyst, Grade AA (excellent expansion, clear inner cell mass, cohesive trophectoderm)**
- **1 blastocyst, Grade AB (good quality)**
- **1 blastocyst, Grade BB (moderate quality)**

The embryology team selects the Grade AA blastocyst for transfer, while the Grade AB and Grade BB blastocysts are cryopreserved. The remaining embryos are not suitable for transfer or freezing.

1. What are the main criteria used to select the best embryo for transfer?
2. What is the importance of embryo morphology in selection?
3. How are cleavage-stage embryos (day 2–3) graded?
4. What is the ideal number of blastomeres on day 3 of development?
5. What features suggest poor-quality cleavage-stage embryos?
6. How are blastocysts (day 5–6 embryos) graded?
7. What is the role of inner cell mass (ICM) and trophectoderm quality in blastocyst grading?
8. What is the significance of embryo fragmentation?
9. What is the role of compaction (morula stage) in embryo assessment?

10. How does embryo development timing (morphokinetics) influence selection?
11. What is the role of time-lapse imaging in embryo selection?
12. What is the role of preimplantation genetic testing (PGT) in embryo selection?
13. How do euploid vs aneuploid embryos differ in implantation potential?
14. What are non-invasive methods of embryo selection (e.g., spent media metabolomics)?
15. What is the impact of female age on embryo selection and implantation rate?
16. How do you decide between single vs multiple embryo transfer?
17. What is the evidence-based recommendation regarding single blastocyst transfer?
18. What are the risks of transferring lower-quality embryos?
19. What are "add-ons" in embryo selection (AI, metabolomics, proteomics)?
20. How do you counsel a couple about embryo selection and transfer strategy?

CASE NO. (21) OVARIAN HYPERSTIMULATION SYNFROME

A 28-year-old woman with polycystic ovary syndrome undergoes controlled ovarian stimulation for IVF. On day 10 of stimulation, ultrasound shows more than 25 developing follicles, and serum estradiol level is markedly elevated. After ovulation trigger and oocyte retrieval, she presents with abdominal bloating, nausea, and rapid weight gain over 48 hours. Clinical examination reveals ascites, enlarged ovaries, and mild shortness of breath. Laboratory investigations demonstrate hemoconcentration and elevated hematocrit.

1. What is ovarian hyperstimulation syndrome (OHSS)?
2. What is the pathophysiology of OHSS?
3. What are the risk factors for developing OHSS?
4. How is OHSS classified (mild, moderate, severe, critical)?
5. What are the clinical features of mild, moderate and severe OHSS?
6. What are the laboratory findings in severe OHSS?
7. What are the possible complications of OHSS?
8. How is OHSS diagnosed clinically and by ultrasound?
9. What is the role of VEGF in OHSS pathogenesis?
10. How can OHSS be prevented in high-risk patients?
11. What is the role of GnRH antagonist protocol in prevention of OHSS?
12. What is the role of GnRH agonist trigger instead of hCG in OHSS?
13. What is the role of "freeze-all" strategy in OHSS risk patients?
14. How is mild, moderate, severe and critical OHSS managed?
15. What is a pigtail catheter and how is it used in OHSS?
16. What is the role of thromboprophylaxis in severe OHSS?
17. What is the prognosis of OHSS for future cycles and fertility?
18. How do guidelines (ESHRE/ASRM) recommend preventing OHSS?
19. How do you counsel a patient at risk of OHSS before starting IVF/ICSI?

CASE NO. (22) LOW RESPONDERS

A 39-year-old woman with a 6-year history of primary infertility is scheduled for IVF. Baseline assessment shows an antral follicle count of 4 and AMH of 0.6 ng/ml, indicating reduced ovarian reserve. Controlled ovarian stimulation is started with high-dose gonadotropins. After 10 days of stimulation, ultrasound monitoring shows only two follicles reaching

maturity, and estradiol levels remain low. At oocyte retrieval, two mature oocytes (MII) are obtained and injected by ICSI. Only one embryo develops to day 3, graded as fair quality, and is transferred to the uterus.

1. What is meant by "poor ovarian response" or "low responder" in IVF/ICSI?
2. What are the Bologna criteria for defining poor ovarian response?
3. What are the limitations of the Bologna criteria?
4. What is the POSEIDON classification, and how does it improve on Bologna?
5. What clinical factors are associated with poor ovarian response?
6. What is the role of age in predicting ovarian response?
7. What is the role of ovarian reserve tests (AMH, AFC, FSH) in identifying poor responders?
8. How do previous cycle outcomes predict low response?
9. What stimulation protocols are commonly used for low responders?
10. What is the role of antagonist protocol in low responders?
11. What is the role of (short agonist) protocol in low responders?
12. What is the evidence for using adjuvants (DHEA, Coenzyme Q10, GH, PRP) in low responders?
13. What is the role of dual stimulation (DuoStim) in low responders?
14. How does oocyte/embryo accumulation strategy help in low responders?
15. What are the success rates of IVF/ICSI in low responders compared to normal responders?
16. How do you counsel a couple with low ovarian reserve about prognosis and options?
17. What alternative options can be discussed (donor oocytes, adoption)?
18. What psychological and emotional support should be provided to low responders?

CASE NO. (23) IVF/ICSI WITH ENDOMETRIOSIS & ADENOMYOSIS

A 34-year-old woman with a 7-year history of primary infertility is diagnosed with stage III endometriosis and adenomyosis. She has undergone laparoscopic surgery for ovarian endometriomas in the past. Despite surgery and medical treatment, conception did not occur, and she is referred for IVF with ICSI. COS is started with gonadotropins. At oocyte retrieval, 7 mature oocytes are collected, and ICSI is performed. Five oocytes fertilize normally, and three good-quality embryos develop to the blastocyst stage. One blastocyst is transferred, and the remaining two are cryopreserved. Due to adenomyosis, prolonged luteal phase support is planned, and the patient is closely monitored for implantation outcome.

1. How does endometriosis affect fertility and IVF/ICSI outcomes?
2. What is the impact of endometrioma on ovarian reserve and oocyte quality?
3. When should surgical removal of endometrioma be considered before ICSI?
4. What are the risks of surgery for endometrioma in women planning IVF/ICSI?
5. What is the role of medical pretreatment (GnRH agonists, dienogest) before IVF/ICSI in endometriosis patients?
6. How does adenomyosis impair implantation and pregnancy rates in IVF/ICSI?
7. What imaging findings suggest adenomyosis in women undergoing IVF/ICSI?
8. What is the role of GnRH agonist pretreatment in adenomyosis before ICSI?

9. What is the role of hysteroscopy in evaluating the uterine cavity in adenomyosis/endometriosis patients?
10. How do endometriosis and adenomyosis contribute to recurrent implantation failure (RIF)?
11. What stimulation protocol is preferred in women with endometriosis undergoing ICSI?
12. What is the role of "freeze-all" strategy in patients with endometriosis/adenomyosis?
13. How does endometriosis affect embryo quality compared to adenomyosis (which mainly affects implantation)?
14. What are the adjuvant therapies that may improve ICSI outcome in adenomyosis patients (e.g., GnRH agonist, LNG-IUS)?
15. How should patients with endometriosis or adenomyosis be counseled regarding success rates of IVF/ICSI?

CASE NO. (24) IVF/ICSI IN PATIENTS WITH CARDIAC DISEASES

A 29-year-old woman with a history of surgically corrected congenital heart disease presents with secondary infertility of 4 years. She has been stable on regular cardiology follow-up and is classified as NYHA functional class II. Pre-treatment evaluation includes cardiology clearance and echocardiography to assess cardiac function. Multidisciplinary planning is arranged between the reproductive medicine team, anesthesiologist, and cardiologist. Controlled ovarian stimulation is initiated with a mild stimulation protocol to reduce the risk of ovarian hyperstimulation syndrome (OHSS) and minimize cardiovascular strain. Oocyte retrieval is performed under conscious sedation with close hemodynamic monitoring. ICSI is carried out using her partner's sperm,

and two blastocysts develop. A single blastocyst transfer is planned to reduce the risk of multiple pregnancy, while the remaining embryo is cryopreserved. Luteal support is initiated, and the patient continues under joint follow-up with the fertility and cardiology teams.

1. What are the risks of ovarian stimulation in women with underlying cardiac disease?
2. How does pregnancy itself increase cardiovascular load in cardiac patients?
3. What pre-treatment cardiac evaluation is necessary before IVF/ICSI?
4. Which cardiac conditions are considered high-risk or contraindications for pregnancy?
5. What modifications are needed in ovarian stimulation protocols for cardiac patients?
6. What is the role of mild stimulation or natural cycle IVF in women with cardiac disease?
7. What are the anesthesia considerations for oocyte retrieval in cardiac patients?
8. How should luteal phase support be managed in women with cardiac disease?
9. What are the risks of OHSS in cardiac patients, and how can they be prevented?
10. What is the role of a multidisciplinary team in managing IVF/ICSI in cardiac patients?
11. How should anticoagulation be managed in women with prosthetic heart valves undergoing IVF?
12. What is the safest embryo transfer strategy in cardiac patients (single vs double embryo transfer)?

13. What counseling should be given regarding maternal and fetal risks in cardiac patients undergoing ART?
14. What are the long-term risks of pregnancy in women with congenital heart disease undergoing IVF/ICSI?
15. How do guidelines (e.g., WHO/ESHRE/ESC) classify maternal cardiac risk in assisted reproduction?

CASE NO. (25) IVF/ICSI IN PATIENTS WITH AUTOIMMUNE DISEASES

A 33-year-old woman with a 5-year history of primary infertility is known to have systemic lupus erythematosus (SLE) controlled with low-dose corticosteroids and hydroxychloroquine. She has a past history of positive antiphospholipid antibodies but no thrombotic events. Pre-treatment evaluation is coordinated with her rheumatologist to ensure disease stability before starting IVF. Controlled ovarian stimulation is carried out with careful dose adjustment of gonadotropins, and low-molecular-weight heparin along with low-dose aspirin are introduced for thromboprophylaxis. At oocyte retrieval, 10 mature oocytes are collected and fertilized by ICSI, resulting in six normally fertilized embryos. On day 5, a single good-quality blastocyst is transferred, and the remaining embryos are cryopreserved. Luteal phase support with progesterone is continued, and the patient is closely monitored throughout early pregnancy in collaboration with her rheumatology and obstetric teams.

1. What are the common autoimmune diseases that may affect fertility or ART outcomes?
2. How does systemic lupus erythematosus (SLE) impact fertility and IVF/ICSI?

3. What are the risks of ovarian stimulation in women with autoimmune diseases?
4. How do autoimmune diseases increase the risk of miscarriage and implantation failure?
5. What pre-IVF workup is required in patients with autoimmune disease (labs, antibodies, organ function)?
6. How does antiphospholipid antibody syndrome affect ART outcomes?
7. What is the role of anticoagulation (aspirin, heparin) in IVF/ICSI cycles for autoimmune patients?
8. What is the role of immunosuppressive therapy in women with autoimmune disease undergoing IVF/ICSI?
9. What are the anesthesia considerations for oocyte retrieval in autoimmune patients with organ involvement?
10. How does lupus nephritis or renal involvement influence ART planning?
11. What is the role of corticosteroid therapy in IVF/ICSI cycles with autoimmune background?
12. How should embryo transfer be planned in patients with high thrombotic risk?
13. What are the pregnancy complications associated with autoimmune disease after IVF/ICSI?
14. How important is disease remission/stability before initiating IVF/ICSI?
15. How do you counsel a couple about the maternal and fetal risks of IVF/ICSI in autoimmune disease?
16. What is the role of multidisciplinary management (rheumatology, hematology, obstetrics, fertility specialist)?

CASE NO. (26) IVF/ICSI IN PATIENTS WITH THYROID DISEASES

A 31-year-old woman with a 3-year history of primary infertility is diagnosed with hypothyroidism and has been on levothyroxine replacement therapy. Pre-treatment evaluation confirms a normal thyroid profile (TSH within target range) before initiating IVF. Controlled ovarian stimulation with gonadotropins is started, and follicular growth is monitored by ultrasound and estradiol levels. At oocyte retrieval, 11 mature oocytes are collected, and ICSI is performed using her partner's sperm. Eight oocytes fertilize normally, and five good-quality embryos are obtained by day 5. A single blastocyst transfer is performed to minimize the risk of multiple pregnancy, and the remaining embryos are cryopreserved. Thyroid function tests are monitored throughout the cycle, and levothyroxine dose adjustment is continued as needed in preparation for early pregnancy.

1. How does thyroid function affect female fertility and ART outcomes?
2. What is the impact of hypothyroidism on ovulation and implantation?
3. How does hyperthyroidism affect fertility and pregnancy outcomes?
4. What is subclinical hypothyroidism and how is it relevant in IVF/ICSI?
5. What is the role of thyroid autoimmunity (anti-TPO, anti-TG antibodies) in infertility and ART failure?
6. What thyroid function tests should be performed before IVF/ICSI?
7. What is the recommended target TSH level before IVF/ICSI according to international guidelines?
8. How is hypothyroidism managed in women planning IVF/ICSI?
9. How is hyperthyroidism managed before IVF/ICSI?

10. What are the risks of untreated thyroid disease during IVF/ICSI and pregnancy?
11. How do thyroid antibodies affect miscarriage and implantation failure
12. What is the role of levothyroxine supplementation in thyroid autoimmunity with normal TSH?
13. How should thyroid function be monitored during controlled ovarian stimulation?
14. What are the anesthetic considerations for oocyte retrieval in uncontrolled thyroid disease?

CASE NO. (27) IVF/ICSI IN PATIENTS WITH HEPATIC DISEASES

A 35-year-old woman with secondary infertility of 6 years is known to have chronic hepatitis B infection. She is under regular hepatology follow-up with stable liver function tests and no evidence of cirrhosis. Prior to initiating IVF, viral load assessment and liver function evaluation are performed, and she is maintained on antiviral therapy. Controlled ovarian stimulation with gonadotropins is started cautiously to avoid excessive estrogen exposure. At oocyte retrieval, 9 mature oocytes are collected, and ICSI is carried out with her partner's sperm. Six oocytes fertilize normally, resulting in four good-quality embryos by day 5. A single blastocyst transfer is performed, while the remaining embryos are cryopreserved. Strict universal precautions are applied in the laboratory to prevent viral transmission, and the patient continues on coordinated follow-up with both the reproductive medicine and hepatology teams.

1. How do chronic liver diseases affect female fertility?
2. What are the common hepatic diseases encountered in women of reproductive age undergoing IVF/ICSI?

3. How does advanced liver disease (cirrhosis, portal hypertension) impact fertility and ART planning?
4. What is the effect of hepatitis B and C infections on fertility and IVF/ICSI outcomes?
5. What infectious disease screening is mandatory before IVF/ICSI in patients with hepatitis?
6. What precautions are required in the IVF laboratory when handling gametes/embryos from HBV/HCV positive patients?
7. What are the possible risks of ovarian stimulation in patients with hepatic impairment?
8. How are gonadotropin doses adjusted in women with liver disease?
9. What is the role of antiviral therapy before IVF/ICSI in patients with hepatitis B or C?
10. How does hepatic dysfunction affect estrogen metabolism during stimulation?
11. What anesthesia considerations should be taken for oocyte retrieval in patients with liver disease?
12. What is the risk of vertical transmission of HBV/HCV during ART and pregnancy?
13. How can the risk of mother-to-child transmission of hepatitis B be minimized?
14. How do you counsel couples regarding fertility treatment in the presence of chronic liver disease?
15. What is the role of a multidisciplinary team (hepatologist, fertility specialist, obstetrician) in managing such cases?

CASE NO. (28) IVF/ICSI IN PATIENTS WITH D.M

A 34-year-old woman with type 2 diabetes mellitus for 8 years presents with a 5-year history of primary infertility. She is on oral hypoglycemic agents but is transitioned to insulin therapy prior to IVF for optimal glycemic control. Pre-treatment evaluation includes HbA1c, renal profile, and fundus examination. HbA1c is optimized to <6.5% before stimulation. Controlled ovarian stimulation with gonadotropins is initiated, and blood glucose is closely monitored throughout the cycle. At oocyte retrieval, 10 mature oocytes are obtained, and ICSI is performed with her husband's sperm. Seven oocytes fertilize normally, producing four good-quality blastocysts. A single blastocyst is transferred to minimize obstetric risk, while the remaining embryos are cryopreserved. Luteal support is provided with progesterone, and the patient continues tight glycemic monitoring under joint care of the fertility and endocrinology teams.

1. How does diabetes mellitus affect female fertility?
2. What are the effects of poorly controlled diabetes on ovarian function and oocyte quality?
3. How does diabetes affect endometrial receptivity and implantation?
4. What are the risks of miscarriage and congenital anomalies in diabetic women undergoing IVF/ICSI?
5. What pre-IVF evaluation should be performed in diabetic women?
6. What is the recommended HbA1c target before initiating IVF/ICSI?
7. How does PCOS with insulin resistance overlap with diabetes in infertility management?

8. What is the role of metformin in diabetic women undergoing IVF/ICSI?
9. How does diabetes affect male fertility (sperm parameters, DNA fragmentation)?
10. What are the risks of ovarian stimulation in diabetic women with vascular complications?
11. What are the anesthesia considerations for oocyte retrieval in women with diabetes?
12. How should blood glucose be managed during controlled ovarian stimulation and early pregnancy?
13. What are the pregnancy-related risks after IVF/ICSI in diabetic women (e.g., preeclampsia, macrosomia)?
14. How should luteal phase support and early pregnancy be monitored in diabetic patients?
15. What counseling should be provided to couples about IVF/ICSI success and risks in diabetes?
16. What is the role of a multidisciplinary team (endocrinologist, fertility specialist, obstetrician) in managing IVF/ICSI in diabetic patients?

CASE NO. (29) FERTILITY PRESERVATION

A 27-year-old woman recently diagnosed with breast cancer is scheduled to begin chemotherapy in three weeks. She is referred for fertility preservation before starting gonadotoxic treatment. To maximize the number of oocytes retrieved in a limited time, a double stimulation (DuoStim) protocol is used. Controlled ovarian stimulation with gonadotropins and letrozole is started in the follicular phase, and a GnRH agonist trigger is given when follicles mature. At the first oocyte retrieval,

8 mature oocytes are collected. Immediately after retrieval, a second stimulation cycle is initiated in the luteal phase using the same protocol. This results in 7 additional mature oocytes, giving a total of 15 oocytes. Eight oocytes are cryopreserved by vitrification, and seven are fertilized with her partner's sperm to create embryos, which are cryopreserved at the blastocyst stage. The patient then proceeds with her oncology treatment plan, preserving future fertility options.

1. What is meant by fertility preservation?
2. What are the main indications for fertility preservation?
3. What are the methods of fertility preservation available for women?
4. What is the role of oocyte cryopreservation and when is it preferred?
5. What is the role of embryo cryopreservation and when is it used?
6. What are the techniques of ovarian tissue cryopreservation?
7. What are the indications for ovarian tissue cryopreservation?
8. What are the fertility preservation options for prepubertal girls?
9. What is the role of GnRH agonists during chemotherapy for ovarian protection?
10. What are the fertility preservation methods available for men?
11. What are the options for prepubertal boys needing fertility preservation?
12. How does cancer treatment (chemo/radiotherapy) affect fertility in both sexes?
13. What is oncofertility and why is it important?
14. What are the ethical issues related to fertility preservation in cancer patients?
15. How successful are pregnancies after oocyte or embryo thawing?
16. What are the risks associated with ovarian tissue transplantation?

17. What counseling should be offered to patients before fertility preservation procedures?
18. What are the social indications for elective oocyte freezing?
19. How does age impact the success of fertility preservation strategies?
20. What is the role of a multidisciplinary team in fertility preservation?

CASE NO. (30) RECURRENT IMPLANTATION FAILURE

A 35-year-old woman with a 7-year history of primary infertility has undergone three previous IVF/ICSI cycles. In each cycle, good-quality blastocysts were transferred, but no clinical pregnancy was achieved. Endometrial thickness was adequate in all cycles, and luteal support was provided with progesterone. Further evaluation is performed, including hysteroscopy, which reveals a normal uterine cavity, and thrombophilia screening, which shows no abnormalities. Endometrial receptivity testing is performed to optimize embryo transfer timing. In the current cycle, preimplantation genetic testing (PGT-A) is used to select euploid embryos for transfer. A single euploid blastocyst is transferred under ultrasound guidance.

1. What is the definition of recurrent implantation failure (RIF)?
2. How many failed embryo transfers are required to diagnose RIF?
3. What are the maternal (uterine) factors contributing to RIF?
4. What are the embryonic factors contributing to RIF?
5. How does advanced maternal age contribute to RIF?
6. What is the role of preimplantation genetic testing (PGT-A) in RIF?
7. How do congenital uterine anomalies contribute to implantation failure?

8. What is the role of hysteroscopy in RIF evaluation?
9. How does chronic endometritis contribute to implantation failure?
10. What is the impact of thin endometrium on implantation?
11. What immune factors may be involved in RIF (e.g., NK cells, thrombophilias)?
12. What is the role of thrombophilia screening in RIF?
13. What adjuvant treatments are proposed for RIF (aspirin, heparin, steroids, immunotherapy)?
14. What is the role of endometrial scratching in RIF?
15. What is the role of intrauterine PRP infusion in RIF management?
16. What is the role of double embryo transfer or blastocyst transfer in RIF?
17. How does sperm DNA fragmentation contribute to RIF?
18. What is the role of time-lapse embryo monitoring in RIF?
19. How should couples be counseled about prognosis after RIF?
20. What do ESHRE/ASRM guidelines recommend for investigation and management of RIF?

CASE NO. (31) ADD-ONS IN IVF/ICSI

A 34-year-old woman with secondary infertility is undergoing her fourth IVF/ICSI cycle after previous failed attempts despite transfer of good-quality embryos. In this cycle, several add-ons are incorporated to potentially improve outcomes. Endometrial scratch is performed in the cycle prior to stimulation. During ovarian stimulation, growth hormone is added as an adjuvant. Sperm selection is carried out using physiological ICSI (PICSI) to choose mature spermatozoa. Embryos are cultured to the blastocyst stage under time-lapse monitoring to assess morphokinetics.

On day 5, preimplantation genetic testing for aneuploidy (PGT-A) is performed, and a single euploid blastocyst is transferred. Remaining euploid embryos are cryopreserved for future use.

1. What is meant by "add-ons" in IVF/ICSI?
2. Why are add-ons commonly used in assisted reproduction despite limited evidence?
3. What is the role of time-lapse embryo imaging as an add-on?
4. What is the role of assisted hatching in IVF/ICSI?
5. How does preimplantation genetic testing (PGT-A) fit as an add-on?
6. What is the role of endometrial scratching in improving implantation rates?
7. How is intrauterine infusion of PRP used as an add-on?
8. What is the role of growth factors (e.g., G-CSF) in thin endometrium cases?
9. What are the immunological add-ons (steroids, intralipids, IVIG) and when are they considered?
10. What is the role of sperm selection techniques (PICSI, IMSI, MACS) as add-ons?
11. What is the use of artificial oocyte activation in IVF/ICSI?
12. What is the role of hyaluronan-enriched embryo transfer medium (EmbryoGlue)?
13. What is the role of endometrial receptivity array (ERA) testing as an add-on?
14. What is the role of mitochondrial supplements or Coenzyme Q10 as add-ons?
15. How do international guidelines (ESHRE/ASRM/HFEA) classify add-ons (green, amber, red) according to evidence?
16. What counseling should be given to couples before offering IVF add-ons?

CASE NO. (32) MYOMA IN IVF/ICSI

34-year-old woman with a 5-year history of infertility is diagnosed with uterine fibroids. Ultrasound reveal one intramural myoma measuring 4 cm that does not distort the endometrial cavity, and one submucosal myoma measuring 2.5 cm that distorts the cavity. She has a history of two failed IVF cycles with good-quality embryos transferred. Before starting a new cycle, she undergoes hysteroscopic myomectomy to remove the submucosal fibroid while the intramural myoma is left in place since it does not affect the endometrial contour. After recovery, controlled ovarian stimulation is initiated, and 10 mature oocytes are retrieved. ICSI is performed, resulting in six normally fertilized embryos. Two blastocysts are developed, one is transferred, and the other is cryopreserved. The cycle is managed with close monitoring to optimize implantation rates following correction of the endometrial cavity.

1. What types of fibroids are most likely to affect fertility and IVF outcomes?
2. How do submucous fibroids impair implantation and pregnancy rates?
3. What is the effect of intramural fibroids on IVF/ICSI success?
4. Do subserosal fibroids usually affect IVF/ICSI outcomes?
5. What imaging modalities are used to assess fibroids before IVF/ICSI?
6. What is the role of hysteroscopy in evaluating submucous fibroids prior to IVF?
7. When is myomectomy indicated before IVF/ICSI?
8. What are the risks of performing myomectomy in infertile women?
9. How long should a patient wait to attempt conception after myomectomy?

10. What is the impact of fibroids on miscarriage rates after IVF/ICSI?
11. What is the role of medical management (GnRH agonists, SPRMs) for fibroids before IVF?
12. How does adenomyosis differ from fibroids in their effect on IVF outcome?
13. What is the effect of fibroid size and number on IVF success rates?
14. How do you counsel a patient with fibroids planning IVF/ICSI?
15. What do international guidelines (ESHRE/ASRM) recommend regarding fibroids and IVF/ICSI?
16. What is the FIGO classification of uterine fibroids and how is it clinically relevant in IVF/ICSI?

CASE NO. (33) CONGENITAL UTERINE ANOMALIES IN IVF/ICSI

A 29-year-old woman with a 4-year history of primary infertility is evaluated for IVF/ICSI after two failed cycles of ovulation induction with intrauterine insemination (IUI). Transvaginal ultrasound reveal a septate uterus. Hysteroscopy confirms the diagnosis, and a hysteroscopic septal resection is performed to restore a normal endometrial cavity. After adequate healing, the patient proceeds with IVF. Controlled ovarian stimulation is started, and 12 mature oocytes are retrieved. ICSI is performed, resulting in eight normally fertilized embryos. By day 5, three good-quality blastocysts develop. A single blastocyst is transferred under ultrasound guidance, and the remaining embryos are cryopreserved. The patient continues luteal support with progesterone, and pregnancy outcome is monitored closely given her history of congenital uterine anomaly.

1. What are congenital uterine anomalies and how common are they in infertile women?
2. What is the embryological basis of congenital uterine anomalies?
3. What are the main types of congenital uterine anomalies (septate, bicornuate, unicornuate, didelphys, arcuate)?
4. Which congenital uterine anomaly is most strongly associated with infertility and recurrent pregnancy loss?
5. How can septate uterus be differentiated from bicornuate uterus?
6. What imaging modalities are used to diagnose congenital uterine anomalies (2D/3D US, HSG, MRI)?
7. What is the role of hysteroscopy in diagnosing and managing congenital uterine anomalies?
8. How does septate uterus affect IVF/ICSI outcome?
9. What is the effect of bicornuate uterus on fertility and ART outcomes?
10. What is the clinical significance of arcuate uterus in infertility?
11. What are the obstetric complications associated with congenital uterine anomalies?
12. What is the role of surgical correction (hysteroscopic metroplasty) in septate uterus?
13. How does surgical correction of uterine anomalies affect IVF/ICSI success rates?
14. What are the risks of surgery for congenital uterine anomalies?
15. How do you counsel a patient with congenital uterine anomaly planning IVF/ICSI?
16. What do ESHRE/ASRM guidelines recommend for evaluation and management of uterine anomalies in infertile women?

CASE NO. (34) HYPOPLASTIC UTERUS IN IVF/ICSI

A 25-year-old woman with primary amenorrhea and primary infertility is diagnosed with hypoplastic uterus. She has a history of delayed puberty and was treated with hormonal replacement therapy to induce menstruation. On transvaginal ultrasound, the uterus is markedly small with reduced endometrial thickness that fails to respond adequately to estrogen stimulation. Ovarian reserve assessment shows normal antral follicle count and AMH levels, indicating preserved ovarian function. Controlled ovarian stimulation is performed, and 11 mature oocytes are retrieved. ICSI is carried out, resulting in 7 normally fertilized embryos. However, due to the poor uterine environment, embryo transfer is not performed. The couple is counseled regarding the option of embryo cryopreservation

1. What is a hypoplastic uterus, and how does it differ from other congenital uterine anomalies?
2. How does a hypoplastic uterus impact implantation and pregnancy outcome in IVF/ICSI?
3. Why is embryo transfer usually not feasible in patients with a hypoplastic uterus?
4. What alternative fertility options can be offered to a woman with preserved ovarian reserve but hypoplastic uterus?
5. What are the potential psychosocial implications for patients counseled about the need for surrogacy?
6. What is the legal and ethical status of surrogacy for patients with hypoplastic uterus, and how does it differ across countries and religious contexts?

CASE NO. (35) ENDOMETRIAL POLYP IN IVF/ICSI

A 33-year-old woman with secondary infertility for 3 years is scheduled for IVF/ICSI. Baseline transvaginal ultrasound reveals a focal hyperechoic lesion within the uterine cavity suggestive of an endometrial polyp measuring 1.5 cm. Hysteroscopy is performed, and the polyp is resected to restore normal endometrial architecture. After recovery, controlled ovarian stimulation is initiated, and 11 mature oocytes are retrieved. ICSI is performed, resulting in seven normally fertilized embryos. By day 5, three good-quality blastocysts are obtained. One blastocyst is transferred under ultrasound guidance, while the remaining two are cryopreserved. Luteal support with progesterone is provided, and the patient is followed up for pregnancy outcome.

1. What is an endometrial polyp and how common is it in infertile women?
2. How do endometrial polyps contribute to infertility?
3. What is the effect of endometrial polyps on natural conception vs IVF/ICSI outcomes?
4. How are endometrial polyps diagnosed (TVUS, saline infusion sonography, hysteroscopy)?
5. What are the typical ultrasound features of an endometrial polyp?
6. What is the gold standard for diagnosis and treatment of endometrial polyps?
7. When should hysteroscopic polypectomy be performed before IVF/ICSI?
8. What is the evidence regarding improvement in pregnancy rates after polypectomy?

9. What is the recurrence rate of endometrial polyps after removal?
10. How do small (<1 cm) polyps affect fertility compared to large polyps?
11. What are the possible complications of hysteroscopic polypectomy?
12. How do endometrial polyps interact with other uterine factors such as fibroids or adhesions in infertility?
13. How should polyps detected during controlled ovarian stimulation be managed?
14. What is the role of frozen embryo transfer (FET) after polypectomy?
15. How do you counsel a patient with an endometrial polyp before IVF/ICSI?

CASE NO. (36) THIN ENDOMETRIUM IN IVF/ICSI

A 35-year-old woman with a 6-year history of primary infertility is undergoing IVF/ICSI. During endometrial preparation, serial ultrasound monitoring shows endometrial thickness persistently below 6 mm despite adequate estrogen supplementation. Various adjuvant therapies are introduced, including low-dose aspirin, vaginal sildenafil, and intrauterine granulocyte colony-stimulating factor (G-CSF) instillation to improve endometrial receptivity. Eventually, endometrial thickness reaches 7 mm, and a single good-quality blastocyst is transferred under ultrasound guidance. Remaining embryos are cryopreserved, and luteal phase support is provided with progesterone. The patient is closely monitored for implantation and early pregnancy outcome due to the history of thin endometrium.

1. What is the definition of thin endometrium in IVF/ICSI cycles?
2. What is the optimal endometrial thickness required for implantation?

3. How does thin endometrium affect implantation and pregnancy rates in IVF/ICSI?
4. What are the causes of thin endometrium (uterine, hormonal, iatrogenic)?
5. How does Asherman's syndrome contribute to thin endometrium?
6. What is the role of inadequate estrogen priming in thin endometrium?
7. How is endometrial thickness assessed and monitored?
8. What is the role of Doppler blood flow studies in thin endometrium assessment?
9. What are the medical treatments available for thin endometrium (estrogen, sildenafil, pentoxifylline, vitamin E)?
10. What is the role of intrauterine G-CSF in managing thin endometrium?
11. What is the role of intrauterine PRP (platelet-rich plasma) in thin endometrium treatment?
12. What are the surgical options for thin endometrium caused by adhesions?
13. What is the role of stem cell therapy in refractory thin endometrium?
14. How should embryo transfer strategy be modified in patients with thin endometrium?
15. What do ESHRE/ASRM guidelines recommend in managing thin endometrium in IVF/ICSI cycles?

CASE NO. (37) ENDOMETRIAL CAVITY FLUID IDENTIFIED DURING IVF

A 36-year-old woman with secondary infertility is undergoing IVF/ICSI. During ovarian stimulation, transvaginal ultrasound on day 9 reveals fluid collection within the endometrial cavity measuring 4 mm in depth. The endometrial lining appears thin and irregular around the fluid

pocket. Further evaluation rules out tubal disease but suggests chronic endometritis as a possible cause of intrauterine fluid accumulation. Due to the negative impact of intrauterine fluid on implantation, embryo transfer is deferred. All good-quality blastocysts are cryopreserved, and the patient is referred for hysteroscopic evaluation and appropriate treatment before planning a frozen embryo transfer cycle in a subsequent attempt.

1. What is meant by endometrial cavity fluid (ECF) in the context of IVF/ICSI?
2. How common is the finding of ECF during controlled ovarian stimulation?
3. What are the possible causes of endometrial cavity fluid during IVF cycles?
4. How does ECF affect implantation and pregnancy rates in IVF/ICSI?
5. How is ECF diagnosed and monitored?
6. What is the significance of transient vs persistent endometrial cavity fluid?
7. What is the role of aspiration of endometrial fluid before embryo transfer?
8. What is the role of antibiotics in managing ECF?
9. What is the impact of recurrent/persistent ECF on IVF outcome?
10. How should embryo transfer be managed if ECF is detected on the day of transfer?
11. When should the cycle be cancelled or converted to freeze-all in cases of ECF?
12. What is the role of treating hydrosalpinx (salpingectomy or proximal tubal occlusion) in preventing ECF?
13. What is the role of hysteroscopy in recurrent endometrial fluid cases?
14. How do you counsel patients about prognosis if ECF is found during IVF treatment?

CASE NO. (38) HYDROSALPINEX IN IVF/ICSI

A 35-year-old woman with a 7-year history of primary infertility is planned for IVF/ICSI. Transvaginal ultrasound and HSG demonstrate bilateral hydrosalpinx with recurrent intrauterine fluid noted during previous cycles. She previously had one failed IVF attempt where good-quality embryos were transferred but implantation did not occur. Given the detrimental effect of hydrosalpinx fluid on endometrial receptivity and embryo implantation, laparoscopic bilateral salpingectomy is performed before starting a new cycle. Following recovery, controlled ovarian stimulation is initiated, and 12 mature oocytes are retrieved. ICSI is performed, resulting in eight normally fertilized embryos. On day 5, two blastocysts of good quality are obtained; one is transferred, and the other is cryopreserved. The patient continues luteal phase support and is followed closely for pregnancy outcome.

1. What is hydrosalpinx and how does it develop?
2. How common is hydrosalpinx in infertile women undergoing IVF/ICSI?
3. How does hydrosalpinx negatively affect implantation and pregnancy rates in IVF/ICSI?
4. What are the proposed mechanisms by which hydrosalpinx fluid impairs embryo implantation?
5. How is hydrosalpinx diagnosed (ultrasound, HSG, laparoscopy)?
6. What is the role of sonohysterography in diagnosing hydrosalpinx?
7. How does hydrosalpinx affect miscarriage rates after IVF/ICSI?
8. What is the impact of hydrosalpinx on ectopic pregnancy risk?

9. What is the role of salpingectomy before IVF/ICSI in patients with hydrosalpinx?
10. What are the alternatives to salpingectomy (proximal tubal occlusion, clipping, aspiration)?
11. What is the evidence from randomized controlled trials regarding salpingectomy and IVF outcomes?
12. When is a freeze-all strategy recommended in women with untreated hydrosalpinx?
13. What are the risks of salpingectomy in terms of ovarian reserve and blood supply?
14. What is the role of antibiotics in management of hydrosalpinx?
15. How do you counsel a patient with unilateral vs bilateral hydrosalpinx before IVF/ICSI?
16. What do ESHRE/ASRM guidelines recommend for the management of hydrosalpinx prior to IVF?

CASE NO. (39) C.S SCAR DEFECT IN IVF/ ICSI

A 37-year-old woman with secondary infertility is scheduled for IVF/ICSI. She has a history of two previous cesarean sections. During baseline transvaginal ultrasound, a cesarean section scar defect (isthmocele) is noted, with a small anechoic fluid collection within the niche. The endometrium appears irregular around the scar area. The patient reports postmenstrual spotting, consistent with the C.S. defect. Because intrauterine fluid and scar defects may impair implantation, hysteroscopic correction of the isthmocele is performed before proceeding with ovarian stimulation. After recovery, controlled ovarian stimulation is initiated, and 10 mature oocytes are retrieved. ICSI is performed, leading

to six normally fertilized embryos. By day 5, three good-quality blastocysts develop, one is transferred, and the remaining two are cryopreserved for future use.

1. What is a C.S scar defect (isthmocele) and how does it form?
2. What is the prevalence of isthmocele in women with previous cesarean delivery?
3. How does a C.S scar defect contribute to infertility?
4. What symptoms are associated with C.S scar defect (e.g., abnormal uterine bleeding, dysmenorrhea)?
5. What is the association between isthmocele and secondary infertility?
6. How does a C.S scar defect affect embryo implantation in IVF/ICSI cycles?
7. What is the relationship between isthmocele and chronic endometritis?
8. How is C.S scar defect diagnosed (TVUS, saline infusion sonography, hysteroscopy, MRI)?
9. What are the typical ultrasound findings of an isthmocele?
10. What is the role of hysteroscopy in evaluation and treatment of C.S scar defect?
11. What are the surgical management options (hysteroscopic resection, laparoscopic repair, combined approaches)?
12. How does correction of C.S scar defect improve IVF/ICSI outcomes?
13. What are the risks of surgical repair of isthmocele?
14. How does the presence of a C.S defect affect pregnancy complications (e.g., scar pregnancy, rupture)?
15. What is the role of medical management, if any, in isthmocele-related infertility?
16. How do you counsel a patient with a C.S scar defect planning IVF/ICSI?

CASE NO. (40) MISSED IVF/ICSI TREATMENT

A 34-year-old woman with primary infertility for 6 years is undergoing IVF/ICSI. After completing controlled ovarian stimulation, she is instructed to administer the ovulation trigger (hCG) 36 hours before oocyte retrieval. By mistake, the patient injects only the diluent (water for injection) without mixing it with the hCG powder. On review, no actual ovulation trigger had been administered. The medical team reassesses the situation, reschedules the trigger injection with the correct preparation, and adjusts the timing of oocyte retrieval. At the new scheduled time, oocyte pickup is successfully performed, and mature oocytes are retrieved for ICSI.

1. What are the common medications used during IVF/ICSI cycles?
2. What happens if a patient misses a dose of gonadotropins during stimulation?
3. How should you manage a missed GnRH antagonist dose?
4. What is the consequence of missing a GnRH agonist dose in the long protocol?
5. What happens if a patient delays or misses the ovulation trigger (hCG or GnRH agonist)?
6. How is cycle cancellation considered in case of missed or incorrect trigger timing?
7. What is the impact of missing luteal phase support medications after embryo transfer?
8. How should a patient be counseled if progesterone doses are missed post-transfer?
9. What are the most critical medications in IVF/ICSI that must not be missed?

10. What tools or strategies can be used to reduce the risk of missed medications (e.g., reminders, apps, nursing support)?
11. What is the role of patient counseling before starting IVF/ICSI to prevent missed treatments?
12. What are the medico-legal implications of missed or incorrectly administered IVF medications?
13. How should the IVF team document and manage incidents of missed doses?
14. How do you counsel a couple about prognosis if a dose was missed and cycle cancellation is required?

CASE NO. (41) ENDOMETRIOMA IN IVF/ICSI

A 32-year-old nulligravida woman presents with chronic pelvic pain, dysmenorrhea, and infertility for 2 years. Her menstrual cycles are regular but associated with severe pain increasing over the last 6 months. On pelvic examination, there is a fixed, tender, left adnexal mass (~5 cm). Transvaginal ultrasound shows a unilocular cyst with homogeneous low-level internal echoes ("ground-glass" appearance) on the left ovary. CA-125 is mildly elevated.

1. What is an endometrioma, and how does it differ from other ovarian cysts?
2. Describe the typical ultrasound features of an ovarian endometrioma.
3. What are the main differential diagnoses for an adnexal mass with "ground-glass" echogenicity?
4. What is the pathophysiology behind endometrioma formation?
5. How do endometriomas contribute to infertility?

6. What are the indications for surgical management of endometrioma?
7. Describe the laparoscopic appearance of an ovarian endometrioma.
8. What are the advantages and disadvantages of cystectomy versus drainage and coagulation?
9. How does surgery for endometrioma affect ovarian reserve?
10. When is IVF or ICSI indicated in a patient with endometrioma?
11. What are the recommendations from ESHRE or ASRM regarding management of endometrioma before IVF?
12. What are the medical treatment options for endometriosis and their mechanisms of action?
13. How can recurrence of endometrioma be prevented postoperatively?
14. What are the malignant transformation risks associated with endometrioma, and which histologic types are most common?
15. What are the key factors influencing the decision between medical and surgical management in endometrioma?
16. How is ovarian reserve evaluated preoperatively in women with endometrioma?
17. What are the histopathological features characteristic of an ovarian endometrioma?

PART 5

DEBATES AND CONTROVERSIES IN IVF/ICSI

1. **IVF versus ICSI**
2. **AMH versus AFC in IVF/ICSI**
3. **High Responders versus Low Responders**
4. **Myomectomy versus Expectant Management prior to IVF/ICSI**
5. **Routine Hysteroscopy versus No Hysteroscopy prior to IVF/ICSI**
6. **Hysteroscopic Metroplasty versus Expectant Management prior to IVF/ICSI**
7. **Mid-Luteal Long Agonist Protocol versus Antagonist Protocol**
8. **Mid-Luteal Long Agonist Protocol versus Short Agonist Protocols**
9. **PPOS Protocol versus Antagonist Protocol**
10. **DouStim Protocol versus Short agonist Protocol**
11. **Mild Ovarian Stimulation versus Conventional Stimulation**
12. **Fixed versus Flexible GnRH Antagonist Protocols**
13. **Cyst Aspiration versus Conservation before Ovarian Stimulation**
14. **Urinary Gonadotropins Versus Recombinant Gonadotropins**
15. **LH Supplementation versus No LH Supplementation in Ovarian Stimulation**
16. **Urinary hCG versus Recombinant hCG**
17. **hCG Trigger versus GnRH agonist Trigger**
18. **Dual Trigger versus Double Trigger**
19. **Dual Trigger versus hCG alone**

20. Follicular Flushing versus No Flushing during Oocyte Retrieval

21. GV versus MI versus MII Oocytes

22. Preimplantation Genetic Testing versus No PGT in IVF/ICSI Cycles

23. PICSI/IMSI versus Conventional ICSI in IVF Cycles

24. Soft versus Rigid Catheter for Embryo Transfer

25. Blastocyst versus Cleavage-Stage Embryo Transfer

26. Single versus Multiple Embryo Transfer

27. Fresh Embryo Transfer versus Freeze-All Strategy

28. Natural versus Medicated Frozen Embryo Transfer

29. TESA Vs. TESE Vs. micro-TESE Vs. PESA Vs. MESA

30. Role of the following in IVF/ICSI:

- Vitamin D
- Low dose aspirin
- Sildenafil Citrate
- Glucocorticoids
- Antioxidants
- Myoinositol
- Metformin
- DHEA
- Co-enzyme Q10
- Growth hormone
- Testosterone
- PRP
- G-CSF
- Intralipids
- LMWH
- Endometrial Scratching
- Time lapse imaging
- ERA Test
- Intrauterine hCG injection
- Varicocelectomy
- DNA Fragmentation Testing

PART 6

VIVA QUESTIONS IN REPRODUCTIVE MEDICINE

VIVA QUESTIONS

<u>Q 1:</u>

A 31-year-old woman with oligomenorrhea, BMI 32, hirsutism, AMH 8 ng/mL.

1. What is the likely cause of her infertility?
2. What diagnostic criteria support your suspected diagnosis in this patient?
3. How would you manage her?
4. What are the long -term sequalae for this patient & how can be they be avoided?

<u>Q 2:</u>

A high responder with 25 oocytes retrieved develops rapid abdominal distension and shortness of breath the next day.

1. What is your suspected diagnosis?
2. What are the risk factors?
3. How would you manage her?
4. What is the role of pigtail catheter in this case?

<u>Q 3:</u>

A 35-year-old woman with 3 failed IVF cycles. Each cycle had good-quality blastocyst transfer (1 or 2 embryos). Her uterus appears normal on ultrasound. Partner's semen analysis is normal. No known medical conditions.

1. What is your definition of RIF in this case?
2. What initial investigations would you request now?
3. Would you recommend hysteroscopy despite normal ultrasound?

4. What is the role of ERA here?
5. If all tests are normal, what would be your next plan?
6. Would you repeat the same protocol or change it?
7. What do you counsel the patient regarding prognosis?

<u>**Q 4:**</u>

A 39-year-old woman, AMH = 0.7 ng/mL, AFC = 4, had 3 mature follicles after high-dose stimulation

1. What is your assessment of this patient's ovarian reserve?
2. How would you classify her response to stimulation?
3. According to Bologna or POSEIDON criteria, how is this patient categorized?
4. What are the main challenges in managing infertility at age 39 with low AMH?
5. What stimulation protocols can be considered for Low responders?
6. What is the maximum gonadotropin dose you would recommend in this scenario?
7. Would you consider adjuvant therapies (e.g. DHEA, CoQ10, GH)? What is the evidence?
8. What are the advantages and disadvantages of using a mild stimulation protocol here?
9. What are the pros and cons of using PGT-A in this patient?
10. How would you counsel her regarding success rates and prognosis?

<u>**Q 5:**</u>

A 28-year-old woman, married for 2 years, presents with secondary amenorrhea for 8 months, hot flashes, and infertility. She diagnosed as Premature ovarian insufficiency (POI), She is very anxious and asks about egg donation as she read it online.

1. What is the definition and diagnostic criteria of Premature Ovarian Insufficiency (POI)?
2. What investigations are required to confirm POI?
3. What are the common causes of POI?
4. What genetic tests would you consider in this patient?
5. What hormone replacement therapy options would you recommend, and why?
6. How does POI affect bone health, and how do you prevent complications?
7. What are the cardiovascular risks associated with POI?
8. How often would you follow up her hormone replacement and bone density?
9. What is the legal and religious position of egg donation in Saudi Arabia?
10. How would you counsel this patient regarding egg donation requests locally?

PART 7

MOCK EXAMS IN REPRODUCTIVE MEDICINE

MOCK EXAM (1)

1- A 30-year-old woman presents with irregular periods and infertility. Her FSH is 45 IU/L, and AMH is undetectable. Her clinical examination is normal, and there is no history of chemotherapy or radiation. What is the most appropriate treatment for this patient?

A. IUI

B. Ovulation induction with clomiphene citrate or Gonadotropins

C. ICSI

D. Ovarian tissue freezing

E. Hormonal Replacement Therapy

2- A 36-year-old woman undergoes her second IVF cycle. The first cycle failed, and the second one was done with controlled ovarian stimulation, resulting in 5 blastocyst embryos. Unfortunately, after transfer, she did not achieve a pregnancy. Her ovarian reserve is low (AMH 0.6 ng/mL), and her partner's semen analysis is normal. What is the most appropriate next step in her management?

A. Repeat IVF with a higher dose of gonadotropins

B. Use preimplantation genetic testing (PGT-A)

C. Switch to egg donation

D. Try a third IVF cycle with the same protocol

E. Perform a hysteroscopy to evaluate the endometrium

3- A 33-year-old woman with known endometriosis and a history of two previous laparoscopies presents with infertility. Her partner has normal semen parameters. She has undergone 2 cycles of IUI without success, and her AMH is 1.1 ng/mL. What is the next best step in her fertility management?

A. Start ovulation induction with IUI

B. Proceed with IVF

C. Laparoscopic excision of endometriosis

D. Use a GnRH agonist for 3 months

E. Advise adoption

4- A 30-year-old woman undergoing IVF with PPOS Protocol has been started on gonadotropins for ovarian stimulation. On Day 11, her estradiol level is 5000 pg/mL, and she has 20 follicles 18-20 mm. She is asymptomatic. What is the next best step in management?

A. Proceed with IUI

B. Cancel the cycle

C. Coasting

D. hCG trigger and fresh embryo transfer

E. GnRH agonist trigger and freeze-all strategy

5- A semen sample shows: 3 mL volume, 7 million/mL count, 50% progressive motility, 8% normal forms. According to WHO, this sample:

A. Oligospermia

B. Normal

C. Asthenospermia

D. Teratozoospermia

E. Oligoasthenoteratozoospermia

6- Which factor does NOT improve IUI outcomes?

A. Controlled ovarian stimulation

B. Ultrasound monitoring of ovulation

C. Use of soft intrauterine catheter

D. Performing IUI after ovulation

E. High number of follicles (>4)

7- A 28-year-old woman presents with primary infertility. Her progesterone level on day 21 of the cycle is 5 nmol/L. What does this indicate?

A. Normal ovulation

B. Luteal phase defect

C. Anovulation

D. Premature ovarian insufficiency

E. Polycystic ovarian syndrome

8- A 35-year-old woman with painful periods and dyspareunia is infertile for 2 years. Ultrasound shows a 3 cm left ovarian endometrioma. Tubes patent. AMH is 0.7 ng/mL. What is the best management strategy?

A. Laparoscopic cystectomy

B. GnRH agonist for 3 months

C. Follow up

D. IVF without surgery

E. Clomiphene Citrate

9. A 32-year-old woman with a 3-year history of infertility and mild pelvic pain undergoes a laparoscopy for unexplained infertility. The findings show minimal pelvic endometriosis and peritoneal adhesions. Her partner's semen analysis is normal. What is the best management option following laparoscopy?

A. Wait and try for 6 months

B. Continue with IUI cycles

C. Start IVF immediately

D. Advise surgical removal of all adhesions and endometriosis

E. Laparoscopic ovarian drilling

10- A couple presents with secondary infertility. Semen analysis shows concentration 3 million/mL, motility 5%, normal morphology 2%. Female partner is 29 with normal workup. What is the best next step?

A. Repeat semen analysis after antioxidants

B. IUI with washed semen

C. IVF

D. ICSI

E. Donor insemination

11- A couple presents with 1 year of infertility. The man's semen analysis shows azoospermia. What is the most appropriate next step?

A. Repeat semen analysis

B. Start ICSI

C. Testosterone therapy

D. Testicular biopsy

E. Karyotyping

12- In patients undergoing IVF/ICSI, hysteroscopy is most indicated in which of the following situations?

A. Mild male factor infertility only

B. Normal ultrasound findings

C. History of recurrent implantation failure

D. Successful previous embryo transfer

E. Normal hysterosalpingogram

13- Which is the most appropriate method for luteal phase support after Oocyte Retrieval?

A. Estrogen tablets

B. hCG

C. Progesterone (vaginal or IM)

D. GnRH antagonist

E. Low-dose aspirin

14- According to FIGO PALM COEIN classification for myomas: a myoma given the number 1 is:

A. Submucosal pedunculated polyp

B. Subserosal pedunculated polyp

C. Intramural but projecting from both serosa and uterine cavity

D. Submucosal with < 50% intramural

E. Submucosal with > 50% intramural

15- Which of the following is an advantage for AMH over AFC in the diagnosis of ovarian reserve:

A. Operator independent

B. Prediction of poor response

C. Prediction of hyper response

D. Prediction of oocyte retrieval

E. All of the above

16- A 36-year-old woman undergoing IVF presents with abdominal pain and ascites 7 days after egg retrieval. What is the most likely diagnosis?

A. Pelvic infection

B. Ectopic pregnancy

C. Ovarian hyperstimulation syndrome (OHSS)

D. Luteal cyst rupture

E. Appendicitis

17- A 34-year-old woman with a history of recurrent implantation failure is undergoing preimplantation genetic testing for aneuploidy (PGT-A).

Which day of embryo development is most appropriate for biopsy to minimize harm and maximize diagnostic accuracy?

A. Day 2 cleavage stage

B. Day 3 cleavage stage

C. Day 5 trophectoderm biopsy

D. Day 6 inner cell mass biopsy

E. Polar body biopsy before fertilization

18- Compared to GnRH antagonist protocol, which of the following is an advantage of PPOS?

A. Higher clinical pregnancy rate per transfer

B. Can be used with fresh transfer in the same cycle

C. Lower cost and oral route for LH surge suppression

D. Shorter cycle length and lower gonadotropin use

E. Higher live birth rate in poor responders

19- Which of the following is the most established method of fertility preservation in women undergoing chemotherapy?

A. Ovarian tissue freezing

B. Oocyte cryopreservation

C. GnRH agonist co-treatment

D. Embryo co-culture

E. Endometrial scratching

20- What is the ideal timing for oocyte retrieval after hCG or GnRH agonist trigger?

A. 34–36 hours

B. 12–14 hours

C. 24–26 hours

D. 40–42 hours

E. 48 hours

21- Which of the following measures is recommended to optimize success during embryo transfer?

A. Full bladder for better ultrasound visualization

B. Use of general anesthesia

C. Avoid use of ultrasound guidance

D. Transfer embryos into the endocervical canal

E. Place patient in Trendelenburg position

22- A 30-year-old woman with unexplained infertility and recurrent implantation failure undergoes hysteroscopy, which reveals a small submucosal fibroid. What is the recommended management?

A. No treatment is necessary

B. Proceed with IVF without intervention

C. Remove the fibroid via hysteroscopic myomectomy

D. Perform laparoscopic fibroid removal

E. Initiate hormonal therapy to shrink the fibroid

23- Which of the following findings on laparoscopy would justify surgical intervention before proceeding with IVF/ICSI?

A. Mild endometriosis with minimal adhesions

B. Hydrosalpinx

C. Polycystic ovaries

D. Unilateral ovarian cyst

E. Bilateral tubal patency on HSG

24- A 29 -year-old Nullipara comes to see you for an infertility evaluation. The patient has been trying to conceive for the past 2 years. her cycles are irregular with oligomenorrhea. Her husband's is semen analysis. On examination her BMI is 33. Initial labs show (LH) of 36 miU/mL,

(FSH) of 8 miU/mL, (TSH) of 1.6, normal (DHEA), and mildly elevated androstenedione and testosterone.

What is the best next step in addressing the patient's infertility?

A. Hysterosalpingography

B. Combined estrogen and progesterone challenge

C. Magnetic resonance imaging of the brain

D. Ovulation induction with Letrozole

E. Pelvic ultrasound

25- With regard to the investigation of the infertile couple:

A. A full hormone profile, tubal patency testing and semen analysis should be completed on all couples attending a referral for primary infertility.

B. A mid-luteal progesterone 0.25 nmol/L confirms ovulation.

C. Semen analysis should be performed as an initial investigation alongside the female partner's basic infertility workup.

D. Laparoscopy can be used to assess tubal patency in all patients.

E. Postcoital test should be done.

26- What is the second common cause of congenital adrenal hyperplasia (CAH)?

A. 17-hydroxylase deficiency

B. 21-hydroxylase deficiency

C. 11-Beta hydroxylase deficiency

D. 3 Beta- hydroxysteroid dehydrogenase deficiency

E. 17 Beta-hydroxysteroid dehydrogenase deficiency

27- Unsuccessful oocyte retrieval following apparently normal ovarian stimulation is more likely due to:

A. Using a large dose of gonadotropins during ovarian stimulation

B. Reduced biological activity in some batches of commercially prepared hCG

C. The use of long agonist protocol

D. Young age of the patient

E. Poor handling the last dose of human menopausal gonadotropin (hMG)

28- Regarding Embryo transfer, the following are true EXCEPT:

A. Outer sheath is designed to protect embryos in the inner sheath

B. Better to be done under ultrasound guidance

C. Outer sheath should not pass the cervical isthmus

D. Embryos are loaded near the tip of inner sheath

E. Air bubble should be in the inner sheath

29. In IVF cycles, the main advantage of the GnRH agonist long protocol:

A. Shorter duration of stimulation

B. Reduced risk of OHSS

C. Lower gonadotropin requirement

D. Suitable for poor responders

E. Better follicular synchronization

30- TVUS: Spot Diagnosis

A. Intramural myoma

B. Endometrial polyp

C. Endometriosis

D. Endometrial Carcinoma

E. Adenomyosis

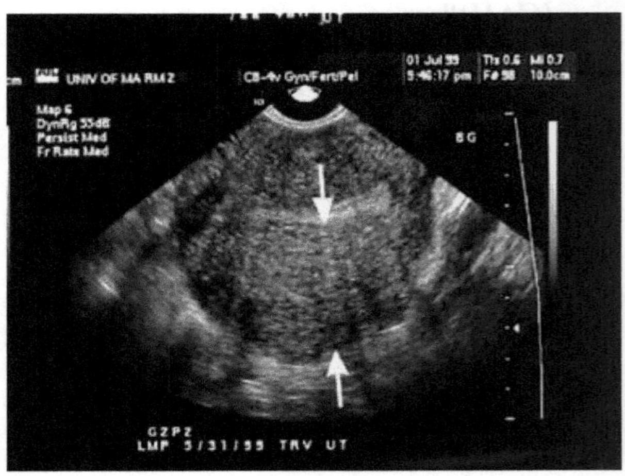

MOCK EXAM (2)

1- In a woman who is at a high risk for severe OHSS; the correct answer is:

A. Basal ultrasound shows AFC > 16

B. Estradiol on day of hCG < 3500 pg/ml

C. Cabergoline is only given if she developed OHSS

D. Long protocol should be the standard

E. ICSI is safer than IVF for her

2- The most common side effect of long protocol is:

A. Low number of follicles

B. Low pregnancy rate

C. Increased incidence of ovarian cysts

D. Increased incidence of asynchronized follicles

E. Injection site abscess

3- A patient aged 25 years was diagnosed as infertile with hypothalamic amenorrhea sought IVF treatment. What is your plan of treatment?

A. Antagonist protocol

B. Gonadotropin only protocol

C. Long protocol

D. Short protocol

E. Low dose step-up protocol

4- The luteal phase is more impaired with:

A. Less ovarian stimulation.

B. More ovarian stimulation.

C. hCG for ovulation triggering than after GnRHa triggering.

D. Progesterone for luteal phase support

E. hCG for luteal phase support

5- Male infertility in a patient with cystic fibrosis is likely to be due to which condition?

A. Congenital absence of testes

B. Congenital absence of vas deference

C. Hypothalamic failure

D. Oligospermia

E. Testicular failure

6- Following an IVF treatment cycle where 16 oocytes were collected three days later patient presented to the clinic with history of abdominal pain, nausea and vomiting, enlarged ovaries with a mean diameter of 10 cm with small amount of ascites. She going to have a new treatment cycle. Which protocol you suggest?

A. Antagonist protocol

B. Long protocol

C. Short protocol

D. Ultrashort protocol

E. None of the above

7- A 17-year-old woman with primary amenorrhea has been investigated with the following results: FSH = 9mIU/ml, LH = 20mIU/ml, estradiol = 200 pg/ml, free testosterone = 5.0 ng/dl (1-4.3ng/dl). Karyotype is 46XY

A. Prolactinoma

B. Premature ovarian failure

C. Polycystic ovary syndrome

D. Hyperthyroidism

E. Androgen insensitivity syndrome

8- Which is the earliest physical sign of puberty in females?

A. Growth spurt

B. Thelarche

C. Adrenarche

D. Pubarche

E. Menarche

9- A nineteen-year-old girl presents to the clinic and reports that she never had a menstrual period. On examination she is short, wide spaced nipples, webbed neck with coarctation of aorta. What is the most likely diagnosis?

A. Mullerian agenesis

B. 5-alpha reductase deficiency

C. Turner syndrome

D. Anorexia nervosa

E. Primary hypothyroidism

10- The most accurate method for diagnosis of intrauterine adhesion is:

A. 3 D TVUS

B. 2 D TVUS

C. HSG

D. Hysteroscopy

E. Sonohystergrophy

11- What is the main purpose of administering hCG in an IVF cycle?

A. Prevent premature LH surge

B. Stimulate endometrial receptivity

C. Mimic LH surge to trigger ovulation

D. Suppress pituitary function

E. Stimulate follicular growth

12- What is the primary benefit of using a GnRH antagonist protocol over a long GnRH agonist protocol in IVF cycles?

A. Higher oocyte yield

B. Reduced medication cost

C. Higher pregnancy rates

D. Shorter cycle duration and lower OHSS risk

E. Easier luteal phase support

13- Which of the following statements about PPOS protocol is correct?

A. It can be used in fresh embryo transfer cycles

B. It is contraindicated in PCOS patients

C. It requires use of GnRH agonist for LH surge prevention

D. It is suitable for oocyte or embryo freezing cycles

E. None of the above

14- What is a common side effect during the downregulation phase of the long protocol?

A. Luteal phase spotting

B. Hot flashes and mood swings

C. Premature ovulation

D. OHSS

E. Hyperthyroidism

15- Which of the following is an advantage of the long protocol compared to antagonist protocol?

A. Shorter duration of stimulation

B. Lower gonadotropin dose requirement

C. Lower risk of OHSS

D. Better follicular synchronization

E. No need for luteal support

16- A 23-year-old woman with a BMI of 50 attends your GP surgery to discuss her fertility problems because she and her husband have been trying to conceive for 18 months. She has irregular periods with a cycle varying from 35 to 42 days and the ovulation predictor kits she has purchased from the chemist indicate that she is not ovulating. Her husband has two children from his previous marriage. Which of the following is the most appropriate piece of advice

A. Continue trying for six more months then you will refer her to infertility clinic

B. . Commence taking folic acid 10 mcg daily

C. . Make an appointment for her husband to arrange a semen analysis

D. . Prescribe clomiphene citrate to be taken on days two to six of the cycle

E. To avoid pregnancy until she has lost weight

17- A 22-year-old student with an 18-month history of non-cyclical intermittent lower abdominal pain and deep dyspareunia. She is tender in both adnexa and the uterus is retroverted, What is the most likely diagnosis:

A. Adenomyosis

B. Appendicitis

C. Chronic pelvic inflammatory disease

D. Endometriosis

E. Uterine fibroids

18- The following statement is not true regarding embryo transfer:

A. Trial transfers allow better preparation for difficult transfers

B. Firm catheters are associated with higher PR than soft catheters

C. Soft catheters cause less trauma to the endometrium

D. The time interval should be minimized (> 120 seconds carry a poor prognosis)

E. After the transfer, the catheter should be inspected for retained embryos

19- The diameter of the needle used for oocyte retrieval with mature follicle is usually:

A. between 6-8 gage

B. between 8-10 gage

C. between 10-12 gage

D. between 10-14 gage

E. between 16-20 gage

20- Following an IVF treatment cycle where 22 oocytes were collected three months patient presented to the clinic with history of abdominal pain, nausea and vomiting enlarged ovaries with a mean diameter of 10 cm with small amount of ascites. She going to have a new treatment cycle. Which protocol you suggest?

A. Ultrashort protocol

B. Long protocol

C. PPOS protocol

D. Short protocol

E. None of the above

21- Ovarian hyperstimulation syndrome (OHSS) is more frequently associated with:

A. Progesterone for luteal phase support

B. hCG for luteal phase support

C. No luteal support

D. Estrogen for luteal phase support

E. GnRHa luteal phase support.

22- Luteal phase support after ART:

A. Starts after the pregnancy test

B. Not essential

C. Has a positive effect on the pregnancy rate compared with no treatment

D. Only needed when the patient has PCOS

E. Not needed for tubal factor infertility patients

23- A pressure that is optimal for a good recovery and exerts no harm on the oocyte cumulus complex when aspirating mature follicles is:

A. Negative pressure of 60-90 mmHg

B. Negative pressure of 90-120 mmHg

C. Negative pressure of 120-150 mmHg

D. Negative pressure of 160-200 mmHg

E. Negative pressure of 200 -250 mmHg

24- The most common side effect of long protocol is:

A. Low number of follicles

B. Low pregnancy rate

C. Increased incidence of ovarian cysts

D. Increased incidence of asynchronized follicles with

E. Injection site abscess

25- A patient aged 29 years diagnosed as infertile with PCOS sought IVF treatment Which is your trigger?

A. Dual trigger

B. hcg trigger

C. GnRHa trigger

D. Kisspeptin trigger

E- Recombinant LH trigger

26- A 30-year-old woman with anovulatory infertility due to polycystic ovary syndrome (PCOS) is started on Letrozole. Which of the following best describes its mechanism of action in inducing ovulation?

A. It blocks estrogen receptors at the hypothalamus, increasing GnRH release

B. It inhibits aromatase, reducing estrogen synthesis and increasing FSH secretion

C. It stimulates FSH receptors in ovarian follicles directly

D. It acts as a dopamine agonist, reducing prolactin secretion

E. It acts as an LH receptor agonist, promoting ovulation

27- A 17-year-old girl presents with primary amenorrhea. She has normal breast and pubic hair development. Pelvic examination reveals a short vagina ending blindly, and ultrasound shows absence of uterus but normal ovaries. What is the most likely diagnosis?

A. Turner syndrome

B. Müllerian agenesis (MRKH syndrome)

C. Complete androgen insensitivity syndrome

D. Hypothalamic amenorrhea

E. Pituitary tumor

28- A 29-year-old woman presents with amenorrhea and galactorrhea. Her serum prolactin level is elevated. MRI of the pituitary is normal. Which of the following is the *most likely cause* of her condition?

A. Primary hypothyroidism

B. Pituitary microadenoma

C. Cushing's disease

D. Sheehan's syndrome

E. Ovarian failure

29- Chromosomal pattern of turner syndrome is:

A. 47/XX

B. 46/XXY

C. 47/XXY

D. 46/X0

E. 45/X0

30- Laparoscopy: Spot Diagnosis

A. Functional ovarian cyst

B. Para Ovarian cyst

C. Endometrioma

D. Myoma

E. Adenomyosis

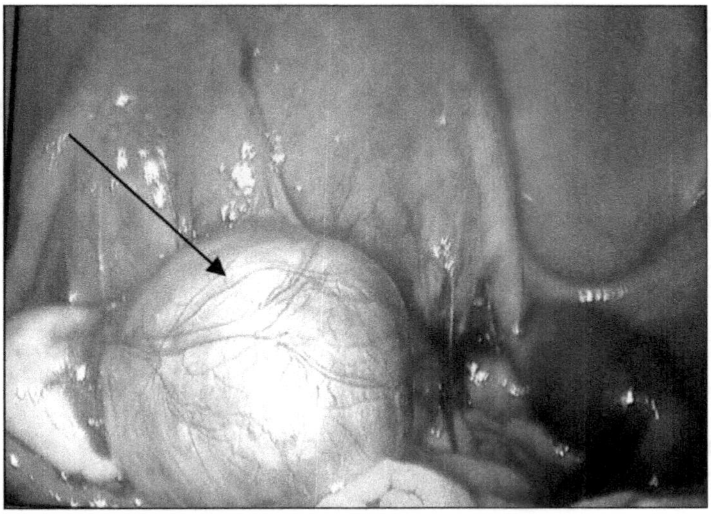

MOCK EXAM (3)

1- Which of the following factors most increases the risk of multiple pregnancy in IVF cycles?

A. Using ICSI technique

B. High BMI in female partner

C. Transferring more than one embryo

D. Controlled ovarian stimulation with antagonist protocol

E. Blastocyst stage transfer

2. In endometriosis, surgery should not be considered when:

A. Medical treatment fails in controlling pain symptoms

B. Cysts larger than 10 cm

C. Ultrasound features become less reassuring.

D. The cyst undergoes a rapid growth

E. Cysts 4 cm in diameter without pain

3- What is the main limitation of current evidence regarding PRP in Low responders?

A. It causes irreversible ovarian damage

B. It is FDA-approved but lacks cost-effectiveness

C. Most data are from small, non-randomized studies

D. It cannot be performed without general anesthesia

E. It has been shown to reduce oocyte quality

4- Which of the following reduces fertility preservation success in patients undergoing cancer therapy?

A. Delayed referral after chemotherapy has started

B. Early referral before gonadotoxic therapy

B. Use of vitrification for egg freezing

D. Hormonal stimulation using letrozole

E. Double stimulation in one cycle (DuoStim)

5- Which factor is most strongly associated with increased clinical pregnancy rates during embryo transfer?

A. Transfer of more than two embryos

B. Use of rigid catheter

C. High operator experience and atraumatic transfer

D. Performing embryo transfer under anesthesia

E. Uterine sounding before every transfer

6- Which of the following is the most common indication for performing a hysteroscopy before IVF/ICSI?

A. Chronic pelvic pain

B. Uterine fibroids causing irregular bleeding

C. Male infertility

D. Recurrent implantation failure

E. Ovarian cysts

7- Which of the following is a common uterine factor associated with recurrent implantation failure?

A. Tubal blockage

B. Ovarian cyst

C. Submucosal fibroid

D. Endometrioma

E. Male infertility

8- Endometrial receptivity array (ERA) testing is used in RIF to:

A. Diagnose hydrosalpinx

B. Identify window of implantation

B. Assess ovarian response

D. Measure embryo quality

E. Detect polyps

9- Oocyte cryopreservation is recommended for social (elective) fertility preservation ideally before what age?

A. 25 years

B. 30 years

C. 35 years

D. 40 years

E. 45 years

10- Which of the following statements about GnRH agonists for fertility preservation is true?

A. They guarantee fertility preservation

B. They are not used in hematologic cancers

C. They are effective in all age groups

D. They reduce the risk of chemotherapy-induced ovarian failure

E. They increase oocyte yield during stimulation

11- Which of the following is the optimal day for embryo transfer to mimic the natural window of implantation?

A. Day 1 post-retrieval

B. Day 2 post-retrieval

C. Day 3 (cleavage-stage)

D. Day 5 (blastocyst-stage)

E. Day 7 post-retrieval

12- What is the recommended endometrial thickness (in mm) on the day of embryo transfer for optimal implantation?

A. < 6 mm

B. 6–7 mm

C. ≥ 8–14 mm

D. ≥ 10 mm

E. Any thickness

13- In patients with recurrent implantation failure, which modification during embryo transfer may improve outcomes?

A. Use of a soft catheter and ultrasound guidance

B. Blind embryo transfer

C. Cervical dilation during transfer

D. Sedation with general anesthesia

E. Using higher pressure to deposit embryos

14- A 39-year-old woman with 2 years of primary infertility is being evaluated. Her Day 3 labs show FSH 12.5 IU/L, AMH 0.7 ng/mL, and AFC is 5. Her partner's semen analysis is normal. Which is the most appropriate next step in her fertility management?

A. Repeat AMH in 3 months

B. Recommend expectant management

C. Start ovulation induction with letrozole

D. Refer for donor egg IVF

E. Counsel for IVF

15- A 40-year-old woman with a history of chemotherapy presents with amenorrhea and infertility. What is the most likely diagnosis?

A. PCOS

B. Endometriosis

C. Hypothalamic amenorrhea

D. Premature ovarian insufficiency

E. Kallman Syndrome

16- In obesity, which of the following statements is correct according the WHO BMI (kg/m2) criteria:

A. A person is obese if BM is ≥ 35 kg/m².

B. A person is obese if BMI is ≥ 30 kg/m².

C. A person is obese if BMI is ≥ 25 kg/m².

D. A person is overweight if BMI is ≥ 30 kg/m².

E. A person is of normal weight if BMI is ≥ 33 kg/m².

17- A 36-year-old, G3P2012 , presents to her primary care physician complaining of several months poor sleep, heat intolerance, newly irregular menses, and decreased libido. She denies recent changes in weight, diet, or activity, and does not use alcohol or illicit drugs. Her obstetric history includes two uncomplicated, full-term vaginal deliveries and one first trimester spontaneous abortion. On examination, she is thin and tired appearing, without exophthalmos or thyromegaly. Vital signs show the following: T 36.8°C, respiratory rate of 17 breaths/min, P 77 beats/min, and BP 142/88 mmHg. Her breasts are nontender, without masses or nipple discharge. Pelvic examination reveals moderately well-estrogenized vaginal mucosa and a small, non-tender uterus with regular contours and no palpable adnexal masses. A urinary pregnancy test is negative. What laboratory values are appropriate to check at this time?

A. Follicle- stimulating hormone (FSH)/luteinizing hormone (LH), prolactin, Thyroid-stimulating hormone (TSH), complete blood count (CBC), basic metabolic panel (BMP)

B. CBC, BMP, serum ferritin/total iron-binding capacity (TIBC)

C. Endometrial biopsy and CT abdomen/pelvis

D. Adrenocorticotropic hormone (ACTH), dehydroepiandrosterone (DHEA), 24-hour cortisol, and memantine challenge

18- What day of a regular 25-day menstrual cycle is a woman likely to ovulate?

A. 4

B. 11

C. 14

D. 20

E. 25

19- What is the most likely histological subtype of ovarian cancer associated with endometriosis?

A. Clear cell carcinoma

B. Serous adenocarcinoma

C. Borderline serous tumour

D. Muscinous cystadenocarcinoma

E. Granulosa cell tumour

20-Gonadotropin Releasing Hormone (GnRH) is what type of Biochemical?

A. Tripeptide

B. Octapeptide

C. Nanopeptide

D. Decapeptide

E. Polypeptide

21- The immediate layer around the oocyte of the tertiary follicle is known as the:

A. Lamina propria

B. Cumulus oophorus

C. Zona pellucida

D. Zona granulosa

E. Theca interna

22- A 37-year-old woman presents to clinic complaining of lower abdominal discomfort. Exam of uterus is enlarged. Biopsy shows normal appearing glands in myometrium. What is the most likely diagnosis?

A. Adenocarcinoma

B. Basal cell carcinoma

C. Leiomyosarcoma

D. Adenomyosis

E. Endometriosis

23- A 24-year-old woman with her 35-year-old partner has been referred to the infertility clinic because of 2 years of primary infertility. The woman has an irregular menstrual cycle every 24 months and her partner's semen analysis is normal. The woman's BMI is 26 and there is no significant past medical history. Investigations have confirmed a diagnosis of polycystic ovary. The couple have not achieved a pregnancy despite a 6 months course of clomiphene citrate with evidence of ovulation based on day 21 progesterone concentration and ultrasound scanning, What is the next Step?

A. In-vitro fertilization

B. Intra-uterine insemination

C. Gonadotropins

D. Intra-cytoplasmic sperm injection

E. Clomiphene citrate

24- A 35-year-old mother of three children is referred to the gynecology clinic because she has not had a period for 4 months and her pregnancy test is negative. During that time, she has experienced rapid growth of facial and body hair, deepening of her voice and increased muscle bulk. She has otherwise been healthy and has not taken any medication. The most likely diagnosis is:

A. Prolactinoma

B. Premature ovarian failure

C. Ashermann's syndrome

D. Polycystic ovary syndrome

E. Androgen secreting tumour

25- When you prescribe clomiphene citrate to a woman with PCOS, you advise the couple to have intercourse every other day:

A. For 5 days starting 7 days after the last tablet of clomiphene

B. For 7 days starting 5 days after the last tablet of clomiphene

C. For 5 days starting 3 days after the last tablet of clomiphene

D. For 7 days starting 7 days after the last tablet of clomiphene

E. For 5 days starting 5 days after the last tablet of clomiphene

26- Oocyte retrieval is generally performed approximately:

A. 36 hours after hCG administration

B. 40 hours after hCG administration

C. 24 hours after hCG administration

D. 30 hours after hCG administration

E. 18 hours after hCG administration

27- A 36 years old woman is diagnosed with mild stage pelvic endometriosis at diagnostic laparoscopy. She has regular cycles. Her partner has normal semen. the couple has been trying to conceive for 2 years. Which of the following management option is the preferred initial treatment choice:

A. GnRH antagonist.

B. Clomiphene Citrate treatment.

C. Laparoscopic excision ablation of peritoneal endometriosis.

D. Selective progesterone receptor modulator.

E. Follow up

28- Poor ovarian Reserve Tests include:

A. AMH > 3.5 ng/ml & AFC > 16 follicle

B. FSH < 5 mIU/L

C. AMH < 1 ng/ml & AFC < 7 follicle

D. E2 > 90 pg/ml

E. AMH < 5 ng/ml

29- A 21-year-old presents to the gynecology outpatient clinic with asymptomatic 3 cm endometrioma, expectant management is decided follow up will be:

A. Every month

B. Every 3 month

C. Every year

D. Every 6 month

E. You have other opinion

30- Spot Diagnosis:

A. Normal HSG

B. Hydrosalpinex

C. Bilateral Distal Tubal Block

D. Bilateral Proximal Tubal Block

E. Unilateral Proximal Tubal Block

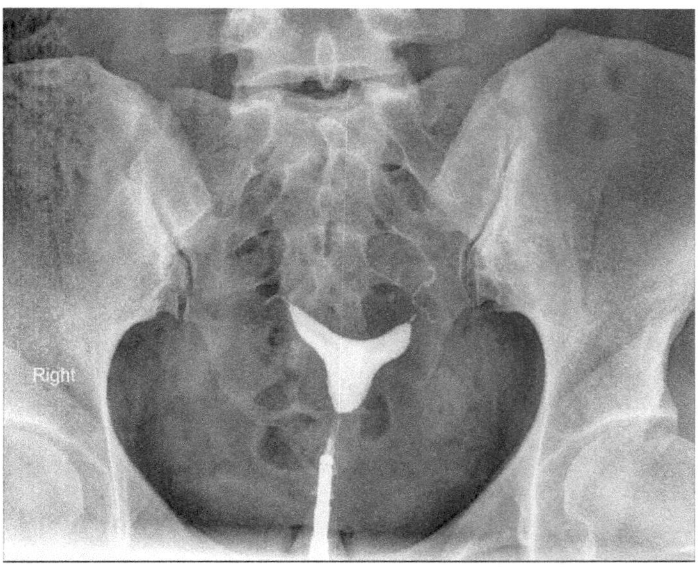

MOCK EXAM (4)

1- The growth factor implicated in mediating the effects of ovarian hyperstimulation is:

A. Insulin-like growth factor

B. Vascular endothelial growth factor (VEGF)

C. Transforming growth factor α

D. Transforming growth factor β

E. Epidermal growth factor (EGF)

2- A 40-year-old woman, who has been trying to conceive for 3 years, is offered IVF as a treatment option by her fertility specialist. Which ONE of the following is an appropriate discussion issue during her clinic counselling?

A. Ovarian volume, ovarian blood flow and inhibin B usefully predict IVF success rate.

B. Preimplantation genetic diagnosis (PGD) of the embryo is required prior to its uterine transfer.

C. Progesterone administration is not required following embryo transfer.

D. Salpingectomy prior to IVF is beneficial in women with hydrosalpinges.

E. The chance of a live birth following IVF treatment increases with rising female age.

3- Which ONE of the following is likely to predict a favourable ovarian response to gonadotrophin stimulation in IVF?

A. Anti-Mullerian hormone ≤ 5.4 pmol/l

B. Follicle-stimulating hormone > 10 IU/l

C. Increased ovarian blood flow on pelvic ultrasound

D. Estradiol (E2) > 500 pmol/L

E. Total antral follicle counts 8-15 on pelvic ultrasound

4- Women with OHSS are especially prone to:

A. Thrombosis of vessels in calf

B. Thrombosis of vessels in upper body

C. Thrombosis of vessels in the spleen

D. Thrombosis of vessels in the kidney

E. Thrombosis of vessels in the liver

5- Measures to predict ovarian response to gonadotrophin stimulation in IVF are all except:

A. Antral follicle count

B. Previous response

C. Anti-Mullerian hormone

D. FSH

E. Ovarian volume

6- In counselling women planning for fertility treatment about the risk of malignancy associated with use of fertility drugs, which of the following statements is true?

A. Aetiology of malignant melanoma, and to a lesser extent that of thyroid cancer, is known to involve endogenous and exogenous hormones; hence, there is a significant association of IVF cycles to non-gynaecological cancers.

B. Most fertility medications are associated with significantly increased risk of breast cancer.

C. There is strong evidence linking infertility treatment with childhood cancers.

D. There is strong evidence to link multiple IVF cycles to development of uterine cancer.

E. When counselling, patients in general should be reassured about the current data: that there is no significant increase in risk of cancer with IVF treatment for them or their offspring.

7- Surgical reversal of tubal sterilization:

A. Is as successful as IVF.

B. NHS funds surgical reversal of tubal sterilization.

C. NHS funds IVF in this patient group.

D. Results are independent of woman's age.

E. Residual tubal length less than 4 cm is a good prognostic factor.

8- Ms XY is 7 weeks pregnant. She has been diagnosed with her 3 consecutive first trimester miscarriages before this pregnancy. She is 28 years old and with the same partner. She is presently on folic acid supplementation. Her miscarriages remain unexplained. Which of the following treatment options are best suited to her?

A. Aspirin

B. Aspirin and LMWH

C. HCG injections

D. Progesterone supplementation

E. Reassurance and expectant management

9- A 36-year-old para 1 is undergoing an IVF cycle. She has egg retrieval and two fresh embryos are transferred. Her initial beta human chorionic gonadotropin is 1600 mIU/ml, and she begins to develop abdominal pain, nausea and vomiting. An ultrasound reveals two gestational sacs and free abdominal fluid. She is not short of breath, her pulse oximetry is 98% on room air and electrolytes and hematocrit and liver function tests are within normal limits. What grade of ovarian hyperstimulation syndrome should she be categorized as having?

A. None.

B. Mild.

C. Moderate.

D. Severe.

E. Critical.

10- A 35-year-old para 0 is in the midst of an IVF cycle. She has undergone egg retrieval following human chorionic gonadotropin administration, and you have just implanted two fresh embryos. What is the chance that she will develop OHSS?

A. 5%.

B. 10%.

C. 20%.

D. 30%.

E. 40%.

11- A 39-year-old male presents to a fertility clinic following a repeat semen analysis for oligoasthenoteratozoospermia. The semen analysis results show semen volume (1.0 ml), sperm concentration (2 × 106/ml), total motility (10%), normal forms (1%) and vitality (10%). What is the appropriate next step in management?

A. Controlled ovarian stimulation with IUI

B. ICSI

C. IVF using donor sperm

D. Natural cycle IUI

E. Induction of ovulation

12- A male patient presents with history of anosmia, azoospermia, bilateral small testes and gynecomastia. What is the best treatment modality?

A. Bromocriptine.

B. Clomiphene.

C. Letrozole.

D. Testosterone replacement.

E. Gonadotropins.

13- After an IVF cycle and a subsequently positive pregnancy test, a patient develops abdominal pain, nausea, vomiting and mild shortness of breath. Further evaluation reveals normal lung sounds, palpable ascites and a pulse oximetry of 97% on room air. A chest x-ray is normal; the hematocrit is 40% and an ultrasound shows ovaries of 9 cm with evident ascites. Which of the following is most consistent with severe OHSS?

A. Shortness of breath.

B. Haematocrit greater than 40%.

C. Palpable ascites.

D. Ovarian size greater than 9 cm.

E. All of the above.

14- A 31 -year- old, G0, with a long history of endometriosis presents to discuss future childbearing. She has no genetic family history complicating her prenatal counseling. Her husband is a nonsmoker with no medical problems. She has used birth control pills in the past to control her menses and pain. She would like to proceed with the best option for her to obtain pregnancy quickly. What would you recommend for this patient?

A. Use depot leuprolide for 6 months and then attempt pregnancy

B. Restart birth control pills for 3 months and then attempt pregnancy

C. Perform laparoscopy with fulguration of endometrial implants and then attempt pregnancy

D. Start clomiphene therapy cycle with next cycle on days 5 to 9

15- In male factor infertility:

A. Cystic fibrosis may be the reason for male infertility.

B. Diagnosed in less than 20% of couples who failed to conceive

C. Needs expensive investigations to be confirmed

D. Only diagnosed in males above the age of 35 years

E. Asthenospermia means abnormal morphology of sperm.

16- Subclinical hyperthyroidism refers to:

A. Low TSH level with a normal both FT3 and FT4

B. High TSH level with normal FT3 and high FT4

C. High TSH level with normal FT3 and FT4

D. High TSH level with high FT3 and FT4

E. Low TSH level with a high FT3 and normal FT4

17- A woman with POI is classified:

A. Class III WHO anovulation

B. Class 1 WHO anovulation

C. Class II WHO anovulation

D. Class IV WHO anovulation

18- Regarding anovulation all the following are true EXCEPT:

A. Anovulation is failure to release a mature ovum

B. Kallmann's syndrome is characterized by hypothalamic amenorrhea and anosmia

C. Anovulation may manifest in a variety of clinical presentations, luteal insufficiency, oligomenorrhoea or amenorrhea

D. Norm-gonadotrophic anovulation represents 10% of all ovulatory disorder

E. Weight related amenorrhea is the most common hypothalamic cause of anovulation

19- The following is not a contributor to impaired fertility related to obesity:

A. Oocyte and embryo development

B. Anovulation

C. Sperm hostility

D. Implantation failure and pregnancy loss

E. Endometrial development

20- Regarding Hyperprolactinemia:

A. galactorrhea is always present

B. commonly associated with hypersecretory endometrial development

C. bromocriptine lowers prolactin level by suppression dopamine

D. can be cause by certain medications

E. can be caused by hyperthyroidism

21- Laparoscopic myomectomy is indicated in:

A. > 3 leiomyomas > 5 cm

B. A uterus > 18 weeks size

C. ≤ 3 intramural or subserous leiomyomas of ≤5 cm

D. Subserous myoma > 7cm

E. Multiple myomas

22- In PCOS infertile women in spite of high ovulation rate with clomiphene citrate pregnancy rates are much lower this is largely because clomiphene:

A. Stimulates androgen production by theca cells of the developing follicles

B. Leads to failure of midcycle LH surge

C. Deplete FSH receptors in the hypothalamus due to its long half life

D. Has an anti-estrogenic effect on the endometrium

E. Interferes with the quality of the ovum

23- The first line pharmacological therapy for treatment hirsutism in women:

A. Spironolactone

B. GnRH analogues

C. COCs

D. Cypreterone acetate

E. flutamide

24- Which of the following is an advantage for AMH over AFC in the diagnosis of ovarian reserve:

A. Operator independent

B. Prediction of poor response

C. Prediction of oocyte retrieval

D. Prediction of hyper response

E. None of the above

25- Bariatric surgery in the treatment of obese infertile women:

A. pregnancy can be attempted 1 year after surgery

B. is associated with increased risk of gestational diabetes, macrosomia hypertensive disorders due to operation induced weight loss

C. recommended as first line fertility treatment for obese women

D. let women avoid the need for a weight reduction diet

26- One of the following is NOT among Rotterdam criteria for diagnosis PCOS:

A. US picture of PCOM

B. Laboratory hyperandrogenism

C. Clinical hyperandrogenism

D. Oligo/anovulation

E. Elevated LH/FSH ratio

27- A 28 years old woman was given 6-month therapy of clomiphene citrate to treat her anovulatory infertility but did not pregnant in spite of timed intercourse and US evidence of ovulation. You decide to start gonadotropin therapy as a second line treatment for her. All the following are true for gonadotropin therapy in the outpatient clinic EXCEPT:

A. The dose is individualized according to response.

B. Minimize the risk of OHSS

C. Opt for singleton pregnancy.

D. Induce multifollicular development

E. Start with the least dose.

28- What follow up is needed after treatment of intrauterine adhesions:

A. None

B. Laparoscopy

C. HSG

D. Second look hysteroscopy

E. HSG

29- Which one of the following is correct in relation to polycystic ovarian syndrome, PCOS?

A. Increased risk of type II diabetes or gestational diabetes

B. Increased risk of uterine polyps

C. No induction of uterine bleeding following 5 days of oral progestogen therapy

D. Resistant to clomiphene citrate ovulation induction in 50 % of cases

E. Virilization is common

30- Hysteroscopy Finding: Spot diagnosis

A. Uterine Septum

B. Submucous Myoma

C. Endometrial Polyp

D. Intrauterine Adhesions

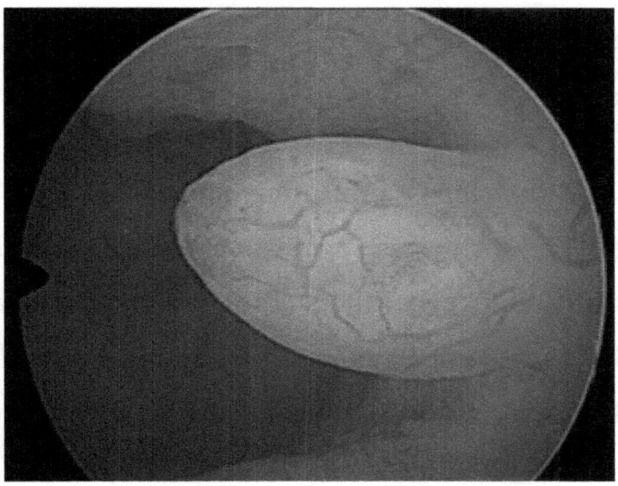

MOCK EXAM (5)

1- Comparing letrozole with clomiphene citrate in patients with polycystic ovarian syndrome, clomiphene citrate is associated with:

A. Lower live birth rate.

B. Lower rate of multiple pregnancy.

C. Lower incidence of ovarian hyperstimulation.

D. Better side effects profile.

E. Higher implantation rate.

2- A 29-year-old with primary subfertility and a BMI of 30 kg/m2 is known to have polycystic ovarian syndrome based on anovulation, transvaginal ultrasound appearances of the ovaries and a raised testosterone. She has remained anovulatory despite increasing doses of clomiphene citrate over six cycles. What is the most appropriate next step in her management?

A. Unstimulated intrauterine insemination.

B. Continue further three cycles of clomiphene citrate.

C. Continue further six cycles of clomiphene citrate.

D. Gonadotropins.

E. Metformin.

3- A 25-year-old athlete with a BMI of 18 presents to the fertility clinic trying for a pregnancy for 2 years. She has oligomenorrhea and her partner's semen analysis is within the normal range. Her gonadotropin level shows a low FSH and LH. estrogen levels are also low, although the androgen, prolactin is normal. What is the best strategy for her ovarian stimulation?

A. Clomiphene citrate.

B. Lifestyle interventions (normalizing weight and exercise) + human menopausal gonadotropins.

C. Pulsatile GnRH.

D. Norethisterone 10 mg for 5 to 7 days and clomiphene citrate 50 mg on days 2 to 6.

E. Recombinant FSH + LH preparations.

4- Ms XY (30 years) and her male partner (26 years) have been trying to conceive naturally for the last 3 years. They have had infertility investigations over the last year. These include a normal semen analysis, normal USS pelvis, normal HSG, normal TSH, prolactin, D3 FSH, LH and normal AMH. Her day 21 progesterone suggest ovulation. Ms XY is rubella immune and has negative swabs for an STI. Her recent cervical smear is normal. Which of the following treatment options are best suited to her?

A. Clomiphene citrate

B. IUI

C. Letrozole

D. IVF-ICSI

E. IVF

5- Which of the following is considered a risk factor for the development of endometriosis?

A. late age of menarche

B. delayed childbearing

C. long menstrual cycle > 30

D. short duration of menstrual flow <5 days

6- Which of the following is accurate about the presentation of endometriosis?

A. Onset of pain usually begins 1-2 days after menses begins

B. The degree of visible endometriosis correlates with the degree of pain and other symptomatic impairment

C. Lateral disease is generally believed to be more painful than midline disease

D. intrapelvic/intra-abdominal adhesions are important determinants of the degree of pain

7- Selection of patients for surgery on endometrioma is dependent on all of the following except:

A. endometrioma growth rate

B. Size of endometrioma

C. Presence of infertility

D. Presence of pain

E. Other opinion

8- Oral contraceptives (OC) and progestins are considered the first-line option for medical therapy of Endometrioma. Surgery should not be considered when:

A. medical treatment fails in controlling pain symptoms

B. the cyst undergoes a rapid growth

C. ultrasound features become less reassuring

D. cysts 4 cm in diameter without pain

E. cysts larger than 10 cm

9- A 23-year-old lady presented with chronic pelvic pain, an ultrasound scan showed a 4 cm endometrioma on her right ovary. What is the best management option?

A. Tricycling of combined oral contraceptive pill

B. Ovarian cyst drainage

C. Oophorectomy

D. Ovarian cystectomy

E. Ovarian Drilling

10- A 30-year-old woman has been trying to conceive for 2 years. Her partner's semen analysis is normal as is her hormonal profile, tubal patency test and pelvic ultrasound. Her luteal phase progesterone is ovulatory. She had deep dyspareunia and mild dysmenorrhea and had a laparoscopy where peritoneal endometriosis was ablated 6 months ago. ASA Stage 1 endometriosis was diagnosed. What should be the next line of management?

A. Clomiphene ovulation induction

B. IUI

C. IUI with clomiphene induction of ovulation

D. IUI with gonadotrophin induction of ovulation

E. IVF- ICSI

11- The possible benefits of the short agonist protocol do not include:

A. Shortening the stimulation time

B. Reducing the amount of agonist used

C. Increasing the cycle success rate

D. Reducing the cost of the cycle

E. Reducing the amount of hMG used

12- The presence of ultrasonically visible hydrosalpinx:

A. Decreases the success rate in IVF/ICSI

B. Has no effect on the pregnancy rate after IVF/ICSI

C. Is associated with endometriosis

D. Affect Oocyte quality

E. Is frequently associated with PCOS

13- 33-year-old woman presents for evaluation of a 7-month history of amenorrhea. Examination discloses bilateral and normal breast and pelvic examinations. Pregnancy test is negative. Which of the following classes of medical use of her condition?

A. Phenothiazines

B. Prostaglandins

C. GnRH analogues

D. Antiestrogens

E. Gonadotropins

14- Choose the correct statement with regards to Clomiphene Citrate:

A. Anti-estrogen

B. Risk of multiple pregnancy is around 8%

C. Ovulation rate 70-85%

D. Pregnancy rate 40-50%

E. All are correct

15- You see a 28-year-old woman in your clinic. She is referred by her GP with a 6- month history of chronic pelvic pain and deep dyspareunia. A pelvic ultrasound scan shows a retroverted uterus, 4 cm endometrioma on the right ovary, normal left ovary and no free fluid in the pelvis. She is using the progesterone-only pill for contraception, and this has helped slightly with the pain. You consent her for laparoscopy and ovarian cystectomy and discuss risks and potential complications associated with these. Which of the following best describes the risk of bowel injury?

A. 15% of bowel injuries might not be diagnosed at the time of laparoscopy.

B. 25% of bowel injuries might not be diagnosed at the time of laparoscopy.

C. 35% of bowel injuries might not be diagnosed at the time of laparoscopy.

D. 45% of bowel injuries might not be diagnosed at the time of laparoscopy.

E. 55% of bowel injuries might not be diagnosed at the time of laparoscopy.

16- Medical management of fibroids is best indicated when:

A. Fibroid is less than 3 cm, not distorting the cavity and asymptomatic.

B. Fibroid is less than 3 cm, distorting the cavity and asymptomatic .

C. Fibroid is less than 3 cm, not distorting the cavity and causing heavy bleeding.

D. Fibroid is more than 3 cm, distorting the cavity and asymptomatic .

E. Fibroid is more than 3 cm, not distorting the cavity and asymptomatic.

17. In GnRH antagonist protocol; all the following are true EXCEPT:

A. Basal ultrasound on cycle day 2

B. Preferred choice for PCOS cases

C. Triggering is done when 3 follicles reach 17 mm

D. Premature LH surge occurs in ~10% of cases

E. Antagonist is superior than GnRH agonist long protocol for pregnancy rates

18- A 20 years-old man underwent semen analysis for infertility. His sperm count was 8 million/ml with 60% motile sperms, no clot formation and 50% normal morphology. The interpretation of this seminogram is:

A. Oligospermia

B. Azoospermia

C. Motility disorder

D. Antisperm antibodies

E. Normal seminogram

19- The best site to deposit the embryos during embryo transfer is:

A. Just below the fundus of the uterus

B. At the level of the internal os

C. The midportion of the uterus, far enough from the fundus and internal os

D. At the right cornu of the uterus

E. Just above the internal os

20. The main advantage of day 5 transfer compared to day 3 is that:

A. Day 5 transfer makes embryo transfer an easier procedure

B. Day 5 transfer is more accepted by the patient

C. Day 5 transfer can avoid multiple pregnancy by transferring 1 blastocyst

D. Day 5 transfer improves pregnancy rate per cycle initiated

E. Day 5 transfer increases number of embryos available for freezing

21- The maximum number of embryos to be transferred according to the ASRM recommendation is:

A. 1 blastocyst for favorable groups of women less than 35 years old

B. 2 blastocysts for favorable groups of women less than 35 years old

C. 3 blastocysts for favorable groups of women less than 35 years old

D. 3 blastocysts for all groups of women less than 35 years old

E. 4 blastocysts for all groups of women less than 35 years old

22. One of the following, if present, is related to aneuploidy:

A. Loss of a part of a chromosome.

B. Duplication of a part of a chromosome.

C. Exchange of genetic material between two chromosomes

D. Transverse division of a chromosome.

E. A missing chromosome

23. Regarding Pre-implantation genetic diagnosis, choose the most correct answer:

A. It is a way of creating designer babies.

B. It is used for sex selection for social reasons in all countries.

C. It is regulated by the common law.

D. It can be applied for screening embryos to ascertain their genetic composition prior to implantation.

E. It improves pregnancy rate.

24- A heterozygous man with neurofibromatosis (an autosomal dominant trait) was married to a normal woman, they ask you about the probability of transmission of neurofibromatosis to their offspring, you correctly answer that neurofibromatosis may affect:

A. 0% of the offspring

B. 25% of the offspring

C. 50% of the offspring

D. 75% of the offspring

E. 100% of the offspring

25- Regarding chromosomes in human reproduction, all of the following are true EXCEPT:

A. 20% of human ova are chromosomally abnormal.

B. The expected chromosomal abnormality rate at fertilization and before implantation is 40%.

C. 50% of first trimester pregnancy losses occur due to chromosomal abnormalities.

D. 10% of 2nd trimester pregnancy losses occur due to chromosomal abnormalities.

E. Most chromosomally lost pregnancies are due to structural chromosomal abnormalities.

26. The commonest chromosomal abnormality in newborn infants is:

A. Down's syndrome

B. Edward's syndrome

C. Cri du chat syndrome

D. Turner syndrome

E. Klinefelter's syndrome

27. The gold standard route for oocyte aspiration is:

A. Trans-abdominal ultrasound-guided oocyte retrieval

B. Trans-vaginal ultrasound-guided oocyte retrieval

C. Laparoscopic oocyte retrieval

D. Trans-urethral ultrasound-guided oocyte retrieval

E. Oocyte retrieval through laparotomy

28. The disadvantages of laparoscopic ovum retrieval (OR) do not include:

A. It has a poor oocyte recovery rate.

B. General anesthesia may be needed.

C. Exposes healthy women to certain risks.

D. Is a technically demanding technique using expensive instruments

E. Unsuitable to performing multiple OR sessions on the same day

29. IVF is indicated in women with PCOS if they failed to get pregnant after:

A- 3 cycles of clomiphene citrate and 1 cycle of gonadotropin therapy

B- 3 cycles of clomiphene citrate and 3 cycles of gonadotropin therapy

C-3 cycles of clomiphene citrate and 6 cycle of gonadotropin therapy

D. 6 cycles of clomiphene citrate and 3 cycles of gonadotropin therapy

E- 6 cycles of clomiphene citrate and 6 cycles of gonadotropin therapy

30- Spot Diagnosis

A. Polycystic ovary syndrome (PCOS)

B. Ovarian hyperstimulation syndrome (OHSS)

C. Ovarian torsion

D. Serous cystadenoma

E. Tubo-ovarian abscess

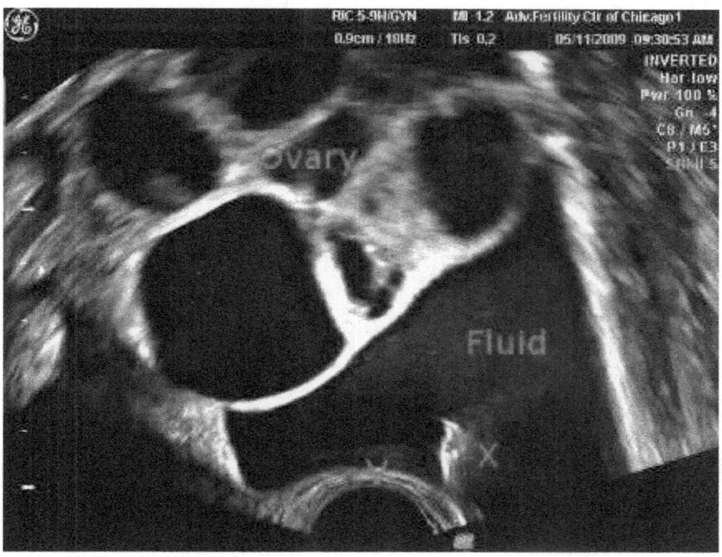

MOCK EXAM (6)

1- A 34-year-old woman, who has been trying to conceive for 3 years, is referred to the infertility clinic for further management. Which ONE of the following is an appropriate discussion issue during her clinic counselling?

A. Altering smoking, alcohol or caffeine intake has no impact on spontaneous or IVF pregnancy success

B. Despite having regular monthly menstrual cycles, a mid-luteal serum progesterone test is recommended in order to confirm ovulation

C. Laparoscopy is the only reliable method to screen for tubal abnormalities

D. Low serum progesterone in the mid-luteal phase of their cycle confirms ovulation

E. There is a need for an endometrial biopsy to exclude luteal phase defect

2- The single largest cause of acquired tubal pathology is:

A. Acinetobacter

B. Bacterial vaginosis

C. Group A streptococcus

D. Chlamydia trachomatis

E. Mycobacterium tuberculosis

3- According to ESHRE recommendation the diagnosis of primary ovarian insufficiency requires:

A. an elevated FSH and LH levels with decreased estradiol and AMH level

B. elevated FSH and LH levels and decreased estradiol levels

C. oligo/amenorrhea for at least 4 month and an elevated FSH and LH levels

D. oligo/amenorrhea for at least 4 month and an elevated FSH level >25 IU/l in two occasions > 4 weeks apart

E. oligo/amenorrhea for at least 4 month and an elevated FSH level and decrease estradiol levels

4- A 30-year-old woman with a history of polycystic ovarian syndrome presents for evaluation of infertility after 1 year of unprotected intercourse. What is the initial step in her evaluation?

A. Anatomic assessment of the female genital tract

B. Serum AMH, FSH and estradiol

C. Laparoscopy

D. Determination of ovulation

5- 25 years old female patient with Primary Infertility 2 years ago, Ovulation was Confirmed, Semen analysis within normal, HSG show Bilateral Hydrosalpinex, what is the best management:

A. Medical Treatment

B. Combined Laparoscopy & Hysteroscopy

C. Antibiotics

D. Salpingectomy

6- A 30-year-old woman has been trying to conceive for 3 years. She has infrequent menstrual cycles. Ultrasound confirms a normal uterus and polycystic ovaries. X-ray hysterosalpingogram has confirmed bilateral patent fallopian tubes. Her partner's semen analysis is reported as within normal limits. Her BMI is 25 kg/m2. She has normal prolactin, FSH, estradiol and testosterone. Of the options listed, which one of the following therapies is considered the most appropriate initial therapy?

A. Bromocriptine

B. Letrozole

C. Gonadotrophin

D. Laparoscopic ovarian drilling

E. Metformin

7- Which of the following is accurate about symptoms and physical examination of patients with endometriosis?

A. Bleeding at the umbilicus, abdominal wall, or perineum is more common than hematuria or hematochezia

B. Patients who are sexually active often report deep dyspareunia that is worst after menstruation

C. Secondary dysmenorrhea is more common in women with endometriosis

D. The hallmark finding on examination is a bluish nodule in the vagina due to infiltration from the posterior vaginal wall

8- Which of the following drugs can be used for the treatment of pain and bleeding of endometriosis:

A. Prednisolone.

B. Mifepristonel

C. Urinary gonadotropins

D. Dydrogesterone

E. Dinoprostone

9- All of the following are causes of premature ovarian failure except:

A. Fragile X syndrome

B. Kallmans syndrome

C. Mumps oophoritis

D. Pelvic irradiation

E. Turner's syndrome

10- Post testicular causes account for the following percentage of male infertility:

A. 10 %

B. 20 %

C. 30 %

D. 40 %

E. 50 %

11- Average pregnancy rated with ICSI (intracytoplasmic sperm injection):

A. 10–15 %

B. 15–25 %

C. 30–40 %

D. 50–60 %

E. 60–70 %

12- Which one of the following statements is correct regarding recurrent miscarriage?

A. Antiphospholipid syndrome, if found to be the cause of recurrent miscarriage, is untreatable.

B. Antiphospholipid antibodies are present in 15 % of women with recurrent miscarriage

C. Cervical weakness (incompetence) is a recognized cause of first-trimester recurrent miscarriage.

D. One of the partners carries a chromosomal abnormality in at least 25 % of couples with recurrent miscarriage.

E. Recurrent miscarriage is defined as the loss of two or more consecutive pregnancies before 24 weeks gestation.

13- Which ONE of the following is correct in relation to the prevalence of the main causes of infertility in the UK?

A. Factors in the male causing infertility (10 %)

B. Fibroids (30 %)

C. Ovulatory disorders (10 %)

D. Tubal damage (50 %)

E. Unexplained infertility (25 %)

14- Which ONE of the following clinical scenarios is considered diagnostic of polycystic ovarian syndrome?

A. Infrequent periods, elevated testosterone

B. Infrequent periods, infertility, low day 21 serum progesterone

C. Infrequent periods, impaired glucose tolerance, obesity

D. Polycystic ovaries, obesity, low day 21 serum progesterone

E. Polycystic ovaries, elevated LH:FSH ratio, obesity

15- A 40-year-old woman, who has been trying to conceive for 3 years, is offered IVF as a treatment option by her fertility specialist. Which ONE of the following is an appropriate discussion issue during her clinic counselling?

A. Ovarian volume, ovarian blood flow and inhibin B usefully predict IVF success rate.

B. Preimplantation genetic diagnosis (PGD) of the embryo is required prior to its uterine transfer.

C. Progesterone administration is not required following embryo transfer.

D. Salpingectomy prior to IVF is beneficial in women with hydrosalpinges.

E. The chance of a live birth following IVF treatment increases with rising female age.

16- Bariatric surgery in the treatment of obese infertile women:

A. Pregnancy can be attempted 6 months after surgery.

B. Is associated with increased risk of gestational diabetes, macrosomia and hypertensive disorders due to operation induced weight loss.

C. Is associated with iron, vitamin A, vitamin B12, vitamin K or calcium deficiencies.

D. Recommended as a first-line fertility treatment for obese women.

E. Let Women avoid the need for a weight reduction diet.

17- Regarding Ovum pick up, one of the following is true:

A. Should be done without anesthesia or analgesia

B. Suction pressure should be between 140-180 gauge

C. Aseptic techniques are not needed

D. Only aspirate follicles more than 18 mm

E. Should be done about 36 hours after hCG administration

18- The following will not help to minimize the occurrence of difficult embryo:

A. Trial transfer

B. A comfortably full bladder

C. Blastocyst stage transfer

D. Use of ultrasound guidance

E. Use of a soft/firm catheter

19- Advantages of abdominal US guided transfer do not include:

A. Facilitate negotiation of cervico-uterine angle.

B. Avoid the need of full bladder

C. Avoid touching fundus.

D. Avoid catheter twisting.

E. Ensure correct location in the uterine cavity

20- Evidence-based guidelines regarding embryo transfer DO NOT include:

A. Effort should be made to avoid "difficult" transfers.

B. Ultrasound guidance will result in easier transfers.

C. Soft catheters should be used when feasible.

D. A few hours bed rest after the procedure is required.

E. Ultrasound guidance will result in improved outcomes

21- Regarding aromatase inhibitors (Letrozole) for induction of ovulation in patients with PCOS:

A. It acts through blocking hypothalamic estrogen receptors

B. The starting dose is 25 mg/day and the maximum dose is 75 mg/day

C. It has a long half-life (2 weeks)

D. It is a second line treatment that is used in clomiphene citrate failure cases.

E. It is associated with less rate of twin pregnancy than clomiphene citrate.

22- The gonadotropin induction protocol recommended to be used in the clinic for women with PCOS that gives the least OHSS rate is:

A. The conventional protocol.

B. The low-dose step down protocol

C. The low-dose step down then up protocol

D. The low-dose step up protocol

E. The ultrashort protocol

23- In laparoscopic ovarian drilling:

A. Best results are obtained in women with higher LH and androgen levels.

B. Bipolar electrode use is recommended

C. The fixed dose method gives higher results than the adjusted dose method.

D. The use of anti-adhesion barriers intraoperative is recommended.

E. Second look laparoscopy shows severe adhesions in 1/3 of patients.

24- According to the WHO, 2010 normal semen parameters, using the strict criteria; the number of NORMAL sperms should be at least:

A. 4%

B. 20%

C. 40%

D. 60%

E. 80%

25- Side effects of GnRH agonist do not include:

A. Hot flashes

B. Headache

C. Vaginal dryness

D. Bone resorption & Osteoporosis

E. Decrease high density lipoproteins

26- Which of the following is a key advantage of the GnRH antagonist protocol compared to the long GnRH agonist protocol in controlled ovarian stimulation?

A. Higher pregnancy rates in all age groups

B. Reduced risk of ovarian hyperstimulation syndrome (OHSS)

C. Improved endometrial receptivity

D. Increased number of retrieved oocytes

E. Longer duration of stimulation

27- Which of the following statements about the Double Stimulation (DuoStim) protocol in assisted reproduction is most accurate?

A. Double stimulation requires a minimum interval of 2–3 menstrual cycles between stimulations.

B. The second stimulation is performed during the luteal phase of the same menstrual cycle.

C. DuoStim is contraindicated in patients with poor ovarian reserve.

D. Double stimulation significantly increases OHSS risk compared to conventional stimulation.

E. The protocol results in lower cumulative oocyte yield compared to a single stimulation.

28- Which of the following statements about endometrial preparation for frozen embryo transfer (FET) is most accurate?

A. In natural cycle FET, ovulation must be suppressed with GnRH agonists to allow endometrial development.

B. Modified natural cycle FET does not require monitoring of ovulation or endometrial thickness.

C. The presence of a corpus luteum in artificial FET cycles reduces the risk of pre-eclampsia.

D. Live birth rates are consistently higher in artificial cycles compared to natural cycles in all patient groups.

E. Artificial (hormone replacement) FET cycles require luteal support because there is no endogenous corpus luteum.

29- Which of the following statements regarding IVF in patients with SLE is most accurate?

A. IVF is absolutely contraindicated in all women with a history of lupus nephritis.

B. Controlled ovarian stimulation in SLE patients should avoid estrogen exposure to reduce the risk of disease flare.

C. Antiphospholipid antibody–positive patients undergoing IVF may require anticoagulation (heparin ± aspirin) to reduce thrombotic risk.

D. IVF significantly increases the risk of permanent SLE flare in all patients, regardless of disease activity.

E. Cyclophosphamide therapy should be continued during IVF to prevent relapse.

30- Identify the instrument shown in the image?

A. Soft embryo transfer Catheter

B. Single Lumen Aspiration Needle

C. Hard embryo transfer Catheter

D. Double Lumen Aspiration Needle

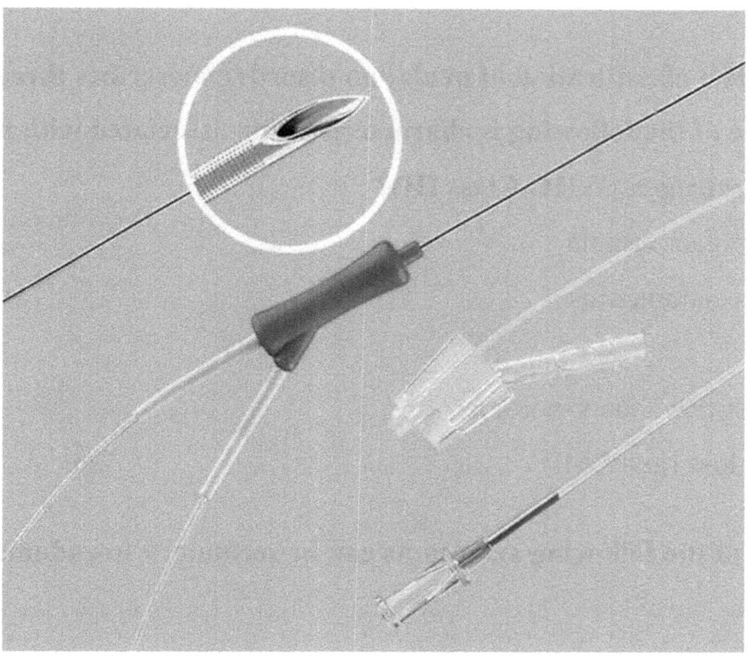

MOCK EXAM (7)

1- The WHO classification of ovulation disorders describes three classes. Which one of the following is characteristically associated with low FSH and low oestrogen (WHO Class I)?

A. Hyperprolactinaemia

B. Ovarian endometriosis

C. Ovarian failure

D. Polycystic ovarian syndrome

E. Weight loss (low BMI)

2- The WHO classification of ovulation disorders describes three classes. Which one of the following is characteristically associated with high FSH and low oestrogen (WHO Class III)?

A. Hyperprolactinaemia

B. Ovarian endometriosis

C. POI

D. Polycystic ovarian syndrome

E. Weight loss (low BMI)

3- Which of the following symptoms can be secondary to endometriosis?

A. Oliguria.

B. Postmenopausal bleeding.

C. Painful laparotomy scar.

D. Anorgasmia.

E. Amenorrhoea.

4- The mother of a 10-year-old girl with beta-thalassemia major seeks consultation in order to enquire about how the fertility prospects of her daughter may be affected due to her medical condition. Which of the following statements would be incorrect to tell her?

A. Her daughter's fertility may be reduced due to iron overload

B. Hormonal contraceptives are contraindicated in these women.

C. Ovulation induction with injectable gonadotrophins may be needed.

D. Prolonged period of iron chelation therapy may be required prior to induction of ovulation and pregnancy.

E. Puberty is often delayed and incomplete in girls with beta-thalassemia major.

5- A 40-year-old man undergoes a semen analysis test. Which one of the following components listed in his test result is considered to be ABNORMAL according to WHO 2010 semen analysis criteria?

A. Progressive motility 25 %

B. Sperm concentration 50 × 106 per ml

C. Total (progressive and non progressive motility) 75 %

D. Total sperm number 200 × 106 spermatozoa per ejaculate

E. Volume 4.0 ml

6- Ms XY is 38 years old and suffers from primary infertility and endometriosis. Her recent TV scan suggests the presence of a 2.5 cm endometrioma. Her pain is well controlled using simple analgesics. She is due to undergo IVF. Which treatment is best suited to deal with her endometrioma?

A. Expectant management

B. Laparoscopic ovarian cystectomy

C. Laparoscopic ovarian cyst aspiration

D. Laparoscopic ovarian cyst fenestration and drainage

E. Laparoscopic salpingoophorectomy

7- A 29-year-old woman who has never been pregnant presents after 2 years of inability to conceive. She has a history of asthma, frequent urinary tract infections and an appendectomy for a ruptured appendix. Her cycles are regular every 30 days. Her partner has two children from a previous relationship. What is the most likely cause of their infertility?

A. Endometriosis

B. Male factor infertility

C. Anovulation

D. Fallopian tubal occlusion

8- A worried mother gets her 16-year-old girl to her GP. She is concerned that her daughter has not as yet commenced her periods. On examination there is poor development of secondary sexual characters, cubitus valgus, evidence of webbed neck and short stature. Which of the following investigations will help you confirm the diagnosis?

A. Estimation of serum FSH: LH

B. Karyotyping

C. MRI of the pelvis

D. Ultrasound of the pelvis

E. X ray of the limbs

9- The mean age of menopause is:

A. 45 years

B. 51 years

C. 55 years

D. 53 years

E. 48 years

10- A 16-year- old is brought into her primary care physician's office because her mother is concerned that her daughter has not starting menstruating yet. In conversation with the teenager, her doctor learns that she has been having low pelvic pain for the past few months. On speculum examination, a dark bulging mass is identified 5 cm from the vaginal introitus, and the hymenal ring is identified distal to the bulging mass. What is the most likely etiology of this patient's condition?

A. Failure of fusion of the paramesonephric duct and the urogenital sinus

B. Failure of fusion of the mesonephric duct and the urogenital sinus

C. Failure of fusion of the paramesonephric duct and the vitelline duct

D. Failure of fusion of the mesonephric duct and the vitelline duct

E. Failure of fusion of the urogenital sinus and the vitelline duct

11- A 15 -year-old sexually active adolescent girl presents with primary amenorrhea. Vital signs are as follows: BP 110/68 mmHg, P 88 beats/min, R 16 breaths/min, BMI 24, and height 5 ' 0". An examination reveals normal external genitalia. A three-dimensional (3D) ultrasound reveals the presence of uterus, tubes, and ovaries bilaterally. On speculum examination, she has an unobstructed vagina and a patent cervical os. Breasts are Tanner stage 2. She has scant axillary hair, Tanner stage 2, which has developed over the past 6 months. Follicle- stimulating hormone (FSH) and luteinizing hormone (LH) are low; Thyroidstimulating hormone (TSH), estrogen, and testosterone levels are all within normal limits. She relates that she has grown 2" in the last 3 months.

What is the most likely diagnosis?

A. Androgen insensitivity syndrome (AIS)

B. Anorexia nervosa

C. Constitutional delay

D. Turner syndrome

E. Congenital adrenal hyperplasia

12- Hypogonadotropic hypogonadism as a cause for male subfertility is seen in:

A. < 1 %

B. 5 %

C. 10 %

D. 15 %

E. 20 %

13- Which of the following statements regarding androgen metabolism in women is not true?

A. In healthy women, 80 % of circulating testosterone is bound to sex hormonebinding globulin (SHBG), 19 % is bound to albumin and 1 % circulates freely in the blood stream.

B. Most of the circulating testosterone is metabolised in the liver into androsterone and etiocholanolone.

C. Of the circulating androgens, only testosterone and DHEA-S are able to activate androgen receptors.

D. Some androgen production occurs in all healthy women and is required for the synthesis of estrogens.

E. Urinary 17-ketosteroids are end products of androgen metabolism.

14- The primary metabolic problem in congenital adrenal hyperplasia is a deficiency in production of:

A. Adrenocorticotrophic hormone (ACTH)

B. Aldosterone

C. Cortisol

D. Corticotrophin-releasing hormone (CRH)

E. Dehydroepiandrostenedione

15- The direct biochemical evidence of hyperandrogenism is obtained by measurement of serum:

A. Androstenedione

B. Anti-Mullerian hormone

C. DHEAS (dehydroepiandrostenedione)

D. Levonorgestrel

E. Testosterone

16- A patient with subfertility is found to have tubal obstruction following an HSG. There are no known additional pelvic comorbidities (such as PID, previous ectopic pregnancy or endometriosis).

A. 10% of patients.

B. 20% of patients

C. 35% of patients

D. 55% of patients

E. 65% of patients

17- A 37-year-old para 0, who has undergone controlled ovarian stimulation for IVF treatment 3 weeks previously, presents with abdominal pain, bloating, nausea and vomiting. She is known to have PCOS and had not ovulated previously with clomiphene citrate treatment. She went on to receive antagonist recombinant FSH protocol and was later given human chorionic gonadotropin to trigger ovulation. Ultrasound has shown evidence of ascites with an ovarian size of 14 cm. Her hematocrit was 46%. The patient was admitted to hospital for inpatient treatment.

What is the recommended regime of thromboprophylaxis?

A. LMWH for the duration of her stay in hospital.

B. LMWH for the duration of her stay + 5 days after discharge.

C. LMWH for the duration of her stay + 7 days after discharge.

D. LMWH for the first 12 weeks of pregnancy.

E. LMWH until her OHSS symptoms subside.

18- A 25 -year-old patient, G0P0, and her husband are planning to start a family. The patient has started prenatal vitamins and neither she nor her husband are smokers. What are the chances that she will become pregnant in the first 3 months?

A. 10% to 15%

B. 20% to 25%

C. 35 % to 45%

D. 45% to 55%

19- A 26-year-old woman, GOPO, presents to the office with the inability to conceive after 12 months of unprotected intercourse. She has regular periods and her husband has one child from a previous relationship. Her medical history is positive for asthma and history of Chlamydia when she was 19 . Surgical history is positive for tonsillectomy. What is the most likely cause of her infertility?

A. Male factor

B. Premature ovarian failure

C. Tubal factor

D. Polycystic ovarian syndrome (PCOS)

E. Diethylstilbestrol (DES) exposure in utero

20- A 24-year-old, G0P0 with a body mass index (BMI) of 34, presents to the office. She has had only three periods in the last year, and she complains of moderate facial hair that she has had treated with laser. She has no recent weight gain or fatigue. She desires pregnancy in the next year. What is the next step in her workup?

A. Refer her for assisted reproductive technology

B. Order transvaginal ultrasound to assess ovaries

C. Order a semen analysis

D. Obtain hemoglobin/hematocrit

E. Order testosterone and dehydroepiandrosterone sulfate (DHEAS)

21- Which of the following is not a feature of polycystic ovary syndrome (PCOS)?

A. Elevated luteinizing hormone (LH) levels

B. Insulin resistance

C. Increased androgen levels

D. Regular ovulatory menstrual cycles

E. Polycystic ovarian morphology on ultrasound

22- A 29-year-old, G l POO l O, presents to your clinic desiring pregnancy. She had one ectopic pregnancy in the past treated with methotrexate. She has not been able to become pregnant despite 2 years of unprotected intercourse. Her husband has a normal semen analysis. She is otherwise healthy and has normal menstrual cycles.

What is the next step in her workup?

A. Magnetic resonance imaging

B. Clomid citrate challenge

C. Hysterosalpingogram

D. In vitro fertilization

23- A 24-year- old, GO, and her husband presents to your office for preconception counseling. She has not attempted pregnancy to date because she is concerned about her future pregnancies and wants to know about preimplantation genetic diagnosis. From her statement you ask her about her other medical history.

Which of the following diagnoses is she likely to have?

A. Polycystic ovarian syndrome (PCOS)

B. Sickle cell anemia

C. Hyperstimulation syndrome

D. Hyperprolactinemia

24- A 30-year-old, G 1 P 1 , presents to clinic with intermittent thin milky discharge from both nipples. The symptoms have been present for the past 6 months. The discharge is non-bloody and is not associated with increased breast tenderness. The patient has also had irregular menses lately. The patient says that up until recently her periods were always very regular. The patient is currently not taking any medications. The pregnancy test in the office is negative. The patient says the discharge occurs spontaneously without manual stimulation and denies any recent changes in bras. On physical examination, the breasts are symmetric and no breast lesions or masses are appreciated. A thin white discharge can be manually expressed bilaterally, Serum prolactin 110 ng/ml

What is the most likely mechanism leading to these findings?

A. Microadenoma of the pituitary gland

B. Excessive stimulation of the nipple

C. PCOS

D. Hyperthyroidism

E. Cushing disease

25- Which of the following best describes the clinical role of the ERA test in assisted reproduction?

A. It measures serum estradiol and progesterone levels to guide luteal support.

B. It identifies the genetic profile of embryos to improve implantation rates.

C. It assesses the window of endometrial receptivity to personalize embryo transfer timing.

D. It predicts the risk of recurrent pregnancy loss in women with thrombophilia.

E. It replaces ultrasound and hormonal monitoring in frozen embryo transfer cycles.

26- A 32-year-old woman with normal ovarian reserve (AMH 3.0 ng/ml, AFC 14) is scheduled for her first IVF cycle. Which of the following is the most appropriate stimulation protocol and starting gonadotropin dose?

A. GnRH agonist long protocol with 450 IU/day gonadotropins

B. GnRH antagonist protocol with 150–225 IU/day gonadotropins

C. Natural cycle IVF with no gonadotropins

D. GnRH agonist flare protocol with 75 IU/day gonadotropins

E. Luteal phase stimulation with 450 IU/day gonadotropins

27- Which of the following statements about the PPOS protocol in IVF is Correct?

A. It uses progesterone during the follicular phase to prevent premature LH surge.

B. It requires GnRH agonist for pituitary down-regulation.

C. Fresh embryo transfer is routinely recommended after PPOS stimulation.

D. It is contraindicated in patients with polycystic ovary syndrome (PCOS).

E. PPOS is less effective in preventing LH surge compared to antagonist protocol.

28- Which of the following immunomodulatory interventions has the strongest current evidence for improving IVF outcomes in women with recurrent implantation failure (RIF)?

A. Intravenous immunoglobulin (IVIG)

B. Corticosteroids (e.g., prednisone)

C. Intralipid infusion

D. Lymphocyte immunotherapy (LIT)

E. None have strong evidence from randomized controlled trials

29- Which of the following is the main proposed advantage of using time-lapse (smart) incubators in IVF compared to conventional incubators?

A. They increase fertilization rates by enhancing sperm–oocyte interaction.

B. They allow continuous embryo monitoring without removing embryos from stable culture conditions.

C. They eliminate the need for embryologists to assess embryo quality.

D. They guarantee higher live birth rates in all patient populations.

E. They shorten the duration of ovarian stimulation required before oocyte retrieval.

30- Identify the instrument shown (spot diagnosis):

A. Wallace Catheter

B. Labotecht Catheter

C. IUI Catheter

D. Cock Catheter

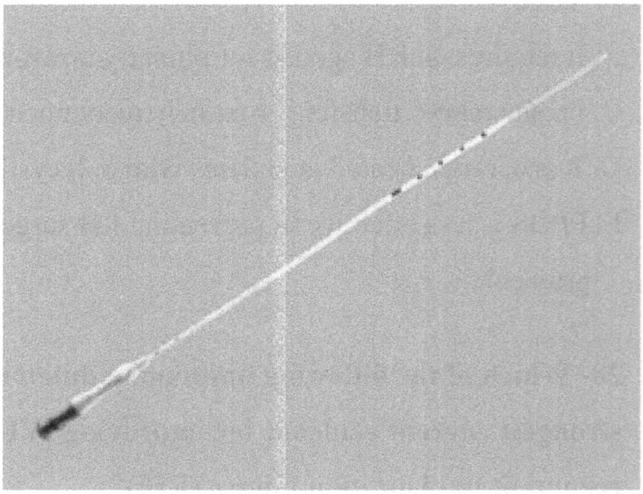

ANSWERS

	MOCK EXAM 1	MOCK EXAM 2	MOCK EXAM 3	MOCK EXAM 4
1	E	A	C	B
2	B	C	E	D
3	B	B	C	E
4	E	B	A	B
5	A	B	C	E
6	E	A	D	E
7	C	E	C	C
8	D	B	B	D
9	B	C	C	C
10	D	D	D	C
11	A	C	D	B
12	C	D	C	E
13	C	D	A	E
14	D	B	E	C
15	A	D	D	A
16	C	E	B	A
17	C	D	A	A
18	C	B	B	D
19	B	E	A	C
20	A	C	D	D
21	A	B	C	C
22	C	C	D	D
23	B	B	C	C
24	D	C	E	A
25	C	C	B	A
26	C	B	A	E
27	B	B	C	C
28	C	A	C	D
29	E	E	D	A
30	E	C	D	C

MOCK EXAM 5

1	A
2	D
3	B
4	B
5	B
6	D
7	E
8	D
9	D
10	C
11	C
12	A
13	A
14	D
15	D
16	C
17	E
18	A
19	C
20	C
21	A
22	E
23	D
24	C
25	E
26	A
27	B
28	A
29	D
30	B

MOCK EXAM 6

1	B
2	D
3	D
4	D
5	C
6	B
7	C
8	D
9	B
10	A
11	C
12	E
13	E
14	A
15	D
16	C
17	E
18	C
19	B
20	D
21	E
22	D
23	A
24	A
25	E
26	B
27	B
28	E
29	C
30	D

MOCK EXAM 7

1	E
2	C
3	C
4	B
5	A
6	A
7	D
8	B
9	B
10	A
11	C
12	A
13	C
14	C
15	E
16	B
17	C
18	C
19	C
20	E
21	D
22	C
23	B
24	A
25	C
26	B
27	A
28	E
29	B
30	D

www.ingramcontent.com/pod-product-compliance
Lightning Source LLC
Chambersburg PA
CBHW061357240926
51846CB00007B/1437
* 9 7 8 6 3 3 9 9 7 0 5 9 7 *